*Signs of dis-ease and imbalance seem to pervade this time in near epidemic proportions. However, what we perceive to be a dis-ease crisis is in truth a healing crisis, characteristically moving back through past trauma, releasing into experience those moments of pain encaged.*

*And though the very concept of medicine itself continues to sustain that which it purports to eliminate, in these times ahead, the practitioner of whole systems in healing will, within the whole of the body of life of which we comprise but individual cells, represent the constructive anabolic forces so profoundly present in all activities of this nature.*

Leslie J. Kaslof

# WHOLISTIC DIMENSIONS IN HEALING
## A Resource Guide

Compiled and Edited by Leslie J. Kaslof
With contributions from over fifty authorities in the field.

A Dolphin Book
DOUBLEDAY & COMPANY, INC.
Garden City, New York
1978

# Acknowledgements

I wish to express my sincere thanks and gratitude to the following individuals whose special assistance helped to facilitate the completion of this work:

To Alick Bartholomew for having the foresight and inspiration to have made the initial contact, and to Patrick Filley for having followed through and maintained confidence in the concept and project. To Judy Skutch, Ilana Rubenfeld, David Bresler, and also to Yoshimo Fujiwara for invaluable contacts and introductions to potential authors.

To Mark Bricklin, Eric Utne, Leonard Jacobs, Marilyn Ferguson, and Jim Sheer, for assistance in soliciting entries. To Alice Bricklin, Richard Heffern, Chris Bird, Harriet Barry, Joyce Prensky, William Staniger, Donal Carter, Leonard Worthington, Neil Whitelaw, Jules Soled, the Association For Humanistic Psychology, and many others, for supplying a substantial portion of the listing information. Very special thanks go to Sandy MacDonald, Phil Lansky, Gene Fellner, Judy Stein, Brandyna Stevens, Arlene Ross, Joan Ann DeMattia, and Kathy Heavey for assistance above and beyond normal consideration, and to Meyer Rosenberg, Aaron Friedland, OD, Burt Sheryll, DC, Yaacov Moshe Schlass, Julio Pereyra, United Communications and Ralph Kaslof for financial assistance during the inbetween periods.

To the various contributors (see Biographies) who trusted in a common dream and gave their limited and valuable time to compile and submit manuscripts for the text. And especially to Norma . . . for holding together when it was really important.

ISBN: 0-385-12628-X
Library of Congress Catalog Card Number: 76-50874

Design Concept: Leslie J. Kaslof and Dan McClain
Design and Production: Andrew Bromberg

# How To Use This Resource Guide

The purpose of this guide is to supply a much-needed resource tool for both the lay public and the practitioner, by indicating where there is interest and receptivity among professionals to implement new ideas within their respective fields.

The material in this guide is divided into topical sections such as INTEGRATIVE MEDICAL SYSTEMS, NUTRITION AND HERBS, and HUMANISTIC AND TRANSPERSONAL PSYCHOTHERAPIES. Each section consists of chapters (or individual modalities, which fall within the general topic of the section). Each chapter is prefaced by an introductory article and followed by a list of groups active in that particular field. Individuals listed only include researchers or representatives of organizations. Each group is given an entry number and in addition to such details as addresses and telephone numbers, the list includes annotations concerning the group's services and activities.

Entries are divided into four classifications: Groups and Associations; Schools, Centers, and Clinics; Journals and Publications; and Products and Services. Where appropriate, a fifth classification, Researchers, has been added. When entries for a particular classification were not available, it was not included.

Within each classification, entries are listed alphabetically by state and city. Canadian and overseas listings follow the last state listing and are listed alphabetically by country and city. Where there are multiple entries for a city, they are alphabetized by name of organization.

Those groups and organizations whose activities made it necessary to include their names in more than one modality section are cross referenced by the means of a main entry number (in parentheses), which refers the reader back to the primary listing.

As a common courtesy and in order to expedite response, when writing for information to any of the organizations listed in the guide, it is suggested that a stamped self-addressed envelope accompany the inquiry.

# Why: wholistic/holistic

The reader will notice that in this text, and in the field of (w)holistic healing in general, *(w)holistic* is spelled both with and without the . . . w.

The word *holistic* is derived from the word *holism*, which is defined in *Webster's Seventh New Collegiate Dictionary*, as "that which emphasizes the organic or functional relations between parts and wholes." A corresponding meaning of *holistic* is defined in the *Random House Dictionary*, 1973, as "the theory that whole entities, as fundamental and determining components of reality, have an existence more than the mere sum of their parts."

Though the word *wholistic* is not defined in the dictionary at this time, a review of its component parts reveals the necessity for its use. *Whole* is defined in Webster's as "a coherent system or organization of parts fitting or working together as one." The suffix *-istic* is defined as "relating to, or characteristic of."

Therefore, as it is the intention of this work to act as a vehicle for the representation and development of integrated whole systems in healing. The word *wholistic* is used throughout the main format of this text, as it suggests the qualities required for *holism* (representing the more subtle and transcendental aspects of the whole) to be realized and applied in practical ways.

It is important to remember that many modalities or techniques referred to as natural or non-toxic operate just beyond the threshold of toxicological response. Such modalities are useful only as long as they are capable of catalyzing a balancing response in the human system. If and when any technique fails to initiate this response, for whatever reason, its usefulness must then be reevaluated without regard for vested interest. If in the light of careful evaluation the technique is deemed obsolete or disruptive, it must then give up its place to another more suitable to the task.

Finally, it must be realized that the ultimate responsibility for health maintenance lies within each of us. By being in contact with our own healing processes, we take the first step beyond the need for the tools of healing—beyond the need for therapy and technique. This guide is a beginning step in that direction.

# CONTENTS

Listing in this resource guide in no way constitutes an endorsement or recommendation.

Annotations regarding groups were condensed and extrapolated from information forwarded by that organization. No additional information substantiation was made other than address verification.

Not all organizations or individuals in each field have been listed. Inevitably, the addresses of some of those listed may have changed since the publication of this guide.

All individuals included either represent organizations or are researchers in their fields.

No glossary of terms has been provided, since many terms used in the fields included do not have generally agreed-upon meanings.

Wherever possible in the annotations to specific entries, the spelling of *wholistic/holistic* used by the particular organization has been retained. However, in the articles which introduce each modality, the spelling *wholistic* has been used throughout. Where this spelling differs from that in the author's original manuscript, the change has been indicated in a footnote.

All addresses have been verified, with the exception of those state and local affiliate associations which were provided by each association's national headquarters. Since these addresses may change from time to time, it is suggested that interested persons contact the national headquarters for the most up-to-date information.

# General Introduction

*Rick J. Carlson, JD*

This book, though greatly needed, was difficult to do. It's needed, first of all, because the public should know what the options are in regard to their health. The day is past when we could confidently turn to modern medicine for all or even many of our health needs. By most estimates, even conservative ones, medicine influences most indices of health only to about 10 percent. The remaining 90 percent is dependent on environmental, social, and cultural factors over which doctors and hospitals have little, if any, control.

The book is also needed because the public is confused, and understandably so, by the sheer volume of alternatives and is further confounded by the recent rapid proliferation of new techniques and programs. In such a climate the consumer of health care services is often at a loss, unable to sort out the options. Yet clearly people are now, to an unprecedented degree, looking for alternatives to what some perceive to be a dinosaur—the modern medical system.

One of the difficulties in preparing this directory was that lately criticism of standard medicine has amounted to overkill. Medicine may be increasingly out of touch with our needs, but most of us would still race to a physician with a sick child—in many cases with good reason. The medical care system does some things very well—principally, emergency and acute care. Accident victims will hardly find comfort in the conviction that wholistic* health is the wave of the future. What they need is good old mechanistic medicine—and fast.

A second difficulty arose from conflicts among the many practitioners of new wholistic approaches. Their philosophies may be wholistic, but often in their attempts to create a market for their wares they put the money-motivated physician to shame. Then, too, some practitioners insist on waging vendettas against the existing monopoly—the allopathic practice of medicine. Perhaps some vendettas are in order. The traditional medical care system has very cannily, often maliciously, undermined its opposition at every turn. That's how monopolies are made. Practitioners of alternative approaches have cause for complaint. Nonetheless, what is to be gained by more negativity? The field *is* loosening up. The public is demanding access to new practices and practitioners. And a few states have even begun to dismantle the medical monopoly. Today, then, is a time to keep pioneering—and to stop looking over our shoulders at injustices of the past.

A final difficulty was that of discrimination. To be truly helpful, a directory of alternative health care services must be more than a yellow pages. Some criteria must be used to decide who and what should be included. However, this process is tricky. As the confining perspectives of the past begin to yield, we must take care not to develop equally delimiting perspectives in their place. Thus, inclusion in this book by no means constitutes an endorsement. As in all areas, the buyer must beware. Obviously, not everyone now promoting the cause of wholistic health is necessarily ''sound.'' It may be that a good many of the standard bearers in today's parade will drop out along the way. Hence, to suggest that every technique listed here is of equal value would be unwise. Nevertheless, Leslie Kaslof deserves nothing but praise for his pioneering and perseverance in organizing and compiling this work. We have, at last, our first wholistic health directory—a major advance over the mystification of the past.

---

*Spelled holistic in original text.

# Need For A More Humanistic Approach To Health

*Leonard A. Worthington, LLB*

From the beginning of life upon this planet mankind has sought to pierce the veil of ignorance that conceals the mysterious workings of universal law from human sight. For eons it has sought to understand better the flow of energies, vibrations, and rays that subtly affect the actions of atoms and organs of humans and animals. Through decades of laboratory research, observing the law of cause and effect, scientists have established certain credible behavior patterns, with which engineers have been able to calculate, with some degree of certainty, the stresses and strains of matter on matter. Occasionally, however, some unknown "X" factor intervenes and precipitates disastrous results. The researchers frantically rush back to their drawingboards, pondering the question "Why?" In contrast to other disciplines in which unseen forces appear to affect results, in the field of mathematics, equations arrived at centuries ago appear to survive the passage of time.

In this complex society of ours, the most important aspects of living include the problem of ensuring survival, improving life expectancy, and maintaining a sound mind and healthy body. It is understandable that the healing profession, encouraged by the unchanging validity of mathematical principles, would adopt similar procedures, based on laboratory experimentation, in the hope of promulgating formulas with reliable results. Thus, the empirical approach to disease, injury, and illness evolved as a mandate to the medical profession, and through trial and error healing agencies have indeed established some very important guidelines for the betterment of the human race.

However, some medical practitioners have completely failed to understand the intervention of the laws of nature and the effect of unseen energies that alter their patterns of action. These effects, plus the influence of new planetary impacts, have produced illnesses which are now threatening to reverse the extended longevity trends that the medical profession has successfully enhanced. As these apparently incurable ailments affect increasingly large segments of society, healing practitioners must once again ask the distressing question "Why?" With no satisfactory answer forthcoming, they can only fund more experimentation, in the hope of coming across a key to the mysterious afflictions now threatening so many with premature extinction.

Faced with this crisis, adventurous souls have probed uncharted areas in which they hope to find solutions, thus goading their associates to reevaluate the empirical position. Such pioneers spawned the wholistic* movement, which holds that human beings are not just flesh and blood but a combination of energies, electrical impulses, mind substance, and a host of other forces, all of which combine in various ways to bring about well-being or its opposite, disease. Those probing this new continent are like miners searching for precious metals; they leave no stone unturned in their attempt to solve the mysteries of the human mind and body, and to observe the action and interaction which takes place between them, for the benefit of mankind.

Throughout history, the fringes of the medical practice have also harbored many charlatans whose sole purpose is to make money at the expense of the aged and the infirm; consequently laws have been enacted to prevent unqualified persons from practicing quackery on an unsuspecting public. In many cases these laws have been salutary and have proved an effective safeguard. However, history has shown that where statutes are enacted as the result of emotional protests or at the behest of any pressure group, they tend to be unreasonably restrictive in their sincere attempt to alleviate an evil. As a result, many unlicensed persons whose knowledge could benefit society are being stifled by threats of prosecution. Though they might reveal ageless wisdom or methods beneficial to future doctors, such activities

---

*Spelled holistic in original text.

are suppressed whenever proposed or attempted.

We live in a world of tremendous change, which requires constant readjustments in our thinking processes and in our way of life. Remedies that in past ages were effective on human beings appear to have reached a saturation point; since the body builds up immunities, remedies that once were effective are now producing undesirable side effects. As new drugs are tried on patients to counter this trend, the unpredictable results have spawned countless malpractice suits, while increasing medical costs. Practitioners are afraid to explore unorthodox methods of treatment for fear of civil litigation or, possibly, jeopardizing their licenses.

The cosmic rays of uncertain origin and ever greater numbers of microwaves that are bombarding the planet's surface, combined with ecological abuses, appear to be having unpredictable adverse effects on the human body. Studies by qualified practitioners on the effect of the mind and other energies on ailments have given startling results. The public is becoming increasingly aware that there are beneficial treatments other than the accepted orthodox methods and that these have been denied them in the past through overly restrictive laws.

Inexplicable as some of these methods may appear, many medical practitioners are now adopting the slogan, "If it works, try it." At the same time, however, they must consider the threat of professional disapproval. Such considerations tend to impede experimental research that might do much to inform medics of additional factors that must be taken into account when treating patients.

Unless such steps are encouraged, the public might do well to demand that other government agencies take over those areas which have not been satisfactorily explored up to the present time. The no-man's-land that now exists between the orthodox medical view and the frontier of the probative pioneer must be explored by all healing agencies, in a cooperative effort to benefit humanity.

# Creating New Roles For Changing Times

*Jerry Green, JD*

I have been studying our rapidly changing understanding of health from various perspectives for the past six years. My inquiries began with, and remain motivated by, my interest in developing a greater understanding of myself. I offer my impressions of some of the broader implications of these changes in the hope that we may find a common understanding on which to base the organization of our social energies.

Until recently, the medical model of health has been considered comprehensive. Our social, political, and economic resources have been directed toward the pursuit of health according to criteria articulated by medical science.

With the expansion of awareness to dynamics of health that are within the control of and are the responsibility of every individual, we are suddenly confronted with a crisis of expectations about medical practice. By examining the cases in controversy in malpractice litigation, I began to understand how this transition in our awareness of health relates to the current medical crisis.

The public has never clearly understood modern medicine. In training and in practice, it is basically a science of pathology geared to determine scientifically valid principles for diagnosing and treating illness, injury, and disease. Our demand for science to deal with diseases has motivated scientific investment in this direction, and medicine has indeed made remarkable achievements in controlling disease. Our desire that medicine provide us with health has led to a common misunderstanding about the role of medicine. Since we wish that science provide us with more than pathological treatment, our unrealistic expectations have gone unfulfilled and found expression in litigation.

The emergence of wholistic* health perspectives offers concepts and practices that may enable us to appreciate medical science better and to derive greater value from it. However, we must exercise caution to avoid invalidating both medicine and wholistic health by our desire to over simplify matters.

In contrast to the medical model, tne wholistic perspective deals with dynamics of health independent from the treatment of disease. This is not to say that wholistic practices are inappropriate in the presence of pathology. In wholistic practice, pathology is seen as a manifestation of stress, weakness or imbalance, and the goal is to fortify the system as a whole, increasing its efficiency for dealing with crisis and interacting with its environment. Wholistic practices complement medicine; their appropriate use will help to ensure the desired result of medical treatment.

Medicine is governed in trainıng and practice by standards that relate to diagnosis and treatment of pathology. Physicians who employ wholistic techniques risk civil liability and professional censure for providing services that vary from accepted practices. Doctors also risk civil and criminal liability when they practice with others not similarly licensed.

These problems and the difficulties in the doctor-patient relationship may be reduced by clarifying the allocation of responsibility in that relationship. The medical role may be identified with the pathological orientation in a manner that both communicates the doctor's specialized work and, at the same time, outlines for the patient the area in which (s)he must exercise his/her own responsibility. An agreement or plan (contract, if you will) may be established by identifying the decisions, judgments, and responsibilities which the doctor—in accordance with the unique nature of his or her practice—chooses to provide.

In the process, doctor and patient objectify a process of reciprocal questioning that both parties might otherwise find threatening and respond to defensively. Against the background of clearly identified medical responsibility, the parties may explore areas of patient responsibility with similar objectivity. Once the individual has identified the dynamics of his or her health that are independent of medical care,

---

*Spelled holistic in original text.*

there is a basis for comprehending a very different professional relationship in order to pursue them.

Seen in this context, wholistic practitioners function to assist individuals in the assumption of responsibility for those dynamics of their health which are within their control. Their work is complementary to medical practice and does not affront medical licensure laws, which should be interpreted in terms relating to pathology.

Wholistic practitioners focus on the client's interest and motivation concerning growth and change in behavior. Their practice should include an equally thorough exploration of allocating responsibility by agreement. How does one determine a client's needs, desires, and expectations? What form of record keeping will document a client's goals and clarify their understanding of relating wholistic practice with medical treatment? Wholistic practitioners should consider what kind of information it would help them to get from a client's physician. Similarly, what information should they convey to the physician, and in what form?

The consumer of healthcare services is the keystone in these professional relationships. It is not enough to recognize and assume individual responsibility for health. As patients and clients, we must take a second look at the criteria of health that we seek to develop, and explore for ourselves the need for medical treatment in relation to other services. Both require recognition of what we want and need, and demand that we ask questions about the services we purchase.

There are three sets of agreements to be created. Each is a plan designed for a specific purpose and using different factors. With our doctors, we can plan for diagnostic aid and treatment services. Our part of that agreement recognizes our own role in the healing process. The central plan then, is with ourselves, to recognize and deal with the criteria of health that ultimately lie only in our control. We may then contract with wholistic practitioners for assistance in the assumption of our responsibilities.

The growing population of physicians interested in employing wholistic practices presents very special problems. The "wholistic physician" must play two roles for his/her patient/client. Medical standards of practice may be preserved only if this distinction is kept clear. More important, however, the patient/client probably has a more difficult job in identifying the area within which his/her own responsibilities lie when the professional provider is wearing two hats. These professionals should also consider whether they compromise their competence in both fields by marketing an expertise in medicine and wholistic practices alike. Separate agreements with the same patient/client may help clarify the different responsibilities in each relationship.

We should take care to recognize that the wholistic health movement originated in an environment of experiential study far removed from medical science. The physician's training and manner of thinking represent formidable barriers to comprehending the perspectives of wholistic practices. Physicians who have taken an interest in learning wholistic therapeutics should be commended for recognizing their value.

On a social level, we have some important choices to make. Proponents of wholistic health are raising a powerful backlash against conventional medical practice. I submit that the appreciation of medical practice for what it can do will be a measure of the fulfillment that we may derive from the wholistic health movement. If professional defensiveness in medicine governs our evolution of standards in wholistic practice, we shall forfeit the values of both.

The wholistic health movement gives us a special lens through which to examine and appreciate medical practice. The fear that wholistic practices, as an "alternative" system, will threaten medicine has already found expression in legislation that licenses acupuncture by nonmedical practitioners in a manner that will evolve standards of training and practice responsive to the medical model.

The alternative is to see wholistic practices as distinct from medicine and allow standards of training and practice to develop in accordance with the principles inherent in this new work. If wholistic practices are judged and regulated by medical standards, they will cease to develop a public appreciation of health destined to relieve the medical profession of the burden of unrealistic expectations.

And we must keep in mind the miracles of modern medical science. Should we divert the energies responsible for today's medical achievements by directing them away from pathological care? And if wholistic practice rests on criteria different from those of medical science, can the medical model offer its growth and development a nourishing environment?

Our current legal structure does not purport to comprehend health practices outside the medical model. Nor does it intend to prohibit them. Our present legal system was designed to offer preservation for standards of training and practice in medicine. Can they be applied to new perspectives on health that evolve outside the medical model?

The wholistic professions should be given time to articulate their own standards of training and practice. New laws will be necessary to establish procedures regulating licensure and competency in practice. Our choice lies between measuring new horizons by yesterday's concepts and developing a new conceptual framework to suit our experiences of today.

# I
# CHILDBIRTH

---

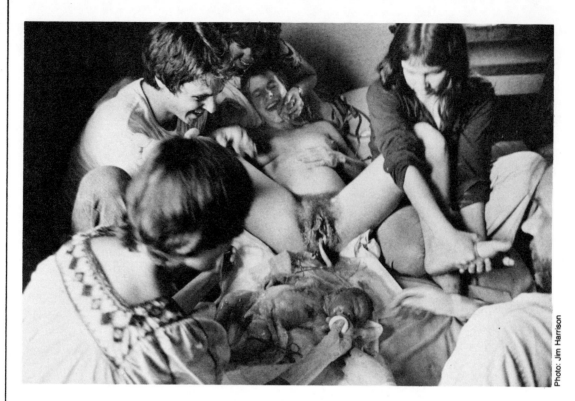

Photo: Jim Harrison

# Childbirth: An Overview
*Ruth T. Wilf, CNM, PhD*

In 1952, when my husband and I told people we were expecting our first child and hoped to have natural childbirth, we were amazed and puzzled by the reactions. Our friends and relatives immediately gave us dire warnings about their childbirth experiences, and ended with strong cautions not to experience the birth process any more than could be helped. Birth was a medical affair, involving the reproductive organs, and the rest of the person should not be involved.

Although we were young and inexperienced, this advice did not square with our perceptions. If raising children was to be a good and worthwhile part of one's life, then, surely, the act of birth, while not necessarily easy, should also be a good act. Also, we strongly believed that whole, sensitive and understanding people should be involved in the helping process, in order to maximize the birth to its fullest potential.

Of course, we were right. Despite poor support, the birth was indeed marvelous, and our positive feelings have been constantly reaffirmed and enlarged upon since. I tell this story because it is typical of so much that has happened in maternity care in this country. Unfortunately, negative conditioning and conditions still exist.

Earlier in this century, when birth took place mainly at home, it was treated in a more "wholesome" manner. At the same time, many mothers and/or babies fell ill or died. In the 1920's and 1930's, great medical advances were made, especially in understanding the role of infection and the importance of good prenatal care. Birth moved largely to the hospital, where women fell into the passive "sick" role, and were "delivered," rather than actively birthing. Usually anesthesia was used, so that the person of the woman was conveniently out of the way. Of course these women could not take care of their babies, who often needed resuscitation, so off the babies went to the nursery. Since the temper of the times dictated strict schedules, breast-feeding just didn't fit in. How easy it is to get off the track, and how hard to get back on again!

Into this confusion came Grantly Dick-Read, the English obstetrician, espousing natural birth in his pioneering book, *Childbirth without Fear*, my own candle in the darkness in 1952. Dick-Read believed that to give birth well, a woman should completely understand the body process and develop the ability (through preparation and practice) to relax and flow with the labor. Simple breathing techniques were taught for greater oxygenation and body harmony. Using the above principles, fear, which had led to tension and pain, was decreased. During labor and birth the woman was supported, helped to give birth actively, and could greet her child with joy.

The second great contribution, the psychoprophylactic method, came to the United States from Russia via France. Dr. Fernand Lamaze observed psychoprophylaxis in Russia in 1951 and began using it in France. However, it wasn't until Marjorie Karmel, an American woman who had her baby in Paris, wrote about it in her inspirational book, *Thank You, Dr. Lamaze*, in 1959, that psycho-prophylaxis became known and popular here. The psychoprophylactic method works on the theory of conditioned response. The woman is trained to respond to specific stimuli, in this case labor contractions, with specific, learned relaxation and breathing responses. At the same time, older, less positive responses toward birth are deconditioned. This is a more active approach than the Dick-Read method.

In the early 1960's significant parent-professional groups were formed to promote the concept that childbearing should be a healthy experience for the whole family, physically, mentally, and emotionally, and to introduce the concept of family-centered maternity care. These organizations have met many needs expressed by parents, which had not been met by the medical profession. They have grown enormously as true consumer movements to the present day, and childbirth classes have literally sprung up everywhere.

According to the concept of family-centered maternity care, the entire family should be involved in the childbearing experience. The goal is to have a healthy mother and baby within the context of the entire experience, suited to this particular family's needs. This experience is designed to strengthen family bonds, promote loving feelings and human growth, and help the family in their parenting task. In the 1960's parents who wished family-centered care were asking for childbirth preparation, which included relaxation and breathing techniques, support in labor and birth from the father as well as professional staff, the right of fathers to participate in the birth, the right of the mother to be "awake and aware" during the birth, rooming-in with the baby, and help with breast-feeding.

Another source of support for family-centered, humanistic care and prepared childbirth is the nurse-midwife. Increasing in numbers throughout the 1960's and 1970's, nurse-midwives are dedicated to the care of the family throughout the entire normal childbearing process, and are especially committed to being responsive to the wishes of the parents being served.

As the 1960's and 1970's progressed, several other childbirth preparation methods and variations appeared. (For instance, the Kitzinger and Bradley methods described herein.) I believe that what all "methods" have in common is far greater than their differences. Moreover, this is a changing field, as childbirth educators learn continually from what works with women in labor and from each other. The goal is a common one: to increase the dignity and meaningfulness of birth through a higher level of functioning and participation.

What of the baby in all this? Parents may now participate in birth and feel a sense of reward, but usually the baby is insensitively whisked away during the first moments of life. Parents become frustrated and babies begin to cry. It is much more natural to put newborns into parents' arms and leave them there. Two important recent developments have helped. Marshall Klaus and John Kennell, pediatricians at Case Western Reserve University School of Medicine, have been documenting the importance of keeping babies and parents together to promote the attachment of the parents to the baby. Simultaneously, Frederick Leboyer, a French obstetrician, has written a book, *Childbirth without Violence*, which has captured the imagination of many parents. He points out that we need to be aware of the infant from the moment of birth as a feeling person and accordingly to treat the baby lovingly and tenderly.

Where do we stand now? As is well known, there have been numerous recent obstetrical advances. These may be valuable and lifesaving when needed, but when applied to all indiscriminately, may interfere with the normal process of labor. This leads to a danger of dehumanizing care and not treating the person as a whole. Parents must be good consumers, ask questions, evaluate individually what is right for them personally and medically and above all, to be sure to give only an "informed consent" to medical procedures. In family-centered maternity care current goals include the right of normal babies and parents to be together from the moment of birth continuously, and for sick babies and/or mothers to be together as much as possible. Other goals are: increasing parent control and responsibility, choice of any support persons for labor and birth, opportunity to labor and birth in the same room in a comfortable bed, support person present in case of cesarean birth, brothers and sisters able to visit mother and new baby, individualized early discharge, and help with parenting on a short- or long-term basis.

The newest concept is that of "alternative birth." There is growing sentiment that for those women who are healthy and responsible there should be an option for giving birth outside the hospital in a birthing center or the home. Hospital facilities should be readily available in case of complications though. Thus birth has come home again, full circle, but this time in a more sophisticated way.

In conclusion, recent research has shown that the affects of a negative birth experience on the parent or child, whether it be through the use of technical procedures or natural causes, does, in many cases, effect the future health of that person. It is, therefore, important to realize that until we make *whole* our beginnings, our future health as a *whole* can only remain uncertain.

# A New Look At Drug Abuse In Childbirth

*Doris B. Haire*

Throughout the ages those who have assisted women in childbirth have sought various means of alleviating the laboring woman's discomfort or pain. Until fairly recently, the safety of the various potions, brews, drugs, and procedures were judged primarily by whether or not the mother and child survived. The placenta was assumed to be a protective barrier, preventing the drugs administered to the mother from entering the baby's bloodstream. As medical technology grew more sophisticated, it became apparent that the placenta is not a protective barrier but, in the words of the late Virginia Apgar, a "bloody sieve" which allows drugs administered to pregnant women to quickly cross the placental membranes and enter the fetal bloodstream, no matter how the drug is administered to the mother.

Until fairly recently, most physicians worried little when an infant was born limp and hypoxic. It was just assumed that if the infant left the hospital in reasonably good condition, it would grow to healthy adulthood. With the development of psychomotor testing of the newborn, it has become apparent that both health professionals and health care consumers must reevaluate the wisdom of traditional American obstetric practices. Let's look at our track record. It is estimated by reliable authorities that:

- One in every thirty-five children born in the United States today will be retarded (in 75 percent of these cases there is no familial, genetic, or sociological predisposing factor);
- One out of every eight children in the United States is learning disabled or has some form of minimal brain dysfunction;
- One in every three newborn infants in the United States admitted to intensive care nurseries comes from a woman who was judged to be completely normal when labor began.

Retardation, minimal brain dysfunction, and learning disability are conditions which cut across the socio-economic and ethnic strata of society. Both American health professionals and expectant parents have been lulled into a false sense of security; they assume that if a drug has been released or approved as "safe and effective" by the U.S. Food and Drug Administration, that drug is in fact safe. A closer look at how the FDA currently regulates drugs produces the disturbing fact that the FDA does *not* guarantee the safety of any drug that that agency approves as "safe and effective." In fact, the FDA does not have a specific definition of "safe." The criteria used by the FDA for determining the relative safety of drugs administered to women during labor and birth does not include a requirement that long-term safety be shown for the mental and neurological development of the child exposed to the drug *in utero*.

There is no drug, whether prescription drug or over-the-counter remedy, that has been proven safe for the unborn child, according to the Committee on Drugs of the American Academy of Pediatrics.

There is no question that obstetric drugs have saved thousands of lives and are essential to the armamentarium of the obstetrician, but the fact remains that any drug (whether necessary or unnecessary) that changes the fetus's intrauterine environment, or changes the mother's or fetus's blood chemistry, can jeopardize the fetus and the integrity of the fetal brain.

Fifty milligrams of meperidine (once considered an innocuous dose), given to the mother at the most optimal time during labor, has now been shown to cause respiratory depression in one out of every four newborn infants. Pudendal block, a common procedure once also assumed to be harmless, has now been shown to have an undesirable effect on both the mother and her newborn infant.

With all our technology, no one knows the degree of maternal hypotension or oxygen depletion an unborn or newborn infant can tolerate before the infant sustains permanent brain damage, dysfunction, or death. Nor do we know the long-term effects of electively inducing or chemically stimulating labor contractions, artificially rupturing the amniotic membranes, confining the mother to bed during labor, applying fundal pressure, or extracting a baby by forceps—all procedures which cause stress to the fetus or newborn infant.

Any drug that slows the mother's respiration, lowers her blood pressure, or increases the need to rupture the amniotic membranes can adversely affect the fetus and newborn infant. The same is true of any procedure that increases the need for fundal pressure, forceps extraction, cesarean section, or resuscitation of the newborn infant. Surely it is unwise to subject the fetus to any unnecessary procedure or drug that could alter the functioning of so complex and vital an organ as the human brain. Even in the hands of a qualified anesthesiologist, analgesics and anesthetic agents are potentially dangerous for the fetus.

Individual differences in the fetus's physiology and metabolism make it impossible for anyone to know the degree of drug toxicity, oxygen depletion, head compression, or traction by forceps that an unborn infant can tolerate before the infant sustains permanent brain damage.

Dr. Yvonne Brackbill of Georgetown University School of Medicine recently cautioned that the human baby is particularly susceptible to the damaging effects of obstetrical drugs because at the time of birth the newborn infant's brain is structurally and functionally incomplete. Because the brain of the fetus and newborn infant is undergoing very rapid change and growth, this intricate developing neurological system is more susceptible to permanent damage. Dr. Brackbill has cautioned that environmental influences can change the direction in which these systems develop, the rate at which they develop, and even the extent to which they develop at all. After the baby is born and must depend on its own bodily functions to detoxify drugs remaining in its system after birth, the rapidly developing nervous system is even more vulnerable to environmental insults which will reroute or alter the neurological development of the child. Dr. Brackbill further warns that many drugs appear to be trapped in the brain and are detoxified only after a relatively long period of time. For example, Valium administered to mothers during labor can still be found in the tissues of their newborn infants ten days after birth.

Those who would justify the use of drugs during labor and birth on the grounds that the electronic monitor will identify deviations in normal fetal physiology should be reminded of or alerted to the fact that *no one knows the long-term or delayed effects of ultrasound, used in electronic fetal monitors, on the physical, neurologic, and mental development of the child*. Evidence drawn from animal studies indicates that ultrasonic radiation can alter the spleen's ability to produce antibodies. Therefore, it would seem commonsense to use ultrasound devices only when medically indicated. Those who contend that ultrasound used for fetal monitoring is harmless should be reminded that many men and women now have iatrogenic cancer as a result of x-ray therapy which at the time it was administered for acne or enlarged tonsils was considered harmless.

Blue hands and feet are seen so frequently in American hospital-born infants after the first hour of life that parents are now told in hospital-based childbirth education classes that such a condition is normal. While American health professionals tend to be satisfied with such "average" or "normal" babies, health professionals in countries that have a better infant outcome than we do tend to put their efforts into seeing that every baby is in optimal condition at birth.

Undoubtedly the home birth movement which has swept across the country has had a beneficial impact on hospital-based maternity care. To attract couples who are determined to have a natural birth, enterprising hospitals have begun to develop communal Labor Lounges and Birth Rooms, where the mother may labor, give birth, and recover surrounded by her family. The new born infant remains in his/her parents' arms as long as the couple wishes. In such an atmosphere the parents feel more in control. There has definitely been a turn for the better.

## Groups and Associations

(1) **ASSOCIATION FOR CHILDBIRTH AT HOME**
National Headquarters
Box 1219
Cerritos, CA 90701

(213) 865-5123

Seeks to give support and encouragement to women who wish to give birth at home, and to educate their families through classes and counseling to provide a basis for responsible decision making in the childbearing process. The Association actively works to support midwifery and various legislation which would facilitate their goals.

**(2) AMERICAN COLLEGE OF NURSE-MIDWIVES**
1000 Vermont Avenue, N.W.
Washington, DC 20005

(202) 628-4642

A professional association of certified nurse-midwives who have completed a standardized postgraduate program in the management and care of mothers and babies throughout the maternity cycle. ACNM publishes the *Journal of Nurse-Midwifery* and is responsible for reviewing university-level, nurse-midwifery training programs **(see 28-41).**

**(3) AMERICAN SOCIETY FOR PSYCHO-PROPHYLAXIS IN OBSTETRICS**
1523 ''L'' Street, N.W.
Washington, DC 20005

(202) 783-7050

*Melba A. Gandy, Executive Director*

A professional association of MDs, registered nurses, and allied health professionals practicing the psychoprophylactic approach to natural childbirth (Lamaze method). There are currently over 2,500 ASPO groups and classes nationwide, and the Society handles over 20,000 referrals in a given year. Among the professional services offered are comprehensive training in psychoprophylaxis leading to ASPO certification, continuing education for ASPO certificate holders, a National Speakers' Bureau, and an extensive collection of literature and audiovisual aids for natural childbirth education classes. The society supports hospital delivery (as opposed to home birth) in a humanistic, homelike hospital setting, and is supportive of the LeBoyer approach. The Society publishes a quarterly newsletter, *Conceptions*, and a ''Professional Bulletin.'' For information on which chapters offer classes in Kitzinger psychosexual birth write to the following:

Northern Illinois Chapter of ASPO
P.O. Box 174
Highland Park, IL 60035

**(4) SOCIETY FOR THE PROTECTION OF THE UNBORN THROUGH NUTRITION**
17 North Wabash, Suite 603
Chicago, IL 60602

(312) 332-2334

*Tom Brewer, MD, President*

Promotes education on the importance of nutrition to pregnant mothers through classes, literature, and audiovisual material. The Society is involved in establishing nutrition centers in metropolitan areas of the U.S. to dispense nutritional supplements and nutritional counseling to pregnant women. Discourages the prescribing of low-calorie and low-salt diets to pregnant women. Founded 1972.

**(5) LA LECHE LEAGUE INTERNATIONAL, INC.**
9616 Minneapolis Avenue
Franklin Park, IL 60131

(312) 455-7730

*Mrs. Clement Tompson, President*

An international organization devoted to supporting mothers who wish to breastfeed their babies. The staff of certified leaders, all experienced nursing mothers, are available to both individuals and maternity centers for consultation. The League is backed by a 34-member Professional Advisory Board, composed of obstetricians, allergists, and pediatricians. Professional seminars for physicians are accredited by the AMA, the American College of Obstetrics and Gynecology, and the American Academy of Family Practice. Nursing mothers with breastfeeding problems can call the above telephone number any time, night or day, for assistance. The League distributes manuals on the subject of breastfeeding in English, French, Spanish, and English and Spanish braille; and publishes a bimonthly newsletter, *Leaven*. Founded 1956.

**(6) NATIONAL ASSOCIATION OF PARENTS AND PROFESSIONALS FOR SAFE ALTERNATIVES IN CHILDBIRTH**
P.O. Box 1307
Chapel Hill, NC 27514

(919) 732-7302

*Lee Stewart, President*

Disseminates information to professionals and the general public on alternatives in childbirth, including family-centered birth in hospitals, childbearing centers, and home birth programs.

**(7) INTERNATIONAL CHILDBIRTH EDUCATION ASSOCIATION**
P.O. Box 20852
Milwaukee, WI 53220

(414) 476-0130

*Jamie Bolane, President*

An international organization dedicated to providing education and other assistance to parents, professionals, hospitals, and other institutions for the establishment of quality family-oriented maternity care. This is accomplished through local classes, regional conferences, a newsletter, a speakers' bureau, and by coordinating and developing literature and other educational aids. The association answers thousands of individual inquiries annually. Information and classes on the Kitzinger psychosexual method also available; contact the regional directors listed below.

**REGIONAL DIRECTORS**

**U.S. SOUTHERN**
c/o Lee and David Stewart
Route 3, Box 23A
Hillsborough, NC 27278

(919) 732-7302

**U.S. MIDWESTERN**
c/o Carolyn Tadge
1819 Sheridan Road
South Euclid, OH 44121

(216) 381-8945

**U.S. EASTERN**
c/o Ann Gray
Drawer Q
McLean, VA 22101

(703) 893-5774

**U.S. WESTERN**
c/o Marie Foxton
8322 Maybelle Lane, S.W.
Tacoma, WA 98498

(206) 588-0814

CANADIAN
c/o Barbara Reid
182 Topcliffe Crescent
Fredericton, New Brunswick
Canada E3B 4P9

(506) 455-2868

## Schools, Centers, and Clinics

### (8) CENTER FOR FAMILY GROWTH
555 Highland Avenue
Cotati, CA 94928

(707) 795-5155

*Anu de Monterice, MD*

Offers workshops in prenatal yoga, postnatal yoga, natural birth control and special groups for new parents. Also specialized workshops and therapy groups for women, as well as other groups in dreams, primal therapy, gestalt, and child and family counseling. In process is a Birth and Death Center to train educators in natural approaches to birth and death. The Center has also opened a holistic prenatal clinic offering herbal family health care, massage for pregnancy, and nutritional counseling. The staff includes Jeannine O'Brien Medvin, author of *Prenatal Yoga and Natural Birth* and a *Natural Birth Control Mandala*, both available from the Center.

### (9) PEOPLE'S SCHOOL OF NATUROPATHIC HEALTH AND INSTITUTE OF THE HEALING ARTS AND COLLEGE OF DOMICILIARY MIDWIFERY
928 Fouth Street
Eureka, CA 95501

(707) 442-8717

Devoted to studying "... micro- and macrolevels of medical-social change to understand cosmic and spatial relationships in the design of a new and evolving medical deliverance system." Provides education and training in nutrition and preventive medicine. Also conducts training programs in natural childbirth, home-birthing techniques, prenatal and postnatal care, and early parenting education.

### (10) DISCOVERY INSTITUTE
1020 Corporation Way
Suite 103
Palo Alto, CA 94303

(414) 969-3800

*Vergal C. Dawson, Director*

Programs in psychological self-healing of mind/body through weekend intensives. Developing education in alternative birthing practices, prenatal awareness, and a holistic approach to childbirth. Techniques employed in therapy include meditation, transactional analysis, gestalt, psychodrama, and group work.

SAN ANDREAS HEALTH CENTER (holistic center)/Palo Alto, CA **(see 101)**

### (11) CHILDBIRTH WITHOUT PAIN EDUCATION LEAGUE, INC.
3940 Eleventh Street
Riverside, CA 92501

(714) 683-9302

Offers preparatory courses for childbirth at the Riverside office and a comprehensive correspondence course. A teacher-training program is available to women who have had babies by the Lamaze method and who have breastfed a minimum of four months. The League has a lending library of volumes on childbirth and related subjects, a comprehensive instructor's guide, a newsletter, and audiovisual materials for the use of teachers and teacher-trainees. Additionally, a Spanish manual is available, covering the Lamaze method, fetal development, and breastfeeding. Workshops and seminars are conducted several times a year. Founded 1965.

SAN DIEGO NATURAL HEALTH CLINIC/San Diego, CA **(see 108)**

### (12) ALTERNATIVE BIRTH CENTER
Room 6J5 OB-GYN
San Francisco General Hospital
1001 Potrero Street
San Francisco, CA 94110

(415) 647-7828

*Judy Goldschmidt, RN, CNM, MA, Coordinator*

Delivery services for women with normal pregnancies. Childbirth preparation classes in Lamaze, Dick-Read, and Bradley methods are offered as part of the program. Founded 1975.

HOLISTIC LIFE UNIVERSITY (childbirth)/San Francisco, CA **(see 111)**

### (13) ENTERPOINT FOUNDATION
P.O. Box 88
San Geronimo, CA 94963

(415) 488-9180

*Lawrence Weiner and Mary Weiner, RN, Co-Presidents*

Offers classes in wholistic, family-centered approaches to childbirth. In planning is the New Life Center, which will train obstetrical associates in meeting the needs of the birthing family in both home and hospital settings. Founded 1975.

AMERICAN ACADEMY OF HUSBAND-COACHED CHILDBIRTH/Sherman Oaks, CA **(see 50)**

ISLA VISTA OPEN DOOR MEDICAL CLINIC/Isla Vista, CA **(see 85)**

INTEGRAL HEALTH SERVICES (holistic clinic)/Putnam, CT **(see 120)**

### (14) HUMAN LACTATION CENTER
666 Sturges Highway
Westport, CT 06880

(203) 259-5995

Seeks to encourage breastfeeding and improve weaning practices in third world areas. At a recent conference a comprehensive review of the literature on breastfeeding was presented, including an overview of economic factors in infant nutrition and importing infant food. Also publishes newsletter.

## (15) HOME ORIENTED MATERNITY EXPERIENCE (HOME)
511 New York Avenue
Takoma Park, Washington, DC 20012

(301) 585-5832

*Esther Herman*

Educates couples on the advantages of home birth and the possibilities for a homelike experience in hospitals. This is accomplished through monthly classes, a home birth manual, individual counseling, and a quarterly newsletter *News from HOME*. The material covers medical and psychological aspects of the home birth experience, breastfeeding, and transition to parenthood. Founded 1974.

## (16) AMERICAN COLLEGE OF HOME OBSTET-RICS
664 North Michigan Avenue
Suite 610
Chicago, IL 60611

(312) 222-1600

*Gregory J. White, MD, Chairman*

A professional association of physicians involved in home birth. Members learn from and teach each other the art of safe supervision of births in the home, ". . . the natural and traditional place for birth throughout the world and the ages."

## (17) MATERNITY CENTER ASSOCIATES LTD.
5411 Cedar Lane #107-B
Bethesda, MD 20014

(301) 530-3300

*Marion McCartney, CNM*

Offers prenatal care, family planning, home birth, and a nurse-midwifery service. Clients attend Lamaze childbirth classes and have an option for a LeBoyer type delivery. The center has two obstetrician-gynecologists serving as medical directors. Founded 1975.

## (18) BIRTH DAY
Box 388
Cambridge, MA 02138

(617) 491-4835

*Gigi Groth Devitt*

An organization of parents and other individuals concerned "with making it possible for women and their mates to choose where, how, and with whom they give birth." Offers an 8-week preparatory class for home birth, holds monthly meetings to discuss home birth and other alternatives, circulates a quarterly newsletter to members, and actively works for legalization of midwifery and development of emergency back-up services for home birth. Birth Day also maintains a speakers' bureau, and makes referrals to doctors and other professionals supportive of home birth.

## AMERICAN COLLEGE OF OSTEOPATHIC OBSTETRICIANS AND GYNECOLOGISTS/Merrill, MI (see 290)

## CHRISTOS SCHOOL OF NATURAL HEALING/Taos, NM (see 135)

## (19) WHOLISTIC BIRTH AND FAMILY CENTER
P.O. Box 421
Midwood Station
Brooklyn, NY 11230

(212) 693-9230

*Harriet R. Barry, Administrator*

Offers workshops in natural childbirth methods (Lamaze, Bradley), in English, French, and Spanish; home birth, breastfeeding, nutrition, and herbal medicine. Classes are also offered in the Alexander technique and a humanistic counseling process. The Center maintains a film and book library on topics related to the birth experience.

## (20) HEALTHORIUM
P.O. Box 59
Lawrence, NY 11559

(212) 471-7308

*Shoshana Margolin, Director*

Offers lectures and workshops in nutrition, weight control, and natural home birth. Maintains a health care referral service.

## (21) MATERNITY CENTER ASSOCIATION
48 East 92nd Street
New York, NY 10028

(212) 369-7300

*Ruth Watson Lubic, General Director*

A national association dedicated to providing quality care to mothers and babies before, during, and after birth. The association's Childbearing Center, serving families in the Bronx, Manhattan and Queens, offers prenatal care, labor and delivery in a homelike setting, and early discharge with home follow-up by the Visiting Nurse Service. Founded 1918.

## THE MOUNTAIN PEOPLES' CLINIC (childbirth)/Hayesville, NC (see 144)

## (22) CENTRE FOR WHOLISTIC BIRTH
934 Washington Street #10
Eugene, OR 97401

(502) 345-3405

The Centre is a nonprofit birth education organization devoted to encouraging a high quality of life through conscious conception and pregnancy, natural and sensitive birth, and creative parenting. "Giving birth is a natural process, and we support parents in creating the experience they choose." Services include prenatal classes and workshops in the wholistic approach to childbirth based on the Leboyer method, film presentations, and other programs including the gentle art of baby massage, conscious conception, prenatal centering yoga, and massage. Information packets and booklets available at nominal fees.

## EUGENE CENTER FOR THE HEALING ARTS (educational center)/Eugene, OR (see 148)

### (23) NATUROPATHIC BIRTH CENTER
671 Southwest Main Street
Winston, OR 97496

(503) 679-6726

*A.M. LaRusch, ND, DC, Director*

Specializes in natural drugless childbirth. Additional work is done with nutritional evaluations accomplished through analysis of both blood and hair; herbology; and orthopedics using xray, physiotherapy, and manipulation.

### (24) BOOTH MATERNITY CENTER
6051 Overbrook Avenue
Philadelphia, PA 19131

(215) 878-7800

A family-oriented maternity center emphasizing natural childbirth. Classes offered for mothers and fathers in childbirth preparation.

### (25) THE MATERNITY CENTER
1119 East San Antonio
El Paso, TX 79901

(915) 533-8142

*Shari Daniels, Director*

Provides delivery services either at the Center or in private homes, prenatal care with emphasis on superior nutrition, and postpartum follow-up consisting of four weekly visits to the center to talk about breastfeeding and early adjustments. A full series of childbirth preparation classes is offered using basic Lamaze techniques with extensive additional material. The Center will assist single mothers in finding families to live with, maintains a baby sitting service, and has a co-op for the purchase of baby clothes and related items. Other services include training programs for midwives, a speakers' bureau, and a 24-hour hotline. Founded 1976.

### (26) THE NATIONAL CHILDBIRTH TRUST
9 Queensborough Terrace
Bayswater, London W23TB
England

Tel 01-229 9319

Offers classes in natural childbirth. Information and classes in the Kitzinger method also available.

### (27) PARAMEDICAL ASSOCIATION FOR CHILD-BIRTH EDUCATION
60 Valley Road
Parktown 2100
Johannesburg, South Africa

Natural childbirth center. Information and classes in the Kitzinger method also available.

**KITZINGER CENTER** (birth center)/Uppsala, Sweden **(see 51)**

*NURSE-MIDWIFERY GRADUATE PROGRAMS UNDER THE SUPERVISION OF THE AMERICAN COLLEGE OF NURSE-MIDWIVES* **(2)**

### (28) YALE UNIVERSITY SCHOOL OF NURSING
Graduate Program in Maternal and Newborn Nursing and Nurse-Midwifery
38 South Street
New Haven, CT 06510

(203) 436-3781

Master's degree programs for RNs and nonnurse college graduates in nurse-midwifery.

### (29) GEORGETOWN UNIVERSITY SCHOOL OF NURSING
3700 Reservoir Road, N.W.
Washington, DC 20007

(202) 625-4373

Graduate program for RNs in nurse-midwifery.

### (30) THE UNIVERSITY OF ILLINOIS AT THE MEDICAL CENTER
College of Nursing
Department of Maternal-Child Nursing
Nurse-Midwifery Program
P.O. Box 6998
Chicago, IL 60680

(312) 996-7800

Graduate program for RNs in nurse-midwifery leading to the Master's degree.

### (31) UNIVERSITY OF KENTUCKY
College of Nursing
Albert B. Chandler Medical Center
Lexington, KY 40506

(606) 258-9000

Graduate program for RNs in nurse-midwifery leading to the Master's degree.

### (32) UNITED STATES AIR FORCE
Nurse-Midwifery Program
Malcolm Grow USAF Medical Center
Andrews Air Force Base, MD 20331

(301) 981-9811

Basic graduate program for RNs in nurse-midwifery.

### (33) THE JOHNS HOPKINS UNIVERSITY
School of Hygiene and Public Health
Nurse-Midwifery Program
615 North Wolfe Street
Baltimore, MD 21205

(301) 955-5000

Graduate program for RNs in nurse-midwifery leading to the Master's degree.

### (34) UNIVERSITY OF MISSISSIPPI
Nurse-Midwifery Program
2500 North State Street
Jackson, MS 39216

(601) 968-5590

Basic graduate and refresher programs for RNs in nurse-midwifery.

### (35) ST. LOUIS UNIVERSITY
Department of Nursing
Graduate Program in Nurse-Midwifery

1310 South Grand Boulevard
St. Louis, MO 63104

(314) 535-3300

Graduate program for RNs in nurse-midwifery leading to the Master's degree.

(36) **COLLEGE OF MEDICINE AND DENTISTRY OF NEW JERSEY**
School of Allied Health Professions
Nurse-Midwifery Program
100 Bergen Street
Newark, NJ 07102

(201) 456-4300

Graduate program for RNs in nurse-midwifery.

(37) **STATE UNIVERSITY OF NEW YORK**
College of Health Related Professions
Nurse-Midwifery Program, Box 1216
450 Clarkson Avenue
Brooklyn, NY 11203

(212) 270-1000

Basic graduate and internship programs for RNs in nurse-midwifery.

(38) **COLUMBIA UNIVERSITY GRADUATE PROGRAM IN MATERNITY NURSING AND NURSE-MIDWIFERY**
Department of Nursing, Faculty of Medicine
Columbia-Presbyterian Medical Center
622 West 168th Street
New York, NY 10032

(212) 280-1754

Graduate program for RNs in nurse-midwifery, leading to the Master's degree.

(39) **SIMPSON CENTER FOR MATERNAL HEALTH**
The Community Hospital of Springfield and Clark County
350 South Burnett Road
Springfield, OH 45505

(513) 325-0531

Refresher and internship programs for qualified nurse-midwives.

(40) **MEDICAL UNIVERSITY OF SOUTH CAROLINA**
Nurse-Midwifery Program, College of Nursing
80 Barre Street
Charleston, SC 29401

(803) 792-0211

Basic graduate program for RNs in nurse-midwifery.

(41) **UNIVERSITY OF UTAH**
College of Nursing
Graduate Major in Maternal and Newborn Nursing and Nurse-Midwifery
25 South Medical Drive
Salt Lake City, UT 84112

(801) 531-7728

Master's degree and refresher programs for RNs in nurse-midwifery.

# Journals and Publications

(42) **BIRTH AND THE FAMILY JOURNAL**
110 El Camino Real
Berkeley, CA 94705

Sponsored by the International Childbirth Education Association (ICEA) and the American Society for Prophylaxis in Obstetrics (ASPO).

(43) **COUNTRY LADY'S DAYBOOK**
Box 7527
Oakland, CA 94601

Monthly magazine with articles on natural agriculture, herbs, home births, and country living.

(44) **KEEPING ABREAST CENTER**
3885 Forest
Denver, CO 80207

(303) 388-4608

*Jimmie Lynne Avery, Editor*

Quarterly journal devoted to supporting the nursing mother and her infant.

(45) **MOTHERING**
P.O. Box 184
Ridgway, CO 81432

(303) 626-5475

*Adeline Eavenson, Editor*

Quarterly journal dealing with all aspects of birth and child-rearing. Articles on alternative education, breastfeeding, home birth, herbal medicine, nutrition, and midwifery.

**HUMAN LACTATION REVIEW** (breastfeeding)/ Westport, CT **(see 14)**

**CONCEPTIONS** (childbirth)/Washington, DC **(see 3)**

**JOURNAL OF NURSE-MIDWIFERY**/Washington, DC **(see 2)**

**NEWS FROM HOME** (childbirth newsletter)/ Washington, DC **(see 15)**

**ALTERNATIVES JOURNAL** (multidisciplinary magazine)/Miami, FL **(see 193)**

**LEAVEN** (La Leche League newsletter)/Franklin Park, IL **(see 5)**

**EAST WEST JOURNAL** (multidisciplinary magazine)/ Brookline, MA **(see 195)**

**NEW AGE JOURNAL** (multidisciplinary magazine)/ Brookline, MA **(see 196)**

(46) **BOOKMARKS**
P.O. Box 70258
Seattle, WA 98107

(206) 789-4444

*Karol Magnuson, Editor*

Published by the International Childbirth Education Association. Reviews books on childbirth, breastfeeding, and related subjects.

## Products and Services

**(47) PHOTOVIEW INSTRUCTIONAL AIDS**
27935 Roble Alto
Los Altos, CA 94022

(415) 948-5832

Distributes 35-mm color slides on childbirth, breastfeeding, infant care, and Mensendieck prenatal exercises, and movement techniques.

**BUTTERFLY MEDIA DIMENSIONS** (multidisciplinary cassette tapes)/N. Hollywood, CA **(see 210)**

**NEW DIMENSIONS FOUNDATION** (multidisciplinary cassette tapes)/San Francisco, CA **(see 212)**

**RAINBOW BRIDGE** (new age books and records)/San Francisco, CA **(see 213)**

**HARTLEY FILM PRODUCTIONS** (multidisciplinary audiovisuals)/Cos Cob, CT **(see 219)**

**(48) CINEMA MEDICA, INC.**
664 North Michigan Avenue
Chicago, IL 60611

(312) 664-6170

Distributes a film on home birth, which was supervised by The American College of Home Obstetrics.

**(49) INTERNATIONAL CHILDBIRTH EDUCATION ASSOCIATION SUPPLIES CENTER**
P.O. Box 70258
Seattle, WA 98107

(206) 789-4444

Issues a directory of films, books and recordings on childbirth. All items are available from the Center.

**TUESDAY ISLAND FARM** (fertility cycle charts)/Nova Scotia, Canada **(see 610)**

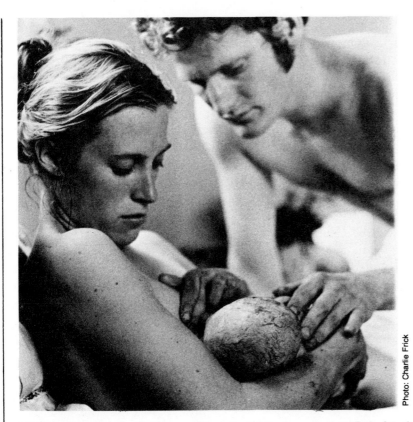

Photo: Charlie Frick

# Husband-Coached Natural Childbirth

*Robert A. Bradley, MD*

Growing up on a dairy farm, I observed that all species of mammals, excluding the human, swim perfectly when entering water, give birth perfectly upon entering labor, and appear to enjoy doing both. At medical school I was horrified by the human approach to the birth experience known as the "knock 'em out, drag 'em out" method. It seemed to me that if humans can be taught how to swim, they could just as easily be taught to give birth.

After trying out my theory on volunteer primiparas, mostly registered nurses, I conceived the idea of using the husband as coach, in continuous attendance throughout the labor. This was not easy, for at that time hospital rules excluded the husband from the delivery room. Finally, after 30 years, we have managed to change these outmoded rules. The Bradley method of *Husband-Coached Childbirth* (Harper and Row, 1974) is now widely accepted, taught, and practiced throughout the world.

The idea of unmedicated, "natural" childbirth, once the object of much derision, gained credence as two new divisions of medicine arose: neonatology and perinatology. Scientific studies have verified the benefits to babies and mothers of the principles I derived by observing nature and instinctual conduct.

All mammalian babies begin to nurse immediately after birth, even though the milk flow is not yet established; thus, it made sense to me to place human babies at the breast, skin to skin with their mothers, right after birth. Moreover, we were warned as children not to take animal babies away from their mothers too soon after birth; their mothers might not accept them back and indeed might even kill them.

In the era of drugged deliveries, separation of mother and child may have been indicated since in their bewildered, hateful state, mothers could not be trusted to care for anything. However, with natural childbirth, thwarting a mother's natural desire to hold her baby to the warmth of her body is nothing short of kidnapping and is deleterious to both baby and mother in many subtle as well as obvious ways. Some modern, humane hospitals now recognize this fact, yet many others, clinging blindly to outmoded practices, continue to "incubate" and separate babies as if their mothers were still being drugged. In desperation young parents have begun to have their babies at home, taking unnecessary chances on the very lives of the mother and baby, for unforeseeable and potentially fatal complications can occur, in birthing as well as swimming. I still say, change the hospitals! Unless there are complications (as in about 10 percent of births), patients can return home within hours.

One of the most important ways to prepare for a safe, natural delivery—aside from studying the Bradley method, attending LaLeche League meetings, and exercising (see Rhonda E. Fleming, *Exercises for True Natural Childbirth*)—is to eliminate drugs from the bodies of both parents at least 2 years prior to conception. All drugs, whether used in obstetrics or passed on through the parents, have deleterious effects on babies, immediate or long-term, obvious or subtle. The drugged mothers of the past generation may very well account for the fact that today increasing numbers of people are resorting to drugs to cope with stress.

Those who advocate and practice true natural childbirth might appropriately be labeled "internal environmentalists." Clearly, hope for the future of this planet lies in cleaning up the pollution in its oceans, lakes, and streams. To accomplish this, we must first clean up the pollutants in the most important streams on earth, the bloodstreams of pregnant women. By giving our children the right to be born drugfree, we may be making way for a better world.

## Associations

(50) **AMERICAN ACADEMY OF HUSBAND-COACHED CHILDBIRTH**
P.O. Box 5224
Sherman Oaks, CA 91413

(213) 788-6662

*Robert A. Bradley, MD, President*

Promotes "The Bradley Method of Husband-Coached Childbirth" developed by its founder, Robert A. Bradley. The Academy trains instructors in the Bradley method and maintains standards for certification and affiliation. It also publishes newsletters, maintains listings of affiliated teachers, and distributes educational and public relations materials.

## Centers

**ALTERNATIVE BIRTH CENTER** (Bradley)/San Francisco, CA **(see 12)**

**WHOLISTIC BIRTH AND FAMILY CENTER** (Bradley)/Brooklyn, NY **(see 19)**

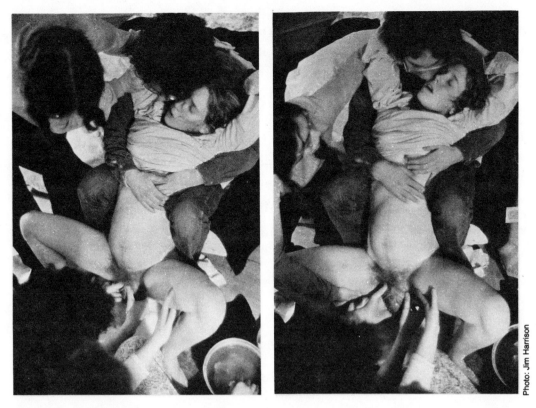

Photo: Jim Harrison

# The Kitzinger Psychosexual Approach To Childbirth

*Sheila Kitzinger, BLitt*

Childbirth should be a profound psychosexual experience rather than a task for which gymnastic exercises have to be learned. This approach to birth, evolved from both Dick-Read and French psychoprophylaxis, stresses that its techniques can be used in conjunction with Lamaze, Bradley, or other methods, and that they are not designed to replace these methods, but to add another dimension of understanding.

Relaxation and body awareness are taught in two ways: touch relaxation, for which a partner gives a signal so that release flows out towards the warmth and pressure of the touching hand; and Stanislavsky relaxation, which Kitzinger developed out of Method acting techniques, using "body memory" and "emotion memory." Breathing in labor is carefully tuned to the intensity and rhythm of each contraction and is called "wave breathing." The woman breathes over the "wave" of each contraction with breath which is always a little lighter than the pressure of the contraction. She does "butterfly breathing," a rapid, light, "mouth-centered" breathing, over the top of difficult first-stage contractions. Breathing is taught using touch relaxation with hand pressure at different levels of the back.

Body awareness includes pelvic floor exercises for increased tone and so that these muscles can be released during the birth process. It is through the action of these muscles that the baby is born, and the woman learns how to open her body and actively *give* birth. The sexual implications of increased awareness of the activity of the vagina and surrounding muscles are fully discussed.

The "gentle" second stage is taught, with no unnecessary straining and no cheer-leading to get the mother to push. The breathing used for expulsion is called the "sheep's breathing."

The psychosexual approach particularly focuses on psychological aspects of childbearing, the women's feelings about her body, the couple's relationship throughout the childbearing cycle and the new parents' changing relationship with their own parents. The emphasis is on the whole woman in the context of her marriage, family, and other social relationships. The psychosexual approach is concerned not only with the act of birth but also with people in relationships of love and interdependence.

## Associations

**ASSOCIATION FOR CHILDBIRTH AT HOME** (Kitzinger)/Cerritos, CA **(see 1)**

**ASPO** (childbirth, Lamaze and Kitzinger)/Highland Park, IL **(see 3)**

**INTERNATIONAL CHILDBIRTH EDUCATION AS-SOCIATION**(Kitzinger) (Regional Directors) /McLean, VA (also South Euclid, OH; Hillsborough, NC; Tacoma, WA; Fredricton and New Brunswick, Canada) **(see 7)**

**THE NATIONAL CHILDBIRTH TRUST** (Kitzinger)/ London, England **(see 26)**

**PARAMEDICAL ASSOCIATION FOR CHILDBIRTH EDUCATION** (Kitzinger)/Johannesburg, South Africa **(see 27)**

## Centers

**HOLISTIC LIFE UNIVERSITY** (Kitzinger)/San Francisco, CA **(see 111)**

**(51) KITZINGER CENTER**
c/o Mrs. Jan Brandt
Bellmansgatan 170
754 28 Uppsala
Sweden

Classes in psychosexual birth.

# II
# INTEGRATIVE MEDICAL SYSTEMS

---

Introduction To Wholistic Healing Groups And Centers

Homeopathy

Homeotherapeutics

Osteopathy

Chiropractic Today

The Posture Of A Profession

Applied Kinesiology

Naturopathic Medicine: A Separate And Distinct
Healing Profession

Cranial Technique

The Position Of The Mandible (Lower Jaw)
As It Relates To Stress In The Human System

Temporomandibular Joint Technique

Developmental Vision Therapy

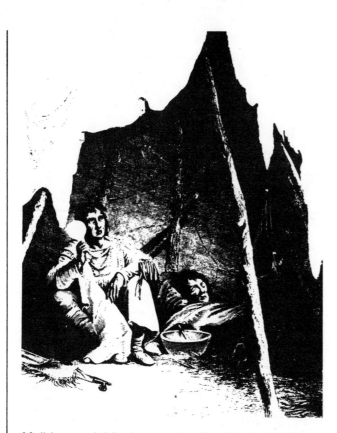

Medicine man administering to a patient, (from Schoolcraft's *History, Condition, and Prospects of the Indian Tribes;* courtesy Univ. of Oklahoma Press, from *American Indian Medicine.* By Vogel, Norman, OK: 1970.

# Introduction To Wholistic Healing Groups And Centers

*Robert M. Giller, MD*

*"Humanistic culture is as important as natural scientific culture for the practice of medicine. As physicians we have to act upon men, and as man is body, mind, and spirit, we cannot limit ourselves to the study of the basic medical sciences . . . we must take into consideration the human spirit, that mysterious power that makes us aware of our uniqueness, our liberty, our creativity, and directs us towards transcendent values."*

Lancet, *September 21, 1957, A. P. Cawadias*

Wholistic* health is a state in which a human being is integrated at all levels of being: body, mind, and spirit. Health is far more than the absence of disease or symptoms, and the concept of a wholistic medicine for the creation of this integrated state of being is far greater than any particular treatment; it is not merely an umbrella for a random collection of "alternative practices." There is no one wholistic therapy, and no one therapy is intrinsically wholistic; rather, there is a wholistic *approach* to creating and maintaining health.

The medical center of the future will be a wholistic healing center that will focus on the whole person, developing a state of health in which the individual is integrated and balanced in all aspects of his or her being. Using a variety of techniques, the center will deal with the causes of disease states, and will actively involve the patient in the healing process. Wholistic therapies do not stand in opposition to traditional health care methods; they are complementary. There is no "old medicine," no "new medicine"—but an integrated approach to the creation of an integrated human being.

---

*Spelled holistic in original text

# Groups and Associations

## (52) HOLISTIC HEALTH ORGANIZING COMMITTEE
Village Design
1545 Dwight Way
Berkeley, CA 94703

(415) 841-6500 Ext. 142

Stresses preventive medicine and health education as well as full recognition and legal protection for all forms of alternative healing and their qualified practitioners. The Committee's activities have included a holistic health retreat (workshops on Chinese medicine, food combining, iridology, and Reichian bodywork), a newsletter, and programs on the legal aspects of holistic health approaches. Formed in 1976.

## (53) QUEST OF CARMEL
P.O. Box 6301
Carmel, CA 93921

(408) 624-8722

*Florence Zellhoefer, MD, Director*

Dedicated to helping individuals become self-healers of the body, mind, and spirit. Conducts research, establishes teaching and healing centers, develops and produces aids to self-healing, and sponsors educational opportunities for the advancement of local and worldwide community services. Sponsors conferences throughout the year on themes related to healing energies, acupuncture, biofeedback, preventive medicine, Jungian psychology, parapsychology, meditation, and other dimensions of holistic therapies.

## (54) THE COMMITTEE FOR FREEDOM OF CHOICE IN CANCER THERAPY
146 Main Street, Suite 408
Los Altos, CA 94022

(415) 948-9475

Information available on alternative cancer therapies.

## (55) NATIONAL HEALTH LAW PROGRAM (NHeLP)
University of California
10995 Le Conte Avenue, Room 640
Los Angeles, CA 90024

(213) 825-7601

*Ruth Galenter, Newsletter editor*

Federally funded legal services back-up center specializing in issues relating to the health of the poor. A staff of six attorneys provides litigation assistance to local legal aid offices in such areas as access to medical care, eligibility for public funding of personal health care services and enforcement of laws designed to protect the public health. Also publishes analyses of proposed administrative regulations, dealing with health issues, and a monthly newsletter. In addition to assisting attorneys in Neighborhood Legal Services offices, NHeLP aids legislators in drafting and evaluating legislative proposals and attempts to work with other organizations concerned with the health of the poor.

## (56) LOTUS CENTRAL
P.O. Box 274
Monte Rio, CA 95462

*Edward Orem, Director*

An information clearinghouse for the natural healing arts, developing contacts among serious students, teachers, and practitioners. Facilitators involved with Lotus Central practice therapeutic massage (polarity, shiatsu, and Esalen), herbology, and teach yoga and martial arts.

**HUMAN DIMENSIONS INSTITUTE—WEST** (heuristic research)/Ojai, CA **(see 588)**

## (57) CENTER FOR INTEGRAL MEDICINE
P.O. Box 955
Pacific Palisades, CA 90272

(213) 459-3373

*David Bresler, PhD, Executive Director*

Founded by a group of physicians and psychologists dedicated to the maintenance of life and health through innovative approaches to healing and a realization of a benevolent universal life force. A central focus of exploration is the power of the mind to affect physiological functioning. Supports investigation of innovative, safer techniques of medical diagnosis, acupuncture, nutrition, hypnosis, guided imagery, biofeedback, and new approaches for treating chronic pain, hypertension, asthma, anxiety, depression, and other disorders. The Center also co-sponsors professional training programs, publishes a quarterly bulletin and a newsletter, coordinates public education programs, maintains a speakers' bureau, and is planning the development of a healing retreat in Northern California. Founded 1974.

## (58) ASSOCIATION FOR HOLISTIC HEALTH
P.O. Box 33202
San Diego, CA 92103

(714) 298-5965

*David Harris, President*

A nonprofit educational corporation dedicated to promoting and supporting holistic health, and to ensure its continued development in professional methods, standards, and ethics. Major projects include the development of a model holistic healing center, a certificate program in holistic health for health professionals, a public education program, and annual conferences covering such areas. Publishes the *Journal of Holistic Health*. Founded 1976.

## (59) THE EAST-WEST ACADEMY OF HEALING ARTS COUNCIL OF NURSE-HEALERS
P.O. Box 31211
San Francisco, CA 94131

(415) 285-9400

Dedicated to expanding the existing body of knowledge relevant to healing modalities in nursing through theory development, research, and practice. Promotes professional support for healing modalities within all cultures. Establishes parameters for the professional practice of nurse-healers. Provides a communication and education network among nurse-healers, the community of nursing and the community at large. Is presently exploring the feasibility of a formal linkage with the American Nurses Association. Founded 1976.

**(60) INSTITUTE FOR THE STUDY OF HUMANISTIC MEDICINE**
1017 Dolores Street
San Francisco, CA 94110

(415) 826-7171

*Naomi Remen, MD, Director*

Believes that effective medicine mobilizes the multiple dimensions of the person who is the patient. The Institute receives HEW support and private grants to develop new thinking, practical techniques, and educational programs of a fully human medicine. Publishes several books on the theoretical bases and practical methods of humanistic medicine. Founded 1972.

**(61) HAWAII HEALTH NET**
2535 South King Street
Honolulu, HI 96814

(808) 955-1555

*W. Stroude, MD, Director*

A communications network to assist individuals in finding viable alternatives to personal health care.

**(62) THE FOUNDATION OF TRUTH, INC.**
3941 Gateway Court
Indianapolis, IN 46254

*Ikot Alfred Ekanem, Chief Executive Director*

3 Holcombe Road
Ilford, Essex
England 1G1 4XF

Tel: 01-554-7467

*Mrs. Billie Mansfield, Founder and President*

Dedicated to uplifting mankind both spiritually and physically, through Positive Health Community Centers. The Centers include medical, nutritional, educational, legal, and spiritual services. Though centralized in the U.S. and England, the primary focus of the Foundation's activities is the development of such Centers in the country of Botswana, Africa. Long-range goals include the proliferation of these facilities throughout southern Africa.

**(63) CHILDREN IN HOSPITALS**
31 Wilshire Park
Needham, MA 02192

(617) 878-7000

*Barbara Popper, Chairperson*

A nonprofit organization of parents and health-care professionals seeking to support and educate parents wishing to remain in close contact with their children during a hospital experience. Personal counseling, a newsletter, information sheets and meetings are available. Also available is a 1972 survey of Boston area hospitals' pediatric and maternity departments' policies toward visiting and rooming-in (50¢, or free with a $2.00 membership). Founded 1972.

**(64) FOUNDATION FOR ALTERNATE CANCER THERAPIES**
P.O. Box 882

Dearborn, MI 48121

(313) 562-4269

Resource information on alternative cancer therapies.

**(65) AMERICAN MEDICAL-PSYCHIC RESEARCH ASSOCIATION**
135 Madison Avenue N.E.
Albuquerque, NM 87123

(505) 265-0221

Aims to unite individuals in the fields of osteopathy, homeopathy, naturopathy, and other therapeutic fields who share common orientations toward healing. Believes that mind-body-spirit integration can best be accomplished through a multidisciplinary cooperation.

**(66) THE EAST/WEST CENTER FOR HOLISTIC HEALTH**
275 Madison Avenue, Suite 500
New York, NY 10016

(212) 689-1321

*Marie Valenta, Director*

Dedicated to promoting effective approaches to total health and wholeness with the recognition of mind-body-spirit unity. Sponsors conferences in holistic health and is in the process of developing a holistic health facility.

**(67) FOUNDATION FOR ALTERNATIVE CANCER THERAPY, LTD.**
P.O. Box HH
Old Chelsea Station
New York, NY 10011

(212) 741-2790

Information and resources on alternative cancer therapies.

**(68) THE INTERNATIONAL INSTITUTE OF INTEGRAL HUMAN SCIENCES**
P.O. Box 1387
Station H
Montreal, Quebec,
Canada H3G 2N3

A network of scholars involved in research in psychophysical and psychospiritual integration. Research is ongoing in such areas as parapsychology, faith healing, acupuncture, biofeedback, mind-brain studies, Kirlian photography, hypnosis, anthropological studies of psychical experience, and the phenomenological study of systems of meditation and religious experience.

**(69) SOUTH PACIFIC FEDERATION OF NATURAL THERAPEUTICS, LTD.**
c/o Mrs. Clare Gulson, Secretary
1, Sage Street
St. Ives, New South Wales 2075
Australia

International association of qualified practitioners of various schools of natural and alternative healing. Full member of IFPNT **(72)**.

**(70) RESEARCH SOCIETY FOR NATURAL THERAPEUTICS**
8 Stokewood Road

Bournemouth, Dorset
England

*M.L. Budd, Secretary*

A research society providing an independent forum for the free exchange of ideas to further the cause of natural therapeutics. Aims of the society are to develop original research, to investigate new or neglected techniques of therapy and diagnosis, and to disseminate such knowledge through courses and seminars. Membership is open to physicians, scientists, and members of the natural therapeutics professions. Members receive the Research Society Journal which is published periodically. Topics covered in the Society's postgraduate courses include acupuncture, cranial osteopathy, radiesthesia, and homeopathy. Other symposia have focused on subjects ranging from psychology to environmental health. Formerly, the Naturopathic Research Group, founded 1959. Name changed 1974.

## (71) HEALTH FOR THE NEW AGE, LTD.
1A Addison Crescent
London, W14 8JP
England

Tel: 01-603-7751

*Marcus McCausland, Director*

Developing model holistic health care center; networking individuals and groups concerned with areas such as consciousness, meditation, and integrative health care. Publishes newsletter on various topics relating to holistic medicine and self-development.

## (72) INTERNATIONAL FEDERATION FOR PRACTITIONERS OF NATURAL THERAPEUTICS
21, Bingham Place
London, W1M 3FH, England

*R.J. Bloomfield, Liason Officer*

European and Australian Federation of groups engaged in all fields of natural and wholistic therapeutics. Holds conferences and symposia on various subjects relating to the field, as well as publishing a newsletter for members to inform them of legal and other developments within the field, in general. A partial list of full and affiliate member organizations includes: Association Francaise de Défense Ostéopathique **(298)**, Australian Chiropractors, Osteopaths, and Natural Physicians Association **(439)**, Australian Institute of Homeopathy **(260)**, Deutscher Verband fur Homöopathie und Lebenspflege (West Germany) **(263)**, Homöopathischer Verein E.V. (West Germany) **(262)**, Israel Naturopathic Association **(442)**, Maidstone Osteopathic Clinic (England) **(362)**, Nederlandse College Voor Naturopathie **(446)**, New Zealand Association of Naturopaths and Osteopaths **(443)**, Society of Osteopaths (England) **(296)**, South Pacific Federation of Natural Therapeutics (Australia) **(69)**.

## (73) THE HEALING RESEARCH TRUST
Field House
Peaslake, Guildford
Surrey, GU5 9SS
England

Exists to support the development of natural therapeutics in the United Kingdom. It is involved in the publication of research findings, promotion of new methods of healing, maintenance of a general research fund, providing bursaries for studies in the healing arts, and creating liasons with academic and professional societies. "The Trust's ultimate overall objective, which it shares with all responsible elements in the healing field, is to secure the recognition of natural therapeutics by the community as an established and honorable profession while at the same time ensuring that the interests of competent nonprofessionally qualified healers are safeguarded." Founded 1974.

# Schools, Centers, and Clinics

**ARE CLINIC** (Cayce)/Phoenix, AZ **(see 833)**

## (74) HEALTH AWARENESS INSTITUTE
1224 East Northern
Phoenix, AZ 85020

(602) 943-8182

*Stephen H. Grunfeld, DC, Director*

Provides natural health care through chiropractic, nutritional guidance, massage therapy, psychological counseling, and clinical hypnosis. Also hosts a lecture series throughout the year on various aspects of health and health care, including a series on yoga.

**WELL-SPRINGS** (holistic center)/Ben Lomond, CA **(see 987)**

## (75) BERKELEY COMMUNITY HEALTH PROJECT (Free Clinic)
2339 Durant Avenue
Berkeley, CA 94704

(415) 548-2570

*Harvey Smith, Coordinator of Outreach*

Preventive and self-help approaches to health are emphasized in all four areas of the clinic: medical, dental, rap center, and switchboard/crisis intervention. The medical section has optional herbal treatment for hepatitis, colds, and other imbalances not treatable by standard medicine. Clients are also offered body work, relaxation techniques, and visualization methods in group classes. Founded 1969.

## (76) BERKELEY HOLISTIC HEALTH CENTER
916 Ensenada Avenue
Berkeley, CA 94707

(415) 845-4430

Offers classes and workshops in many areas of holistic healing, stressing unity of mind, body, and spirit. These include homeopathy, massage, meditation, nutrition, iridology, polarity, herbology, bioenergetics, dreams, acupressure, reflexology, and weight control. The Center also maintains a speakers' bureau, and circulates a newsletter to members. Regular membership is $10 for six months. Founded 1976.

## (77) BERKELEY WOMEN'S HEALTH COLLECTIVE
2908 Ellsworth Street
Berkeley, CA 94705

(415) 843-1437

Provides extensive informational, educational, medical, and referral services for women in the Bay Area. Mental health counseling, pregnancy counseling, self-help groups are available. The Collective's gynecology, general medical, and pediatrics clinic are prevention oriented, and use herbs and vitamins in addition to traditional Western methods. Services are provided on a sliding scale of fee donation. Other programs include a menopausal rap group, childcare for workers and clients, and a speakers' bureau. Founded 1970.

## (78) THE PSYCHOSOMATIC MEDICINE CLINIC
2510 Webster Street
Berkeley, CA 94705

(415) 549-1228

*Kenneth R. Pelletier, PhD, Director*

A staff of medical doctors and other professional practitioners provide treatment through acupuncture, clinical biofeedback, cancer counseling and visualization therapy, orthomolecular and dietary medicine, relaxation and meditation methods, and psychotherapy. Professional education seminars in these fields are also available, accredited through the State of California's Medical Association, Continuing Education Category.

**ESALEN INSTITUTE** (multidisciplinary center)/Big Sur, CA **(see 1051)**

## (79) INSTITUTE FOR RESEARCH INTO WHOLISTIC THERAPEUTIC ENERGIES
c/o University of the Trees
P.O. Box 644
Boulder Creek, CA 95006

(408) 338-3855

*Steven Langer, MD, Director*

Programs include the relationship between color and personality, aura balancing, toning and chanting, specialized meditation for children and senior citizens, dream analysis, and "creative conflict": a growth process facilitating communication and emotional awareness. Faculty derived from the University of the Trees, a consciousness research school. Founded 1977.

**CENTER FOR FAMILY GROWTH** (childbirth)/Cotati, CA **(see 8)**

## (80) BIOLOGY OF THE MIND/BODY
Department of Behavioral Biology, School of Medicine
University of California
Davis, CA 95616

(916) 752-3259

*Jim Polidora, PhD, Instructor*

P.O. Box 709
Davis, CA 95616

An extensive course series offered to medical students which covers such areas as neurophysiology, nutrition, Eastern philosophy, yoga, transpersonal psychology, and bodywork. For those unable to join the class, eighteen two-hour recordings are available at no charge. Individuals desiring this information should submit blank 120-minute cassette tapes for each session desired.

## (81) NATIONAL ARTHRITIS MEDICAL CLINIC
13630 Mountain View Road
Desert Hot Springs, CA 92240

(714) 329-6422

*Robert Bingham, MD, Medical Director*

A nonprofit community clinic dedicated to the treatment of all forms of arthritis. Following a complete modern medical diagnosis, the patient at the clinic is treated with hot mineral water therapy, physical therapy, ultrasound, and a natural foods diet. The clinic has pioneered the use of Yucca plant saponin as a food supplement for arthritis, uses antiprotozoal drugs in research programs, and has developed an arthritis vaccine. Treatment programs are individually tailored to each patient.

## (82) VITAL HEALTH CENTER
17200 Ventura Boulevard, Suite 305
Encino, CA 91316

(213) 990-9270

*Gary R. Robb, DC, Director*

Provides chiropractic treatment with dietary, herbal, and homeopathic supplementation. For diagnosis of many conditions, the Center makes use of aura field testing, a process of observing a person's muscular response to foods, herbs, or medicines being placed within his/her field. A variety of holistic health educational programs are also offered.

## (83) MEDICINE HOLISTICS
364 South Clovis Avenue
Fresno, CA 93727

*Dave Edwards, MD, Medical Director*

A treatment facility which accepts referrals from health professionals and offers classes to the community. Specialized programs include a holistic approach to curbing smoking behavior and use of biofeedback. Founded 1976.

## (84) WHOLISTIC MEDICINE AND PERSONAL GROWTH CENTER
11633 South Hawthorne Boulevard
Suite 401
Hawthorne, CA 90250

(213) 973-7830

*Richard L. Ferman, MD, Medical Director*

Provides a comprehensive program of outpatient counseling services and an adult voluntary admission inpatient mental health care unit. Individualized treatment includes Organic Nutritional Therapy, biofeedback, yoga, Assertion Training, hypnosis, meditation, and pharmaceutical services. Special individual and group programs are offered in sexual reeducation, substance abuse treatment (drugs, alcohol, cigarettes), weight control, art therapy, and psychological testing and evaluation. Fees for therapy are on a sliding scale. The Center is affiliated with the South Bay Therapeutic Clinic and Memorial Hospital of Hawthorne. For 24-hour psychiatric emergency service call (213) 679-3321, Ext. 250.

## (85) ISLA VISTA OPEN DOOR MEDICAL CLINIC
970 Embarcadero del Mar
Isla Vista, CA 93017

(805) 968-1511

*Wendy E. Asrael, Administrator*

Supplements traditional general medical practice with herbal medicines, iridology, nutritional counseling, and a general preventive approach. Also provides detoxification counseling, pregnancy counseling, and a clinical library. Founded 1971.

## (86) COLLEGE OF NATURAL THERAPEUTICS
1434 Fremont Avenue
Los Altos, CA 94022

(415) 967-1232

*Roy B. Oliver, ND, Dean*

Nonaccredited, correspondence courses offered in homeopathy, naturopathy, nutrition, and magnetic healing.

## ASHTON SCHOOL OF PHYSIOHYDROTHERAPY/
Los Angeles, CA (see 235)

## (87) BARAKA
11110 Ohio Avenue, Suite 204
Los Angeles, CA 90025

(213) 473-0881

*Lee Baumel, MD*

A holistic center for therapy and research. Forms of treatment available include chiropractic, psychiatric counseling, faith healing, massage, and herbal and nutritional remedies. Baraka is interested in all forms of healing from ancient to new age.

## (88) FEMINIST WOMEN'S HEALTH CENTER
1112 South Crenshaw Boulevard
Los Angeles, CA 90005

(213) 936-7219

A nonprofit corporation dedicated to providing quality medical care to women at modest prices. Offers counseling in pregnancy, abortion, and birth control, as well as community educational programs in related areas.

## (89) A HEALING PLACE
2476 South Overland Avenue
Suite 307
Los Angeles, CA 90064

(213) 204-0111

R. Frank Hoffman, MD, Medical Director

Staffed by an MD, a rabbi, and a clinical psychologist, A Healing Place is dedicated to "the exploration of consciousness-expanding vehicles, our resistance to making full use of them, and their utilization in dealing with emotional, physical, and spiritual dis-ease."

## (90) THE HOLISTIC HEALTH CENTER
9201 Sunset Boulevard
Suite 501
Los Angeles, CA 90069

(213) 278-8231

*Griffith Page, MD, Medical Director*

A treatment and education center for the whole person. A staff solely of accredited practitioners provide treatment through massage, acupressure and acupuncture, art and dance therapy, relaxation methods and autogenic training, nutritional counseling, biofeedback, psychotherapy, and traditional Western medicine. The health of clients is evaluated by a holistic "assessment team," which uses a traditional medical workup including laboratory and xray tests, a personal lifestyle inventory, nutritional-exercise-stress evaluation, and psychospiritual interviews to fully diagnose the health of the client. Treatment goes beyond getting better, and aims for a fully integrated state of "wellness." The center also offers classes in psychology (including basic professional training in psychosynthesis), movement, meditation, and Jin Shin Jyutsu, a form of acupressure massage. Special integrated education and treatment programs deal with holistic approaches to arthritis, longevity, and body weight normalization. The Center also maintains a speakers' bureau.

## (91) INSTITUTE OF REALITY AWARENESS
8217 Beverly Boulevard, Suite 7
Los Angeles, CA 90048

(213) 658-8600

*Leslie J. Kent, DD, Director*

A nonprofit, holistic healing arts organization. Services include counseling, meditation, transactional analysis, Intensive Journal, psychodrama, nutritional care, and chiropractic.

## (92) KHALSA MEDICAL AND COUNSELING ASSOCIATES
8733 Beverly Boulevard, Suite 400
Los Angeles, CA 90048

(213) 652-2101

*Jas Want Singh Khalsa, MD, MA, Director*

A nonprofit holistic healing center, balancing treatment and training in kundalini yoga with traditional Western medicine, homeopathy, kinesiology, anthroposophic medicine, acupuncture and acupressure, hypnotherapy, nutrition, and spinal manipulation. A staff of clinical psychologists provides individual and group psychotherapy. Founded 1976.

## (93) WHITE CROSS SOCIETY
Punita
Box 576
Lucerne Valley, CA 92356

(714) 248-6163

Offers classes and experiential training in massage, herbology, nutrition, tissue salts, and homeopathy.

## (94) INSTITUTE FOR CREATIVE AGING
P.O. Box 142
Malibu, CA 90265

(213) 456-6297

*Evelyn Mandel, Director*

Seeks to enrich the lives of persons 65 years and older, and to reestablish this period of life as a time of richness and productivity. A select group of practices are used in the program for body-mind self-improvement and growth. These include acupressure, Jin Shin Jyutsu, biofeedback, counseling, deep breathing, yoga, massage, meditation, T'ai Chi Ch'uan, and art and music therapy. The group is presently in the process of extending its program to geriatric centers and educating geriatric professionals in its implementation. Founded 1975; formerly SAGE, Los Angeles.

## (95) McCORNACK CENTER FOR THE HEALING ARTS
499 Howard Street
Mendocino, CA 95460

(707) 937-5834

*Peter H. Barg, MD, Director*

A multidisciplinary holistic health treatment facility. A staff of eighteen, including medical doctors, homeopaths, chiropractors, herbalists, and massage therapists provide diagnosis and treatment. Among the therapeutic modalities used are acupressure and acupuncture, nutritional guidance, polarity therapy, and traditional Western medicine and surgery. Workshops in meditation, yoga, and T'ai Chi are offered to the public. Founded 1974.

**HEART HAUS CENTER** (holistic center)/Mill Valley, CA **(see 1056)**

## (96) WELLNESS RESOURCE CENTER
42 Miller Avenue
Mill Valley, CA 94941

(415) 383-3806

*John Travis, MD, Director*

Defining "wellness" as a state of health beyond the mere absence of illness, the Center assists people to take charge of their own lives and to experience greater levels of aliveness and satisfaction. The process occurs over three phases. In Phase I, a Wellness Evaluation of the client includes a Health Hazard Appraisal, a Nutritional Survey, a Purpose in Life Survey, and biofeedback testing. Phase II is an individualized stress-reduction program, including biofeedback training and structural awareness. Phase III is an ongoing process of intermediate and advanced biofeedback training, participation in transactional analysis, gestalt, "lifestyle evolution" groups, and optional use of Bates method counseling for vision improvement and visual stress reduction. A professional training program in "well medicine" is available.

## (97) WHOLISTIC HEALTH AND NUTRITION INSTITUTE
150 Shoreline Highway
Mill Valley, CA 94941

(415) 332-2933

*Richard Shames, MD, Medical Director*

Provides medical care, herbal treatment, nutritional guidance, hypnosis, biofeedback, and somatic psychology for the wholistic care of the whole person. Courses and workshops are also offered in such areas as reflexology, iridology, herbology, meditation, naturopathy, T'ai Chi, Jungian surgery. Workshops in meditation, yoga, and T'ai Chi are offered to the public. Founded 1974.

## (98) AUTOGENIC HEALTH CENTER
6401 Broadway Terrace
Oakland, CA 94618
(415) 658-5913

*Vera Fryling, MD, Director*

Uses a holistic approach to personal growth and stress re-

duction using Autogenic Training, visual imagery, and "graduated hypnosis." Also offers biofeedback training, art and movement therapy, nutritional appraisals, workshops in body alignment and "sports consciousness," and programs for weight and smoking control.

## (99) OAKLAND FEMINIST WOMEN'S HEALTH CENTER
2930 McClure Street
Oakland, CA 94609

(415) 444-5676

Provides a self-help clinic for women. Women learn about vaginal/cervical self-examination with a plastic vaginal speculum, breast self-examination, Pap smears, bimanual pelvic examination, and other skills. "Self-help is the experience of a woman learning to be totally familiar with her own body as a well woman."

## (100) OPEN EDUCATION EXCHANGE
6526 Telegraph Avenue
Oakland, CA 94609

(415) 655-6791

*Bart Brodsky, Coordinator*

A nonprofit organization, making available noncredit adult education courses serving the Greater Bay Area. Courses pertaining to health and growth include iridology, fasting, natural birth control, Reichian therapy, hypnosis, reflexology, yoga, biofeedback, gestalt, and different forms of humanistic psychology. Founded 1974.

## (101) SAN ANDREAS HEALTH COUNCIL
531 Cowper Street
Palo Alto, CA 94301

(415) 324-9350

*Susan Harman Stuart, President*

A group of health professionals offering a variety of techniques for attaining and maintaining optimum health. Through both classes and individual work, therapists provide rolfing, gestalt therapy, Reichian therapy, yoga, massage, nutritional counseling, psychosynthesis, T'ai Chi, vision therapy, holistic childbirth preparation, psychic awareness, self-hypnosis, dance therapy, chiropractic, acupressure, work with the Intensive Journal, and "humanistic medicine." Specific programs are coordinated through a Biofeedback Center, a Counseling Center, the Passage Program (ongoing groups for senior citizens), and the LITE Program (Life-threatening Illness: Therapy and Education). Membership is open to the general public. Founded 1973.

## (102) THE LIFE AND HEALTH MEDICAL GROUP
511 Brookside Avenue
Redlands, CA 92373

(714) 824-1750

*Bruce W. Halstead, MD, Director*

Concerned with treatment of chronic degenerative diseases, especially atherosclerosis, senility, cardiovascular diseases, and arthritis. Pharmaceutical methods are avoided, and natural methods including nutritional programs, exercise, hydrotherapy, chelation therapy, and hyperbaric medicine are used. All patients are treated on an outpatient basis.

## (103) SACRAMENTO MEDICAL PREVENTICS CLINIC, INC.
2811 "L" Street, Suite 205
Sacramento, CA 95816

(916) 452-7011

*Howard Greenspan, DO*

A wholistic clinic, using computer diet evaluation, hair analysis, thermography, treadmill electrocardiograms, comprehensive blood analysis, and physical examinations. Treatment modalities may include chelation for heavy metals toxicity as well as generalized detoxification programs, hyperbaric oxygen, chelation for arteriosclerosis, biofeedback, megavitamin therapy, auricular therapy, colonics, fasting, and homeopathic and herbal remedies.

## (104) AGE OF ENLIGHTENMENT CENTER FOR HOLISTIC HEALTH
3545 Revere Street
San Diego, CA 92109

(714) 270-4600

*Harold H. Bloomfield, MD, Director*

An integrative clinical facility centered around the Transcendental Meditation program as taught by Maharishi Mahesh Yogi. Other clinical services include individual and group psychotherapy, acupuncture and acupressure, biofeedback training, physiotherapy and massage, hydrotherapies, natural and homeopathic remedies, nutritional counseling, an optimal weight program, and social and community services.

## (105) BEACH AREA COMMUNITY CLINIC
3705 Mission Boulevard
San Diego, CA 92109

(714) 488-0644

*Juanita Hollisey, RN, Outreach Coordinator*

Staffed by physicians, nurses, trained health workers, and volunteers. Provides general medical services, an outreach program, counseling, and a women's clinic to the community. The emphasis is on taking personal responsibility for one's health. Classes are offered in personal health maintenance and in yoga. Founded 1971.

## (106) THE NATIONAL CENTER FOR THE EXPLORATION OF HUMAN POTENTIAL
6731 Barnhurst Street
San Diego, CA 92117

(714) 278-8210

*Herbert A. Otto, PhD, Chairperson*

A nonprofit educational organization conducting training programs in wholistic healing. Summer programs are offered in transpersonal psychology, parapsychology, and body work. Courses are offered for college credit. Founded 1968.

## (107) THE PHOENIX INSTITUTE
976 Chalcedony Street
San Diego, CA 92109

(714) 488-0626

*Kathryn Breese-Whiting, DD, Founder and President*

Offers classes, workshops, and seminars in the inner crea-

tive action of science, art, and religion. The Institute is licensed by the State of California to give degrees. There is also a farm for research in experimental agriculture, a research and circulating library, a book and art shop, a printing and publishing service, and a counseling center. In planning is an intentional community to be located on the Institute's property. Specialized areas of study focus on the mathematical harmonics of nature, dance movement, mime, and meditation.

## (108) SAN DIEGO NATURAL HEALTH CLINIC
4459 Morrell Street
San Diego, CA 92109

(714) 274-2482

*John Caldwell Luly, DC, Director*

A holistic natural clinic. Diagnostic methods include xray, blood, urine, and hair analysis, sclerology, medical astrology, iridology, radiesthesia (pendulum) testing, physical exams, and biofeedback. Physical therapies include ultrasound, sine wave, acupuncture, shiatsu, reflexology, psychic healing, color therapy, magnetic healing, polarity massage, rebirthing, and postural integration. Detoxification therapies include supervised fasting, transitional vegetarian, fruitarian, and sproutarian dieting, natural chelation therapy, herbal remedies, and wheatgrass colonic irrigations. Counseling approaches involve nutritional, spiritual, psychological, and metaphysical; exercise, yoga, Bates method of eye correction, hypnosis, and natural birth control. Founded 1975.

## (109) CHURCH OF GENTLE BROTHERS AND SISTERS
486 Clipper Street
San Francisco, CA 94114

(415) 824-4422

*Gerry Bronstein, MD*

". . . a New Age Family dedicated to serving humanity through the healing arts." Maintains a holistic medical practice, and offers classes, workshops and seminars in astrology, body awareness through sound, hand analysis, Tarot, and yoga. Individual counseling is offered, as well, drawing from the aforementioned tools, gestalt, and massage. The work of the group aims to bring about a "more dynamic spiritualization of planetary consciousness." The Church publishes a regular newsletter highlighting its activities. Founded 1971.

## (110) EAST WEST ACADEMY OF HEALING ARTS
P.O. Box 31211
San Francisco, California 94131

(415) 285-9400

*Effie Poy Yew Chow, Ph.D., R.N., C.A., President*

The Academy takes a systems approach to Holistic Health/Cultural Practices, in health education public policy issues and in interpreting Holistic Health as it is related to cultural-socio systems. Has provided consultation to educational institutions and service agencies, and offers coursework for health care professionals. The long-term training program on Holistic Health and Accupressure has approval of the AB1503 Committee. Organized the Council of Nurse Healers. The Academy welcomes general membership.

**ESALEN INSTITUTE** (educational center)/San Francisco, CA **(see 1051)**

### (111) HOLISTIC LIFE UNIVERSITY

Holistic Life Foundation
1627 Tenth Avenue
San Francisco, CA 94122

(415) 665-3200

*William Staniger, President*

Consists of four programs for the training of ''life-support professionals,'' holistic health, holistic childbirth, yoga, and life-death transition. Each program is approximately two years, and includes experiential as well as didactic aspects.

*The Holistic Health Program* involves training in nutrition, centering practices and body work, with an overall emphasis on sensitivity and personal responsibility for one's own health. Specific courses are in acupuncture, biofeedback, autogenic training, legal aspects of holistic health, iridology, kinesiology, homeopathy, and chiropractic. Graduates of the program are not trained to be healers or practitioners, but rather as educators who can work through schools and seminars, and with practitioners in a clinical setting.

*The Holistic Childbirth Educators Program* trains teachers to work with expectant parents both in classes and on an individual basis. Preparation includes work in psychological, sociological, consciousness-related, and biological aspects of the birth experience. Trainees also receive instruction in T'ai Chi or yoga, or both.

*The Yoga Teacher Training Program* prepares professional-level yoga teachers who have a basic knowledge in the anatomy and physiology of yoga, as well as in the practice and teaching of asanas (postures), pranayama (breath control), and the psychology and philosophy of meditation. It attempts to integrate traditional knowledge of the East with recent scientific research of the West.

*The Life-Death Transitions Institute* trains guides to assist the dying person to prepare for the life-death transition as a positive growth experience. Texts used include the *Tibetan Book of the Dead* and the *Egyptian Book of the Dead.*

Interdisciplinary research is also done. The first major study is a systematic blood biochemical analysis of persons engaged in yoga and other practices.

### (112) NURSE CONSULTANTS AND HEALTH COUNSELORS

1931 Union Street
San Francisco, CA 94123

(413) 346-1526

Counselors and therapists provide services to individuals and groups in various modes of holistic healing. Individual counseling and classes are provided in acupressure, reflexology, polarity, and nurturing massage, nutrition, meditation, yoga, biofeedback, autogenic training, psychic unfoldment, chromotherapy, tarot, and astrology. The office is staffed by nursing specialists and health counselors trained in specific fields. Founded 1973.

### (113) SAN FRANCISCO WOMEN'S HEALTH CENTER

3789 24th Street
San Francisco, CA 94114

(415) 282-6999

Educational center dedicated to teaching women concepts and methods for self-health care. Women are taught cervical and breast self-examination, the hormonal cycle, patients' rights, and the political aspects of health care, birth, and menopause. Also prints literature and makes referrals. Founded 1971.

### (114) ASSOCIATED PSYCHOLOGISTS OF SANTA CLARA

160 Saratoga Avenue, Suite 38
Santa Clara, CA 95050

(408) 296-5600

A group of eight holistically oriented psychologists dedicated to the client's psychological-structural-nutritional integration, and his or her realization of optimal well-being and satisfaction. Services include herbal, orthomolecular, and nutritional treatment, hair analysis, biofeedback, bioenergetics, hypnosis, acupressure, sex and family therapy, and weight loss groups for men and women.

**GARDEN OF SANJIVANI** (herbal school)/Santa Cruz, CA **(see 543)**

### (115) UNIVERSITY OF CALIFORNIA EXTENSION

Santa Cruz, CA 95064

(408) 429-2971

*Carl Tjerandsen, PhD, Dean*

Offers courses for both nurses and laypersons in acupressure and healing energies, laying on of hands, the healing power of sound (including both mantras and sounds of nature), and the role of stress in disease. Other offerings include T'ai Chi, dance therapy, and Jungian psychology. The University Extension also has sponsored major workshops and symposia featuring leading authorities in the fields of consciousness and holistic health. These have included a birth and rebirth conference, a myth and dream workshop, and programs in the medical and psychotherapeutic applications of biofeedback and autogenic training. A current schedule of courses and symposia may be obtained by writing to the above address.

### (116) FAMILY PRACTICE CENTER

3325 Chanate Road
Santa Rosa, CA 95402

(707) 527-2826

*Roger D. Snyder, PhD, Director*

A staff of medical doctors and behavioral scientists provide an interdisciplinary family systems approach to medicine. Modalities include hypnosis, relaxation techniques, meditation, biofeedback, individual and family therapy, and nutrition. Founded 1969.

**(117) COSMIC JOY FELLOWSHIP**
Box 792
Sausalito, CA 94965

(415) 924-6611

*Stanley E. Russell, Director*

Workshops in sexual tantra and clearing from Hindu, Taoist, and Buddhist perspectives. Also uses biofeedback training in a clearing process, designed to bring areas of "unknowingness" to view. These techniques are supplemented with advising in health and body rejuvenation and nutrition.

**(118) MANN RANCH SEMINARS**
P.O. Box 570
Ukiah, CA 95482

(707) 462-3514

*Larry T. Thomas, Director*

Offers seminars by leading individuals in the fields of psychology, consciousness, and wholistic healing. Seminars are offered both in residence at the ranch and abroad.

**(119) COMMUNITY FREE SCHOOL**
Box 1724
Boulder, CO 80302

(303) 447-8734

Holds ongoing seminars and workshops in holistic healing modalities. These have included auric healing, rolfing, herbology, yoga, massage, and color and light therapy. Recently sponsored (1976) the First Annual Rocky Mountain Healing Festival.

**(120) INTEGRAL HEALTH SERVICES, INC.**
245 School Street
Putnam, CT 06260

(203) 928-7729

*Sandra McLanahan, MD, Director*

Associated with the Satchidananda Ashram which is under the direction of Sri Swami Satchidananda. Provides individual and family health care services with emphasis on preventive medicine and yogic philosophy. A staff of medical doctors, chiropractors, massage therapists and nutritionists provide comprehensive exams, treatment of acute and chronic illness, pediatric care, gynecological and obstetrical services, acupressure, polarity, and reflexology massage, chiropractic, and nutritional counseling. Psychological counseling is provided by clinical psychologists. In addition, workshops in childbirth preparation, weight control, massage, and meditation are offered. Founded in 1975.

**(121) THE STAMFORD CENTER FOR THE HEALING ARTS**
The First Congregational Church
Walton Place
Stamford, CT 06901

(203) 323-0200

*Gabe Lewis Campbell, Minister*

Provides training programs in prayer and meditation from a Judeo-Christian perspective, therapeutic touch, nutrition,

herbs, reflexology, and cooking. Special programs are offered in the applications of biofeedback to meditation and prayer, and in the transition from bodily life to life in the next dimension.

**INSTITUTE OF PNEUMOLOGY** (acupuncture)/
Washington, DC **(see 638)**

**(122) MANKIND RESEARCH FOUNDATION, INC.**
1640 Kalmia Road, N.W.
Washington, DC 20012

(202) 982-4001

*Carl Schleicher, PhD, Director*

Provides information and educational programs in suggestology, biofeedback as a treatment for hypertension, Oriental medicine, moxibustion, yoga and meditation for alcohol and drug rehabilitation, and color and music therapy. Conducts research on Kirlian photography and ESP phenomena. The MRF affiliate organization, Center for Preventive Therapy and Rehabilitation, offers specific therapies including chelation therapy, biofeedback, "bioenergizing," acupuncture, and two cancer therapies: "pulsed magnetic fields" and ultraviolet blood radiation. Also conducts experimental treatment programs for Parkinson's disease, arthritis, and heavy metal poisoning.

**(123) YES EDUCATIONAL SOCIETY**
1035 31st Street, N.W.
Washington, DC 20007

(202) 338-7676

*Lee Lewis, Coordinator*

Offers a selection of 5- to 10-week courses at low cost with emphasis on holistic healing. Course offerings have included T'ai Chi, yoga, shiatsu, massage, homeopathy, kinesiology, Bach flower remedies, healing with color, art, dance, music, meditation, nutrition and herbology. Weekend workshops and lectures are also offered in such areas as auric healing, and biofeedback. A newsletter is published listing current course offerings and upcoming workshops. Founded 1974.

**(124) CORNUCOPIA CENTERS, INC.**
5808 Northeast Fourth Court
Miami, FL 33137

(305) 758-9000

*Gary Schwartz, MA, and Deborah Schwartz*

Educational programs and classes in such areas as T'ai Chi, acupressure, reflexology, nutrition, spiritual healing, vision training, and holistic health applications of altered states of consciousness. Founded 1973.

**THE ROUNDTABLE OF THE LIGHT CENTERS**
(consciousness development)/Miami, FL **(see 785)**

**BIOFEEDBACK MEDITATIONAL TRAINING CENTER**/Glenview, IL **(see 737)**

**(125) HIMALAYAN INSTITUTE COMBINED THERAPY CENTER**
1505 Greenwood Road
Glenview, IL 60025

(312) 724-2273

*Richard M. Ballentine, MD, Director of Therapy Programs*

A branch of the Himalayan Institute founded by Swami Rama, the Center provides a quiet setting for patients who come for ten-day to three-week intensive treatment. Therapeutic modalities include yoga asanas and breathing. exercises, cleansing techniques, biofeedback, videofeedback, and Ayurvedic, homeopathic, and modern Western medicine. Residents have access to the Himalayan Institute's lectures on mediation and tape library on yogic sciences. Founded 1975; Himalayan Institute founded 1971.

**WHOLISTIC HEALTH CENTER** (psychotherapy)/ Hinsdale, IL **(see 1086)**

**(126) CENTERS FOR HEALTH AND LIFE, INC.**
Des Moines Center
2600 Harding Road
Des Moines, IA 50310

(515) 277-6155

*Kenneth G. Brockman, DC, and Robert L. Burns, DDS, Directors*

A wholistic treatment facility dedicated to educating, treating, and preventing disease, sickness, and illness through natural-biologic means. Services offered include pastoral counseling, nutritional guidance, biofeedback, massage, osteopathy, and chiropractic. Founded 1976.

**SELF ACTUALIZATION INSTITUTE** (growth center)/New Orleans, LA **(see 1087)**

**(127) MARTIN BUBER INSTITUTE**
The Meeting House
5885 Robert Oliver Place
Columbia, MD 21045

(301) 730-6044

*Rabbi Martin Siegal*

Offers courses and workshops in New Age alternatives to Western medicine, such as massage, homeopathy, yoga, nutrition, meditation, gestalt, structural patterning, and rebirthing. Additional work is offered in the teachings of Martin Buber and the Bible as a source of healing. Academic credit for some of the courses is available through a special arrangement with Loyola College. The Institute is also preparing a directory of holistic healing resources in the Washington-Baltimore area.

**(128) THE INSTITUTE FOR PSYCHOENERGETICS**
126 Harvard Street
Brookline, MA 02146

(617) 738-4502

*Buryl Payne, PhD, Director*

Offers an integrated program of mind-body balancing which includes bioenergetics, therapeutic massage, rolfing, yoga, biofeedback, dehypnosis, and meditation. Research is conducted in the transformation of orgone, solar, planetary, and life energies. Work includes study of auras and psychic phenomena. Support for research comes from the sale of biofeedback instruments and from seminars and training programs. Founded 1972.

**(129) LAWRENCE II**
The Lawrence Academy
Groton, MA 01450

(617) 448-3344

*August Jaccaci, Project Director*

An alternative school within Lawrence Academy, dedicated to "holistic healing through individual and group life-planning and through developing models for learning based on General Systems principles of growth and synergy." The Lawrence Project, a program of Lawrence II, is a series of workshops open to secondary school teachers and students to plan and design new curricula. Its seminars include such subjects as cosmology, holistic health, and brain-mind development.

**(130) ACUPUNCTURE CENTER OF MASSACHUSETTS**
93 Union Street
Newton, MA 02164

(617) 965-3306

*James Doyle, DO, Director*

Wholistic treatment center utilizing acupuncture, osteopathy, nutrition, and ancillary bioenergetic psychotherapy.

**(131) INTERFACE**
63 Chapel Street
Newton, MA 02158

(617) 965-4491

*Rick Ingrasci, MD, Co-Founder*

". . . a freeform association supporting creative individuals and groups who reflect a holistic awareness of the evolutionary process." Offers workshops in consciousness technology, healing, art and music therapy, bioenergetics, color therapy, group video therapy, and Sufi dancing. Currently in the process of organizing a holistic treatment clinic, video library, and research groups. Founded 1975.

**WOMANKIND** (growth center)/Minneapolis, MN **(see 1110)**

**(132) NATURO-NUTRIC-BIONICS**
Box 24
Mound, MN 55364

*Kenneth Brockman, DC, and Robert L. Burns, DDS*

Offers a seminar in preventive health care focusing on the development of a Health Recommendation Plan. The seminar, which is offered to all health professionals, instructs how to normalize and balance cellular, biochemical, physiologic, neurologic, and psychologic function to restore health as optimally as possible.

**(133) THE FEATHERED PIPE RANCH**
2409 Colorado Gulch
Helena, MT 59601

(406) 442-8196

A retreat, associated with the Holistic Life Foundation in San Francisco, offering programs on holistic health, yoga, and meditation.

(134) **DESERT LIGHT FOUNDATION, INC.**
P.O. Box 40147
Albuquerque, NM 87106

(505) 268-2156

*Harold Cohen, MD, President*

Maintains a holistic health clinic (with one medical doctor and one chiropractor) with individual counseling services. Classes are offered in I Ching, T'ai Chi, yoga, massage, iridology, alternative cancer therapy, astrology, nutrition, polarity, herbology, colonic irrigation, and meditation. Also publishes a newsletter, *Illuminations*. Incorporated 1976. (Formerly P.S.I. Center of New Mexico, Inc.)

(135) **CHRISTOS SCHOOL OF NATURAL HEALING**
P.O. Box 1503
Taos, NM 87571

*William LeSassier, ND, Founder and Director*

Counseling in the areas of nutrition, natural birth, and body release therapies. Operates a Wholistic Clinic which makes available treatment in herbal medicine, massage, color healing, etc. Courses available periodically on most subjects involving a natural approach to healing.

(136) **THE PEOPLE'S HEALTH CENTER**
438 Claremont Parkway
Bronx, NY 10457

(212) 583-8010

*John Lichtenstein, MD*

A community-patient-health worker controlled nonprofit care facility. A staff of physicians, dentists, nurses, and assistants provide a full range of traditional medical and dental services to poor people in the South Bronx area. A 40-week course on medical skills and emergency techniques is offered free of charge to 40 community residents per cycle. Founded 1969.

(137) **INSTITUTE FOR SELF-DEVELOPMENT**
50 Maple Place
Manhasset, NY 11030

(516) 627-0048

Makes available a course in self-development, including studies in yoga, meditation, T'ai Chi Kung, Chinese acupuncture, Korean massage, chirotherapy, nutrition, pulse diagnosis, and Chinese herbal medicine. Use of biofeedback equipment and a taped relaxation exercise series are also available.

(138) **ARTHRITIS MEDICAL CENTER**
320 West End Avenue
New York, NY 10023

(212) 595-1503

*J. Sheridan Bell, MD, Medical Director*

Offers a threefold treatment program for arthritis sufferers consisting of hormonal treatments, nutritional supplements and counseling, and special exercises.

(139) **HEALTH MAINTENANCE CENTER**
1370 Avenue of the Americas
New York, NY 10019

(212) 489-0855

A preventive medicine clinic, with a computerized diagnos-
tic system called "automated multiphasic testing." Latent malfunctions are pointed out in addition to problems which are already manifest.

(140) **ODYSSEY ASSOCIATION**
333 East 49th Street
New York, NY 10017

(212) 751-5239

*Jodi Desmond and Edna B. Kucher, Founders*

Sponsors teachers of spiritual, parapsychological, and esoteric systems which are supportive of the spiritual/psychic/physical growth of the whole person. Examples of courses and workshops offered are auric healing, psychic massage, music as a healing experience, and Kirlian photography. Speakers are selected for their individual integrity; no particular belief systems are selectively supported by Odyssey Association. Founded 1976.

(141) **REILLY'S ON 34TH STREET**
120 East 34th Street
New York, NY 10016

(212) 684-1472

*Stanley Kestenbaum, PhT, Director*

Specializes in the application of colonic irrigations, therapeutic massage, exercises, paraffin baths, and other physical therapy treatments.

(142) **TREE OF LIFE**
101 West 125th Street
New York, NY 10027

(212) 850-0900

*Kanya Kekhumba, Founder*

Offers workshops in such areas as astrology, herbology, psychic awareness, nutrition, yoga, and meditation.

(143) **THE ALTERNATIVE HEALTH EDUCATION CENTER**
715 Monroe Avenue
Rochester, NY 14607

(716) 442-5480

*Thaddeus Bukowski, Coordinator*

Disseminates information to the community through workshops and lectures on such topics as nutrition, homeopathy, yoga, and fasting. Maintains a reference library on subjects in wholistic medicine, and a store selling books, Bach flower remedies, dowsing equipment, homeopathic remedies, Schuessler tissue cell salts, and charts and posters pertaining to alternative healing systems. A women's coalition, "dealing with women's needs in wholistic ways," is also a part of the center.

(144) **THE MOUNTAIN PEOPLES' CLINIC**
Eagle Street
Hayesville, NC 28904

(704) 389-6091

*Jim Campbell, MD, Director*

A clinic in a country farmhouse. Services include gentle general medicine, home childbirth, acupuncture, herbals, and simple remedies, homeopathy, and space therapy.

Home and hospital calls available. Office hours by appointment.

### (145) P.S.I. CENTER
(People Seeking Illumination of the
Physical, Spiritual and Intellectual)
Endicott Building, Room "M"
Cincinnati, OH 45218

(513) 742-2266

*Robert J. Rothan, DDS*

A clinical, educational, and research facility for the treatment of the whole person. A staff of medical doctors, chiropractor, dentist, therapist, nutritionist, and others provide a multidisciplinary approach to health care. Modalities used include standard traditional medicine, nutrition and fasting counseling, biofeedback, homeopathy, herbs, spinal adjustments, yoga, hydrotherapy, meditation, reflexology, silent retreats, and massage. The Center also maintains a health food store, restaurant, book store, and a nutrient supplement center.

### (146) CENTER FOR HIGHER CONSCIOUSNESS
P.O. Box 18406
Cleveland Heights, OH 44118

(216) 932-0723

*Ronald F. Headley, Director*

Offers classes and groups in autogenic training, self-hypnosis and hypnosis, acupressure massage, meditation, psychic investigation, applied metaphysics, and positive awareness programs designed to increase consciousness and love of self and others.

### (147) MERETA GROUP
Box 14191
Columbus, OH 43214

(614) 846-1187

*William J. Strandwitz, Deputy Director*

A group of professional counselors, therapists, and teachers interested in the physical, mental, and spiritual aspects of healing. Offer pastoral counseling, iridology, nutritional guidance, handwriting analysis, and polarity and reflexology massage. Lectures are offered in such areas as natural healing, marriage, and mind sciences.

### (148) EUGENE CENTER FOR THE HEALING ARTS
1045 Monroe Street
Eugene, OR 97402

*Steve Hitchcock, Coordinator*

A center for holistic health education with offerings in massage, homeopathy, macrobiotics, nutrition, fasting, T'ai Chi, astrology, polarity therapy, and radiesthesia. Also organized study groups for natural birth control and Leboyer-style natural childbirth.

### (149) THE INSTITUTE OF PREVENTIVE MEDICINE
6171 Southwest Capitol Highway
Portland, OR 97201

(503) 246-7616

*Mark J. Tager, MD, Director*

Offers individual holistic medical and dental counseling.

Includes consultation about diet, and use of polarity therapy and massage as treatment modalities. Workshops and classes in yoga, T'ai Chi, vegetarian cookery and nutrition, massage, herbology, and bioenergetics. A special holistic program in health care for the elderly is also offered.

### (150) CLYMER HEALTH CLINIC
R.D. 3, Clymer Road
Quakertown, PA 18951

(215) 536-8001

*G.E. Posenecker, ND, DC, Director*

A total natural treatment facility with inpatient accommodations if desired. A complete range of natural treatments are offered including chiropractic and osteopathic manipulations, homeopathic medicines, herbs, massage, fasting, natural dentistry, herbal colonics, and chelation for removal of cholesterol and calcium deposits. Special programs are offered in dynamic weight reduction and control, emotional counseling, and neuromuscular rehabilitation.

**AMERICAN MEDICAL SYMPOSIA** (nutrition)/Dallas, TX **(see 506)**

### (151) THE ESOTERIC PHILOSOPHY CENTER, INC.
523 Lovett Boulevard
Houston, TX 77006

(713) 526-5998

*William David, Executive Director*

Provides a community educational program aimed at formal integration of personality as well as spiritual and self-awareness. Specific classes include astrology, vibration, sound and color, meditation, tarot and qabalah, yoga, palmistry, massage, reflexology, hatha and kundalini yoga, reincarnation, gestalt, and dream and bible symbolism. William David, the executive director, offers workshops in other cities in vibrations, and sound and color healing.

### (152) THE COMMUNITY HEALTH CENTER
260 North Street
Burlington, VT 05401

(802) 864-6309

A community-based health clinic offering services either free or at minimal cost. The staff physician here is interested in herbal and massage therapy as a "means of getting and staying healthy." Founded 1971 as The People's Free Clinic.

### (153) ASSOCIATION FOR BIOCOSMOLOGICAL RESEARCH, INC.
Box 9545
Rosslyn Station
Arlington, VA 22209

(703) 751-5776

Sponsors conferences and seminars in various natural healing modalities.

### (154) ATLANTIC UNIVERSITY (Association of Learning)
P.O. Box 595
Virginia Beach, VA 23451

(804) 428-3588

Offers in-depth study opportunities in small intentional

communities at a variety of locations, integrated into a "balanced lifestyle" approach. "The Association of Learning is not a place; it is an approach to learning based on the principle that all we may know or become already exists within each of us, waiting to be awakened and unfolded." Two-week to three-month programs are offered focusing on meditation, dreamwork, creativity, education, prayer, self-awareness, comparative religion, and counseling. Chartered in 1930; active since 1971.

## (155) HOME CENTER
2100 Mediterranean Avenue
Virginia Beach, VA 23451

(804) 425-1170

*Paul R. Thompson, DC, Director*

A medical education center aimed at prevention. Includes classes and therapeutic sessions in meditation, self-hypnosis, nutrition, yoga, T'ai Chi, herbology, colonic irrigation, astrology, acupressure, massage, and reflexology. Includes staff of medical doctors, chiropractors, and dentists. A library is available for study of natural healing techniques. Works with health readings of various psychics and the Edgar Cayce readings on request.

## (156) PREVENTIVE MEDICINE CLINIC
800 156th Avenue, N.E.
Bellevue, WA 98008

(206) 746-4024

*James C. Johnston, MD, Director*

Holistic medicine practice founded on the belief that each individual is a unique being based on spiritual-emotional life with nutritional-biochemical and structural-anatomical expressions. Complete medical examination is correlated with additional diagnostic systems, including applied kinesiology, iridology, reflexology, and mineral analysis. Therapeutic emphasis is on educational and understanding; therapeutic modalities include nutritional consultation, massage, and manipulation.

## (156.1) SUNSHINE MEDICAL SHOW
2316 Northeast 85th
Seattle, WA 98115

(206) 524-8083

*Charles Thompson, MD*

A holistic clinic comprised of a medical doctor, an acupuncturist psychotherapist, and a Reichian breathing therapist. The skills of the three individuals involved are integrated into holistic methods of diagnosis and treatment.

## (157) THE PAIN AND HEALTH REHABILITATION CENTER
Route 2, Welsh Coulee
LaCrosse, WI 54601

(608) 786-0611

*C. Norman Shealy, MD, Director*

A holistic healing center emphasizing treatment of severe, chronic pain. Treatment modalities include external electrical stimulation, acupuncture, biofeedback, autogenic training, massage, progressive relaxation, guided imagery, nutritional counseling, Cayce techniques, heat and ice applications, and physical exercise such as yoga and aerobics.

Diagnostic methods include traditional medical and psychological tests, hair analysis for trace minerals, and use of clairvoyants. Pastoral counseling is also available. Founded 1971.

## (158) PINE FREE CLINIC
1985 West Fourth
Vancouver, British Columbia
Canada V6J 1M7

(604) 736-2391

Follows a "whole-person" approach to medical (especially gynecological) problems.

## (159) SERENITY HEALTH EDUCATION CENTRE
P.O. Box 4886
Vancouver, British Columbia
Canada V6B 4A6

Provides classes and correspondence courses in nutrition, reflexology, color therapy, herbal remedies, yoga, spiritual healing, natural birth control, Oriental medicine, and related subjects.

**RENAISSANCE REVITALIZATION CENTER** (resort spa)/Nassau, Bahamas **(see 176)**

## (160) LATIN AMERICAN MISSION PROGRAM (LAMP), INSTITUTO NATURISTA ADVENTISTA
Box 228
Antigua, Guatemala
Central America

*Lon Cummings, Co-Director*

An education center clinic sanitarium based on Christianity and "God's principles of health." Advocates vegetarian diet, cleanliness, plenty of sun and fresh air, and exercise. Specifics taught and practiced are anatomy and physiology, agriculture, massage, chiropractic, hydrotherapy, herbology, dentistry, first aid, nutrition, and environmental design. Founded 1970.

## (161) RAMANA HEALTH CENTRE, LTD.
Ludshott Manor Hospital, Bramshott
Liphook, Hants, England

Tel: Liphook 722993

*W. Gibson, Hospital Secretary*

A hospital for alternative medicine, with research and post-graduate teaching programs. Uses such wholistic medical systems as homeopathy, Chinese medicine, Ayurvedic (Indian) medicine, Unani (Moslem) medicine, and osteopathy. Allied therapies include acupuncture, hydrotherapy, physiotherapy, yoga, Bates exercises, spiritual healing, and Alexander technique. Both orthodox and unorthodox (radiesthesia) techniques are used in diagnosis.

**WREKIN TRUST** (parapsychological and spiritual center)/Hertfordshire, England **(see 799)**

## (162) THE 3-L BHAVAN
"Bucklands"
36 Merrilocks Road
Blundellsands
Liverpool 23, England

Tel: 051-924-5848

*Dr. Gopal Puri, PhD, and Mrs. Kailash Puri, BA*

"Rehoboth"
Station Road
Ottringham
Hull, England

Tel: 09644-2945

*N. Edwards, Principal*

4, Chestnut Walk
Healing
South Humberside
England DN37 7NT

Tel: 0472-88-3259

*Margaret Bannister and Mr. F. Bannister, Directors*

Practitioners of Yoga-Eco-Psychica, which incorporates yogic concepts of breath, asana, and meditation into a community system of preventive therapy. Also uses nutrition, herbs, sex, and spiritual counseling into a total "non-medical" therapeutic milieu. In addition to private consultations, the group conducts research into new therapies of stress relief, conducts forums, seminars, and conferences, publishes a newsletter, and explores the relationships between meditation and the arts.

**ROYAL PUMP ROOM** (hydrotherapy)/Warwickshire, England **(see 237)**

(163) **WESTBANK HEALING AND TEACHING CENTRE**
Strathmiglo
Fife, KY14 7QP
Scotland

*Major Bruce and Patricia MacManaway*

Therapeutic practices used at the center are healing, including the laying on of hands, deep muscle therapy, and spinal adjustments. In addition, clients are provided with instruction and counseling in psychosynthesis, organic horticulture, vegetarian cooking, yoga, dowsing, and ESP training. Teaching groups in these same subjects are also held. Founded 1959.

**ITA-WEGMAN-KLINIK** (anthroposophical clinic)/ Arlesheim, Switzerland **(see 813)**

**LUKAS KLINIK** (anthroposophical clinic)/Arlesheim, Switzerland **(see 814)**

**SANATORIUM SONNENECK** (anthroposophical clinic)/Badenweiler, Switzerland **(see 815)**

**GEMEINNÜTZIGES GEMEINSCHAFTSKRAN-KENHAUS HERDECKE** (anthroposophical clinic)/West Germany **(see 818)**

**PARACELSUS-KRANKENHAUS** (anthroposophical clinic)/West Germany **(see 822)**

**SANATORIUM FÜR DYNAMISCHE THERAPIE STUDENHOF** (anthroposophical clinic)/West Germany **(see 823)**

## Resorts and Spas

(164) **LUKATS' PREVENTION REGENERATION RESORT**
Route 1, Box 955
Safford, AZ 85546

(602) 428-2881

*Alexander L. Lukats, DC, ND, Director*

A resort using fasting, physical therapy, colonic irrigations, chiropractic, nutrition, hot springs, sunbathing, and spiritual healing as techniques for prevention and regeneration. Founded 1945.

(165) **PHILADELPHIAN INSTITUTE, INC.**
401 Patterson Street
P.O. Box 98
Sulfur Springs, AR 72768

(501) 298-3362

A Christian fellowship and rejuvenation resort. Features homelike cottages, natural sulfur spring baths, and organic meals.

**ESALEN INSTITUTE** (multidisciplinary workshops)/Big Sur, CA **(see 1051)**

(166) **HIDDEN VALLEY HEALTH RANCH**
Route 1, Box 52
Escondido, CA 92025

(714) 749-2727

*Bernard Jensen, DC, Director*

The goal is prevention of disease. Teaches that health education is just as important as the treatment itself. Fundamentals of proper selection and preparation of food and balanced nutrition are taught. Treatments include fresh air and sunshine, rest, supervised exercise, recreation programs, individualized diet and fasting with supervision, hydrotherapy, herbs, packs, manipulation, and adjusting.

(167) **MEADOWLARK**
c/o Friendly Hills Fellowship
26126 Fairview Avenue
Hemet, CA 92343

(714) 927-1343

*Evarts C. Loomis, MD, Director*

A residential growth center, rejuvenation resort, and treatment center for the whole person. The program includes individual discussion and counseling, time for personal art work and listening to music, use of an Intensive Journal, polarity massage, and body work. Facilities include a medical office, services of a physical therapist, a swimming pool, chapel, library, sauna, and natural foods kitchen. Classes are offered to residents in meditation and natural foods cooking.

(168) **HARBIN HOT SPRINGS**
P.O. Box 82
Middletown, CA 95461

(707) 987-3747

*Robert F. Hartley, Secretary*

Over 1000 acres with natural hot baths of minimum sulfur

content on Indian (Pomo) holy ground. Lodging and vegetarian meals available. Hosts wholistic healing conferences and schools.

### (169) THE HUMAN POTENTIAL CAMP FOR KIDS AND THE GROWTH CENTER FOR ADULTS AT THE VILLAGE OF OZ
P.O. Box 86
Point Arena, CA 95468

(707) 882-2449

*Lawrence S. Kroll, PhD, and Margot A. Kroll, Directors*

A small learning community in northern California, introducing big and little kids (aged 9-90) to country living, tree houses, consciousness raising, wilderness survival, organic gardening and cooking, yoga, massage, herb walks, dream labs, T'ai Chi, hot baths, sauna, the Lilly sensory exploration tank, wind and solar energy, hayrides, capture the flag, and more. Program introduces selected exercises from Esalen, EST, Arica, and other disciplines in game form over an earthy base of farm/country living.

### (170) ORR SPRINGS ASSOCIATION
(Orr's Hot Springs)
Star Route 1, Box 7
Ukiah, CA 95482

(707) 462-6277

A community retreat of 23 persons. Visitors are welcome to bathe or spend time in meditation, massage, and workshops. Facilities include a large communal hot tub, private tubs, a cold mineral water swimming pool, an organic garden, and a sauna. Workshops are offered in herbal medicine, massage, vegetarian diet, country living, and meditation. Both individuals and groups are accommodated. Founded 1974.

### (171) STEWART MINERAL SPRINGS, INC.
Route 1, Box 1093
Weed, CA 96094

(916) 938-7955

*Carol and Winston Goodpasture, Proprietors*

A spa centered around natural, mineral-water baths. Massage is available. Other facilities include a natural foods restaurant, trout fishing, and swimming.

WILBUR HOT SPRINGS/Wilbur Springs, CA (see 1071)

GOULD FARM (resort rest home)/Monterey, MA (see 1104)

PAWLING HEALTH MANOR (resort)/Hyde Park, NY (see 508)

### (172) NEW AGE HEALTH FARM
Neversink, NY 12765

(914) 985-2221/2

*Elza and Graeme Graydon, Directors*

Services offered range from simple weight reduction to restoration of health for persons who suffer from problems of nutrition or stress. Programs include nutritional therapy using liquid diets of fresh fruit and vegetable juices, meditation, yoga, breathing techniques, biofeedback, energy massages, herbal beauty treatments, gourmet health foods, health food education, astrology, spiritual nutrition, and

seminars in health, psychology and metaphysics.

### (173) BULGARIAN TOURIST OFFICE
50 East 42nd Street
New York, NY 10017

(212) 661-5733

Information on resorts, spas, mineral waters, hospitals and clinics in Bulgaria.

### (174) HEALTH AND PLEASURE TOURS, INC.
165 West 46th Street
New York, NY 10036

(212) 586-1775

Travel agents specializing in tours to the various health spas throughout Europe. Has extensive files and information on which spas are best suited for certain disorders.

### (175) YUGOSLAV STATE TOURIST OFFICE
509 Madison Avenue
New York, NY 10022

(212) 753-8710

Information on resorts, thermal springs, and spas in Yugoslavia.

VEGETARIAN HOTEL/Woodridge, NY (see 509)

### (176) RENAISSANCE REVITALIZATION CENTER
Cable Beach, PO Box N4854
Nassau, Bahamas

(809) 32-78441-2

*Elliot Goldwag, PhD, Executive Director*

Comprised of 15 professionals including three medical doctors, Renaissance is a revitalization center for young and old, combining rest and relaxation in a resort atmosphere. Some of the various therapeutic modalities used include thalasotherapy (sea water therapy in spray, shower, sea mud pack and vapor form), and embryonic cell therapy to revitalize old tissue. Accommodations are available at the nearby Ambassador Beach Hotel by special arrangement with the Center.

### (177) TYRINGHAM NATUROPATHIC CLINIC
Newport Pagnell
Bucks MK16 9ER
England

Tel: Newport Pagnell 610450
STD code 0908

A registered medical nursing home for all patients except those with infectious or terminal illnesses. Therapeutic techniques include acupuncture, balneotherapy (mineral waters), breathing exercises, vegetarian diet, fasting, hydrotherapy, massage, herbal and homeopathic preparations, physiotherapy, osteopathy, yoga, and psychological counseling. Founded 1966.

### (178) SHALIMAR HEALTH HOME
First Avenue
Frinton-On-Sea
Essex, England

*Keki R. Sidhwa, ND, DO, Founder*

An educational institution and rejuvenation clinic emphasizing natural hygiene, fasting, relaxation, and exercise. Postural training, including the Alexander technique, chiropractic and osteopathic manipulations and psychological counseling are also available. A library of 2,000 volumes pertaining to natural healing is open to patients. Founded 1960.

**VILLA VEGETARIANA HEALTH SPA**/Cuernavaca, Mexico **(see 510)**

**PORT OF HEALTH INTERNATIONAL NATURO-PRACTIC HEALTHATARIUM**/Guadalajara, Mexico **(see 444)**

**(179) RIO CALIENTE, S.A.**
APDO 1-1187
Guadalajara, Jalisco, Mexico

A holistic living and health center located on an ancient healing and spiritual center in the mountains outside Guadalajara. Vegetarian diet, yoga, meditation, workshops and classes in nutrition, art, and movement therapy are offered. Founded 1962.

**(180) BIRCHER-BENNER PRIVATKLINIK**
Keltenstrasse 48
CH-8044 Zürich
Switzerland

Tel: 01/32 68 90

*D. Liechti-von Brasch, MD, Medical Director*

Located in a beautiful chalet setting, the clinic provides a total environment for medical treatment of digestive and metabolic disorders. Physical treatments include massage, herbal baths, mud packs, and gymnastics. Founded 1897.

**(181) OTTO BUCHINGER CLINIC**
Forstweg 39
Bad Pyrmont, D3280 West Germany

Tel: 05281-19011

*Otto Buchinger, MD, Director*

Uses diet cures, prolonged fasting, hydrotherapy, massage, physiotherapy, homeotherapy, and psychotherapy. Founded 1920.

## Journals and Publications

**MEDICAL RESEARCH BULLETIN**—ARE (Cayce)/ Phoenix, AZ **(see 833)**

**(182) INTERNATIONAL NEW AGE**
Box 1137
Harrison, AR 72601

Monthly journal containing features on meditation, consciousness, and healing.

**(183) MEDICAL SELF-CARE MAGAZINE**
P.O. Box 718
Inverness, CA 94937

*Tom Ferguson, MD, Editor*

Reviews of books and tools in the areas of self-care, preventive medicine, and women's health. Founded 1976.

**(184) BRAIN/MIND BULLETIN**
P.O. Box 42211
Los Angeles, CA 90024

(213) 257-2500

*Marilyn Ferguson, Editor*

Professional newsletter covering information and newsworthy events in the fields of psychology, medical research, and new medicine. Sample copy available by writing to the above address.

**UNI-COM FOUNDATION** (psychic newsletter)/Palo Alto, CA **(see 801)**

**(185) JOURNAL OF HOLISTIC HEALTH**
P.O. Box 33202
San Diego, CA 92103

(714) 298-5965

Annual journal on holistic medicine, publishing transcripts of talks and seminars held by the Association for Holistic Health **(58)**. The 1976-1977 journal is a transcription of the Healing Center of the Future Conference held in San Diego in September 1976.

**(186) WELL-BEING MAGAZINE**
Box 7455
San Diego, CA 92107

(714) 224-4422

*David Copperfield, Publisher*

Shares information on staying healthy and centered through balanced living and ecological lifestyle. Features articles on herbs, nutrition, massage, and natural healing. Each issue has a national directory of natural healing schools.

**(187) COMMON GROUND**
461 Douglass Street
San Francisco, CA 94114

(415) 922-5300

*Andy Alpine, Editor*

A directory (newspaper format) containing profiles of groups and persons in the San Francisco Bay area who are engaged in all aspects of self-growth, consciousness-raising, and holistic medicine.

**NEW REALITIES** (psychic magazine)/San Francisco, CA **(see 802)**

**(188) YOGA JOURNAL**
1627 Tenth Avenue
San Francisco, CA 94122

Bimonthly journal dealing with yoga techniques and philosophy, often in the context of holistic medicine.

**(189) LEAVES OF HEALING**
P.O. Box 5688
Santa Monica, CA 90405

(213) 396-5164

*Blanche Leonard, Editor and Publisher*

A small bimonthly newspaper blending news of natural health and healing with New Age spiritual topics.

**(190) THE CO-EVOLUTION QUARTERLY**
Box 428
Sausalito, CA 94965

(415) 332-1716

*Stewart Brand, Editor*

Published by POINT, a California nonprofit organization. The Quarterly contains information on systems theory, natural agriculture, alternative technology, and alternative medicine. Many of the staff, including Stewart Brand, were responsible for publishing the "Whole Earth Catalog" series.

**(191) THE MONTHLY EXTRACT**
New Moon Communications
P.O. Box 3488
Ridgeway Station
Stamford, CT 06905

(203) 348-8529

Bimonthly. Carries information about women's self-help clinics and gynecological self-care.

**(192) PUBLIC CITIZEN HEALTH RESEARCH GROUP**
2000 "P" Street, N.W.
Washington, DC 20036

(202) 872-0320

Publishes consumers' guides to the practical economics of psychotherapy, dentistry and medicine.

**(193) ALTERNATIVES JOURNAL**
350 Northeast 82nd Street
Miami, FL 33138

(305) 758-4126

*Chick Shank, Editor*

Monthly publication featuring articles on New Age subjects, concepts, and methods that offer alternatives.

**(194) SUNSPARK PRESS**
Box 6341
St. Petersburg Beach, FL 33736

Publishes a *Guide to Alternative Periodicals* containing names and addresses with prices, subscription information, and brief annotations.

**JOURNAL OF NATURAL MEDICINE** (naturopathy)/
Boise, ID **(see 447)**

**(195) EAST WEST JOURNAL**
233 Harvard Street
Brookline, MA 02146

(617) 738-1760

*Sherman Goldman, Editor*

Monthly magazine carrying articles on macrobiotics, natural medicine, country living, and consciousness.

**(196) NEW AGE JOURNAL**
32 Station Street
Brookline Village, MA 02146

(617) 734-3155

*Peggy Taylor, Editor*

Unique monthly journal of New Age phenomena; consciousness, spirituality, music, food, and new medicine.

**(197) NEW ENGLAND JOURNAL OF MEDICINE**
1172 Commonwealth Avenue
Allston, MA 02134

(617) 734-9800

One of the few truly innovative "traditional medical" publications. Contains articles on all aspects of the field of "new medicine," which would include acupuncture, effects of light on health, and much more.

**(198) THE HEALTHVIEW NEWSLETTER**
Box 6670
612 Rio Road West
Charlottesville, VA 22906

(804) 973-1395

*Samuel Biser, Editor and Publisher*

Articles on biological medicine, nutrition, and other preventive approaches.

**(199) THE NEW SUN**
807 Avenue "N"
Brooklyn, NY 11230

(212) 627-0620

*Elliot Sobel, Editor*

Monthly magazine with New Age articles on spiritual masters, consciousness transformation, and wholistic health opportunities. Advertising and articles are oriented to a New York City readership. Founded 1976.

**(200) HEALTH/PAC BULLETIN**
17 Murray Street
New York, NY 10007

(212) 267-8890

Bimonthly journal focusing on the political dimensions of health care.

**(201) HEALTH RIGHT**
175 Fifth Avenue
New York, NY 10010

(212) 674-3660

Quarterly newsletter of Women's Health Forum. Articles pertaining to implementation of women's health care.

**OSTEOPATHIC PHYSICIAN** (multidisciplinary journal)/New York, NY **(see 376)**

**(202) SEEKER**
179 Ninth Avenue
New York, NY 10011

*Jon Mundy, Editor*

Devoted to the concept of centering and opening higher levels of awareness in body and mind. Maintains listings of growth centers, psychical research societies, avant-garde religious movements, psychologists, and academic institutions involved in these fields.

**(203) HUMAN DIMENSIONS**
5695 Main Street
Williamsville, NY 14221

(704) 839-2336

Quarterly journal focusing on consciousness, meditation, parapsychology, Kirlian photography, and healing.

**(204) THE MOTHER EARTH NEWS**
P.O. Box 70
Hendersonville, NC 28739

(704) 692-4256

*John Shuttleworth, Editor*

Bimonthly magazine with articles on country living, alternative lifestyles, natural foods, and natural healing.

**(205) PREVENTION MAGAZINE**
33 Minor Street
Emmaus, Pa 18049

(215) 965-9881

*Mark Bricklin, Editor*

One of the pioneering publications in the field of health and nutrition. Contains articles on all aspects of nutrition and wholistic health maintenance.

**(206) AQUARIAN RESEARCH FOUNDATION NEWSLETTER**
5620 Morton Street
Philadelphia, PA 19144

(215) 849-1259

*Art Rosenblum, Editor*

Monthly newsletter of the Aquarian Research Foundation, dedicated to investigations of healing, natural birth control, and psychic development. Founded 1969.

**(207) UNITED FOCUS JOURNAL**
Box 5019
Seattle, WA 98014

Contains articles on meditation, healing, and consciousness. Bimonthly.

**JOURNAL OF THE RESEARCH SOCIETY FOR NATURAL THERAPEUTICS** (multidisciplinary)/ Dorset, England **(see 70)**

**IFPNT NEWSLETTER** (natural healing)/London, England **(see 72)**

## Products and Services

**HAPPINESS PRESS** (do-in, tapes and books)/Magdia, CA **(see 847)**

**(208) CELESTIAL ARTS**
231 Adrian Road
Millbrae, CA 94030

(415) 692-4500

Publishes an extensive line of significant literature relating to holistic health, psychology, and related fields.

**(209) HEALTH RESEARCH**
Box 70
Mokelumne Hill, CA 95245

Reproduces many hard to get antiquated and public domain works and also many unique original publications. Most books are spiralbound and fairly reasonable in price considering their general inaccessibility.

**(210) BUTTERFLY MEDIA DIMENSIONS**
13047 Ventura Boulevard
North Hollywood, CA 91604

(213) 995-0700

Distributes recordings of conferences, seminars, and lectures in the fields of consciousness, holistic medicine, and transpersonal psychology.

**(211) CENTER FOR HEALTH EDUCATION**
P.O. Box 2553
Palos Verdes, CA 90274

(213) 377-1178

In cooperation with UCLA, distributes cassette tape recordings of workshops and symposia on preventive medicine, biofeedback, hypnosis, and other aspects of mind-body interactions.

**(212) NEW DIMENSIONS FOUNDATION**
519 Montgomery Street
San Francisco, CA 94111

(415) 398-0338

A nonprofit educational organization dedicated to fostering communications on human change and social transformation. Principal activities include producing weekly public radio programs for regional and national dissemination, distributing audiotapes of programs produced, and providing. communication support services to other affinity groups. The tapes cover such subjects as consciousness, Leboyer approach to natural childbirth, yoga, spiritual healing, and all aspects of holistic medicine.

**(213) RAINBOW BRIDGE**
3548 22nd Street
San Francisco, CA 94114

(415) 826-3640

Distributes books and records on Sufism, yoga, childbirth, herbalism, and other subjects related to holistic healing and consciousness. Catalog available on request.

**GENERAL MEDICAL INDUSTRIES** (acupuncture, instruments)/Santa Barbara, CA **(see 656)**

**(214) COGNETICS**
P.O. Box 592
Saratoga, CA 95070

(408) 252-5754

Distributor of cassette tapes on biofeedback, acupuncture, Kirlian photography, parapsychology, and related subjects.

**BIG SUR RECORDINGS** (multidisciplinary audiovisuals)/Sausalito, CA **(see 1135)**

(215) **QUINTESSENCE UNLIMITED**
Consciousness Catalog
P.O. Box 366
Boulder, CO 80302

Publishes a catalog of tools for the natural growth of consciousness. Items include altered states of consciousness induction devices (ascids), earth furniture, geodesic domes, yoga pants, orgone blankets, musical instruments, massage tables, Kirlian photography equipment, and acupuncture charts. Also provides a service whereby individuals may have equipment and ideas custom-made by the manufacturing division.

(216) **SHAMBHALA PUBLICATIONS, INC.**
1123 Spruce Street
Boulder, CO 80302

(303) 449-6111

Publishing house dedicated "to exploring and mapping the inner world of human beings, and to expressing creatively the potential of man's inner evolution, through the medium of books of quality." Publishes books in the fields of comparative religion, philosophy, and psychology, and books dealing with man's relationship to his body and environment. A catalog is available free on request.

(217) **AURORA BOOKS**
Box 5852
Denver, CO 80217

Supplies books by mail order on health, energy, and related fields.

(218) **NUTRI-BOOKS CORP.**
Box 5793
Denver, CO 80217

(303) 778-8383

Wholesale distributor of health-related books.

(219) **HARTLEY FILM PRODUCTIONS**
59 Cat Rock Road
Cos Cob, CT 06807

(203) 869-1818

Producers of high-quality New Age films on healing and spiritual growth, such as biofeedback and indigenous medicine.

(220) **THE WHITE SHOP**
43 College Street
New Haven, CT 06510

(203) 624-2624

Retail and mail order medical books and equipment.

(221) **SMITHSONIAN SCIENCE INFORMATION EXCHANGE, INC.**
Room 300
1730 "M" Street, N.W.
Washington, DC 20038

(202) 381-4211

Extensive computerized data search service in many areas of physical and life sciences, including medicine, psychology, and biology.

(222) **DAVID D. PEDERSON**
1200 Meadowbrook Drive
Mason City, 1A 50401

(515) 423-8434

Distributes cassette tapes for arthritis therapy, relaxation, pain control, weight control, and breast development.

(223) **NATIONAL LIBRARY OF MEDICINE, NATIONAL INSTITUTES OF HEALTH**
8600 Rockville Pike
Bethesda, MD 20014

(301) 656-4000

*Dr. Martin Cummings*

Houses the most comprehensive collection of health science literature in the world in the forms of books, journals, technical reports, pamphlets, microfilms, and prints. The collection includes historical materials dating from the eleventh century and extensive audiovisuals. The library's resources, including computerized research services, can be used by writing to the above address or to the Regional Medical Libraries listed below. Founded 1836.

Covers Virginia, West Virginia, Maryland, District of Columbia, and North Carolina.

**REGIONAL MEDICAL LIBRARIES**

Center for Health Sciences
University of California
Los Angeles, CA 90024

(213) 825-4321

Covers Arizona, California, Hawaii, and Nevada.

A.W. Calhoun Medical Library
Emory University
Atlanta, GA 30322

(404) 329-6123

Covers Alabama, Florida, Georgia, Mississippi, South Carolina, Tennessee, and Puerto Rico.

John Crerar Library
35 West 33rd Street
Chicago, IL 60616

(312) 225-2526

Covers Illinois, Indiana, Iowa, Minnesota, North Dakota, and Wisconsin.

Francis A. Countway Library of Medicine
10 Shattuck Street
Boston, MA 02115

(617) 734-8900

Covers Connecticut, Maine, Massachusetts, Rhode Island, and Vermont.

Wayne State University Medical Library
4325 Brush Street
Detroit, MI 48201

(313) 577-1088

Covers Kentucky, Michigan, and Ohio.

University of Nebraska Medical Center
42nd Street and Dewey Avenue
Omaha, NE 68105

(402) 541-4000

Covers Colorado, Kansas, Missouri, Nebraska, Utah, and Wyoming.

New York Academy of Medicine Library
2 East 103rd Street
New York, NY 10029

(212) 870-8200

Covers New York and northern New Jersey.

Library of the College of Physicians
19 South 22nd Street
Philadelphia, PA 19103

(215) 561-6050

Covers Pennsylvania, Delaware, and southern New Jersey.

University of Texas Southwestern Medical School at Dallas
5323 Harry Hines Boulevard
Dallas, TX 75235

(214) 688-3111

Covers Arkansas, Louisiana, New Mexico, Oklahoma, and Texas

University of Washington Health Sciences Library
Seattle, WA 98195

Covers Alaska, Idaho, Montana, Oregon, and Washington.

(206) 543-2100

**(224) W. G. BAZAN**
Professional Books
P.O. Box 125
O'Fallon, MO 63366

(314) 272-2959

Buyer and seller of antique books on osteopathy, chiropractic, naprapathy, naturopathy, natural hygiene, and bloodless surgery.

**(225) SUN PUBLISHING COMPANY**
P.O. Box 4383
Albuquerque, NM 87106

(505) 255-6550

Publisher and distributor of holistic health and consciousness-oriented books, as well as newspapers in the same field.

**(226) SWAN HOUSE PUBLISHING COMPANY**
P.O. Box 170
Brooklyn, NY 11223

(212) 336-0531

Publisher of quality books related to wholistic healing. Subjects vary from macrobiotics to herbs to traditional Jewish approaches to wholistic healing, and have included innovative works on significant phenomena such as clay therapy and biological transmutations.

**(227) ASI PUBLISHING COMPANY**
127 Madison Avenue
New York, NY 10016

(212) 679-5676

Publishers of books on acupuncture and distributors of a large number of books in the field of wholistic medicine.

**(228) LUMISCOPE COMPANY, INC.**
836 Broadway
New York, NY 10003

(800) 221-5746

Distributors of a professional home blood pressure monitoring kit.

**ALTERNATIVE HEALTH EDUCATION CENTER**
(herbal preparations)/Rochester, NY **(see 143)**

**(229) GREAT EARTH HEALING, INC.**
East Montpelier, VT 05651

PO Box 549, Station N
Montreal, Quebec, Canada H2X 3M6

Distributors of the "Ma Roller," a (wooden) spinal correction and awareness development device.

**(230) THE HERITAGE STORE**
P.O. Box 444-D
Virginia Beach, VA 23458

(804) 428-0100

A retail and mail order outlet for solarama products, food supplements, Cayce remedies, homeopathic supplies, and herbal tonics. Also carries a wide range of books on color therapy, aura, Cayce, homeopathy, and psychic phenomena.

# Physio- and Hydrotherapies

*The following is a listing of groups, centers and clinics engaged in or making use of physio- and hydrotherapies. Physiotherapy, as the name implies, is the use of physical measures in the treatment of disease and mechanical disorder. At one time grouped under this heading was an array of treatments which included electricity; biomagnetics; all forms of radiant energy including xray; radium; ultraviolet ray; infrared ray; visible light; exercises, mechanotherapy and hydrotherapy. Today the physiotherapist confines his/ her activities to the use of some light treatments but mostly uses massage and manipulation, exercises, mechanotherapy, colonics, and some hydrotherapy.*

*Hydrotherapy is the application of water in various forms to the surface of the body for the modification of physiological and pathological processes. If the application is made in the form of a still bath or pack it is simply one method of applying conductive heat or cold. If on the other hand the water is forced against the part or is made to circulate about it the result is obtained by mechanical as well as thermal means. Moderate to short applications of cold water have the effect of lessening the activities of the structures with which the cold comes in contact. This is followed by a state of increased vital activity which is higher than that existing prior to the application of cold. Prolonged applications of water at a temperature above 100° F diminish muscular excitability and capacity for muscular work.*

*On the other hand very short hot applications are the best means to counteract muscular exhaustion due to prolonged exercise. Hot baths are excitive or exhaustive to the nervous system according to the mode of application.*

*The various combinations of hot and cold water to different parts of the body are too numerous to mention here, but properly used, hydrotherapy can be an important adjunct to more standard but non-toxic therapies.*

## Groups and Associations

**(231) GOLDEN STATE PHYSICAL THERAPY ASSOCIATION**
809 Chapala Street
Santa Barbara, CA 93101

(805) 966-3344

*Merlin Kemp, LPT, and Ronald L. Kemp, DC*

Teaches quarterly workshops in physical therapy. Founded 1952.

**(232) NATIONAL ASSOCIATION OF PHYSICAL THERAPY**
P.O.Box 367
West Covina, CA 91793

(213) 332-7755

*Robert F. Robinson, PhD, Executive Director*

Techniques and approaches used in this national organization of 5,000 members include rehabilitative exercise, corrective manipulation, ultrasonic, moist heat, whirlpool, electrostimulation, and pressure point techniques. Publishes a newsletter, *The Independent Practitioner.* Founded 1961.

**(233) NEW JERSEY STATE PHYSICAL THERAPY SOCIETY, INC.**
8A Barberry Avenue
Lakewood, NJ 08701

(201) 367-1841

*Patrick Trotta, PHT, President*

Maintains list of members practicing in New Jersey.

**(234) NEW YORK STATE SOCIETY OF PHYSIOTHERAPISTS, INC.**
37 Bellewood Avenue
Centereach, NY 11720

(516) 981-6021

*Howard G. Krebaum, Jr., PhT, Secretary*

Maintains list of members practicing in New York State.

## Schools, Centers, and Clinics

**LUCATS' PREVENTION REGENERATION RESORT**/Safford, AZ **(see 164)**

**NATIONAL ARTHRITIS MEDICAL CLINIC**/Desert Hot Springs, CA **(see 81)**

**HIDDEN VALLEY HEALTH RANCH** (resort)/ Escondido, CA **(see 166)**

**MEADOWLARK** (resort)/Hemet, CA **(see 167)**

**(235) ASHTON SCHOOL OF PHYSIOHYDROTHERAPY**
630 South Wilton Place
Los Angeles, CA 90005

(213) 387-2737
*-G. Ashton, DC, ND, Director*

Provides clinical treatments and instruction in colon hydrotherapy, therapeutic massage, and xray technology.

**HARBIN HOT SPRINGS** (resort)/Middletown, CA **(see 168)**

**HUMAN POTENTIAL CAMP** (children and adults)/ Point Arena, CA **(see 169)**

**SACRAMENTO MEDICAL PREVENTICS CLINIC**/ Sacramento, CA **(see 103)**

**AGE OF ENLIGHTENMENT CENTER FOR HOLISTIC HEALTH** (holistic clinic)/San Diego, CA **(see 104)**

**SAN DIEGO NATURAL HEALTH CLINIC**/San Diego, CA **(see 108)**

**(236) FAMILY SAUNA SHOP**
1214 Twentieth Avenue
San Francisco, CA 94122

(415) 681-3600

Offers private sauna bathing facilities and massage by appointment.

**ORR SPRINGS ASSOCIATION** (resort)/Ukiah, CA **(see 170)**

**WILBUR HOT SPRINGS** (psychotherapy center)/Wilbur Springs, CA **(see 1071)**

**BOULDER SCHOOL OF MASSAGE THERAPY** (also hydrotherapy)/Boulder, CO **(see 861)**

**DESERT LIGHT FOUNDATION** (holistic clinic and educational center)/Albuquerque, NM **(see 134)**

**BULGARIAN TOURIST OFFICE** (resort and spa information)/New York, NY **(see 173)**

**REILLY'S ON 34th ST** (center and clinic)/New York, NY **(see 141)**

**YUGOSLAV STATE TOURIST OFFICE** (spa and resort information)/New York, NY **(see 175)**

**PSI CENTER** (clinic and educational center)/Cincinnati, OH **(see 145)**

**CLYMER HEALTH CLINIC** (wholistic clinic)/ Quakertown, PA **(see 150)**

**HOME CENTER** (clinic and educational center)/Virginia Beach, VA **(see 155)**

**RENAISSANCE REVITALIZATION CENTER** (resort spa)/Nassau, Bahamas **(see 176)**

**LATIN AMERICAN MISSION PROGRAM, INSTITUTO NATURISTA ADVENTISTA** (wholistic clinic)/Guatemala, Central America **(see 160)**

**TYRINGHAM NATUROPATHIC CLINIC** (wholistic)/Bucks, England **(see 177)**

**RAMANA HEALTH CENTRE** (wholistic hospital)/ Hants, England **(see 161)**

(237) **ROYAL PUMP ROOM**
Warwick District Council
Amenities Department
10 Newbold Terrace
Leamington Spa, Warwickshire
England

Tel: Leamington 27072 (Ext. 282)

Provides physiotherapeutic services and hydrotherapy to patients referred by the National Health Services. Treatments include vortex bath, diathermy, ultrasound, ionization, massage, spinal traction, and ultraviolet and infrared light treatment.

**PORT OF HEALTH INTERNATIONAL NATURO-PRACTIC HEALTHATARIUM** (spa and workshops)/ Mexico **(see 444)**

**ITA-WEGMAN-KLINIK** (anthroposophical clinic)/ Arlesheim, Switzerland **(see 813)**

**FILDERKLINIK** (anthroposophical hospital)/West Germany **(see 816)**

**GEMEINNÜTZIGES GEMEINSCHAFTSKRAN-KENHAUS HERDECKE** (anthroposophical hospital)/ West Germany **(see 818)**

**KLINIK ÖSCHELBRONN** (anthroposophical clinic)/ West Germany **(see 820)**

**LUKAS KLINIK** (anthroposophical)/West Germany **(see 814)**

**OTTO BUCHINGER CLINIC** (wholistic clinic)/West Germany **(see 181)**

**PARACELSUS-KRANKENHAUS** (anthroposophical rest home)/West Germany **(see 822)**

**SANATORIUM FÜR DYNAMISCHE THERAPIE STUDENHOF** (anthroposophical clinic)/West Germany **(see 823)**

## Products and Services

(238) **GENERAL THERAPHYSICAL, INC.**
2018 Washington Avenue
St. Louis, MO 63103

(314) 231-9643

Distributes full line of physical therapy equipment.

**HEALTH AND PLEASURE TOURS, INC.** (spas)/New York, NY **(see 174)**

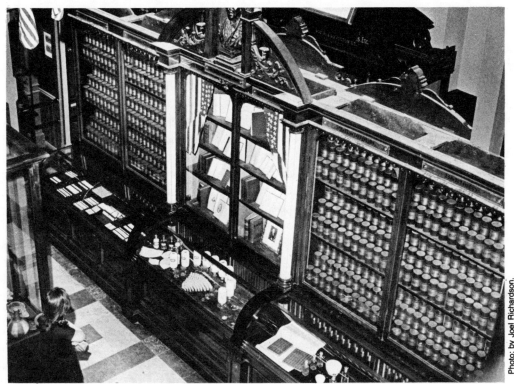

Boericke and Tafel homeopathic display at the Smithsonian Institute Washington, DC.

# Homeopathy

*Harris L. Coulter, PhD*

*"Our only health is the disease*
*If we obey the dying nurse*
*Whose constant care is not to please*
*But to remind of our, and Adam's curse,*
*And that, to be restored,*
  *our sickness must grow worse.*

*The whole earth is our hospital*
*Endowed by the ruined millionaire,*
*Wherein, if we do well, we shall*
*Die of the absolute paternal care*
*That will not leave us*
  *but prevents us everywhere."*
                    *T. S. Eliot*

Originated by Samuel Hahneman (1755-1843), homeopathy* made its first pronounced impact on American and European medical thought during the Asiatic cholera epidemic of 1832; many observers noted that the homeopaths had a far higher incidence of recovery than the allopaths (thus in Paris in 1832 the price of the homeopathic medicine for Asiatic cholera increased a hundredfold). Other epidemic diseases in which homeopathic practitioners distinguished themselves were scarlet fever, dysentery, meningitis, and yellow fever. The nineteenth-century homeopathic records are full of cases of the successful treatment of these diseases.

Perhaps the best evidence of the efficacy of homeopathic medicines is the fact that many have been subsequently adopted by orthodox physicians. In fact, many of these same medicines are still in the allopathic pharmacopoeia and still used in daily practice. Perhaps the best example is nitroglycerine for certain heart conditions. This substance was first used in angina pectoris in the early 1850s by Constantine Hering (1800-1880), known as the father of American homeopathy for his many therapeutic and other contributions. Even the major revolution in therapeutics effected by Louis Pasteur was only a further application of the basic homeopathic principle of cure through "similars."

The fundamental homeopathic tenet is that the remedy for any case of disease or illness is the substance that, when administered systematically to a healthy person, yields precisely the symptomology (symptom pattern) of this case. Substances are "proved" on healthy persons (from the German

---

*Spelled homoeopathy in original text.

47

*Pruefung,* ''trial'' or ''test''), and comprehensive records are kept. (The homeopathic works on materia medica, listing symptoms for each of the thousand or more medicines commonly used in homeopathic practice, are extensive—Constantine Hering's *Guiding Symptoms of Our Materia Medica,* for instance, runs five thousand pages.) Homeopathy holds that when the patient receives the one remedy whose symptomatology most perfectly matches his or her own symptoms, the whole disease is removed, root and branch.

When seeking the remedy whose symptomatology is precisely similar to the symptoms of the patient, the homeopath must isolate one single remedy from the thousand-odd remedies in the homeopathic materia medica. This demands a very precise matching of the patient's symptoms with those in the books. Many remedies, after all, have approximately similar symptomatologies, but only the one ''most similar'' remedy will act curatively in the given case. (An incorrectly selected remedy will usually have no effect at all on the patient or, at most, will alter symptoms without acting curatively.)

Thus, homeopathic prescription, demanding both time and individualized attention, is out of step with the socioeconomic determinants of modern medical practice. Today allopathic physicians may see up to fifty or sixty patients a day, spending from eight to twelve minutes with each; much of their work is allocated to nurses and paramedical personnel. It is not surprising that allopathic medicine has again entered one of its periodic phases of overmedication and polypharmacy, stressing ''broad spectrum'' drugs designed to treat a multitude of different states.

The factors of time and efficiency aside, homeopathy would demand of modern physicians trained in the analytical, reductionist tradition a total turnabout in approach. Since homeopathy aims to treat, systematically, the whole person of the patient, a radically different method of diagnosis is required. Treating the whole person means being guided by the unique aspects of his or her physical and mental life, and, in homeopathy, by the peculiar symptoms that he or she manifests.

Thus, homeopathy, like allopathy, might be called ''symptomatic.'' However, modern allopathy is based on the internal pathological changes characteristic of a given diseased state—that is, the *least* common denominators of the various people suffering from this particular ''disease.'' In the homeopathic method, it is not the symptoms that the patient has *in common* with others that are the guides to treatment, but rather those which *distinguish and differentiate* him or her from any other patient in the world with a similar complaint. Pathological data, homeopaths feel, are too crude, as well as too changeable, to be a good basis for therapy. Symptoms, however, provide fine and other subtle distinctions among diseased states, and, when observed with the necessary accuracy, are also more reliable. This fact might explain why observations made 150 years ago in homeopathic practice are still valid today.

# Homeotherapeutics
*Wyrth Post Baker, MD*

Homeotherapeutics (homeopathy) is a therapeutic method based on the Principle of Similars, from the Latin *"Simila similibus curentur"* ("Likes cure likes"). Hippocrates was probably the first to suggest that superimposition of a similar illness upon an existing pathological process might actuate homeostasis in the disordered body and result in cure. Paracelsus and von Stoerck expressed similar thoughts, but no practical therapeutic application was attempted until 1798, when Samuel Hahnemann proposed a definite methodology which he designated "Homeopathy."

The Principle of Similars is based on the following premises: (1) normal health depends on the ability of the body to maintain homeostasis; (2) recovery from illness is dependent on the inherent vital force of the body, i.e., the basic pattern of health; (3) most disorders or diseases of the human body produce symptoms which are emotional, mental, and/or physical in nature; (4) a substance that is capable of evoking certain symptoms when administered to an apparently healthy human being under controlled conditions may become a potentially effective therapeutic agent when it is prepared according to the standards of the Homeopathic Pharmacopoeia of the United States and administered in accordance with the principles of homeotherapeutics.

Homeopathic treatment is individualized and directed wholistically at the total symptom complex of the patient, not directed at a diagnosis or disease entity. Homeotherapeutic physicians first obtain the customary diagnostic history of the patient, then assemble pertinent objective laboratory, radiological, and ancillary diagnostic data in order to secure a detailed wholistic* (homeopathic) history, which will permit accurate individualization of each patient according to the symptom complex as presented. Recognizing that diagnosis is only a single facet of the total picture necessary to predict whether the disorder is functional, organic, progressive, degenerative, or malignant in nature, they determine whether it is likely to respond to medical treatment in general and homeotherapeutics in particular. Having adequate knowledge of these principles and of the pathogenicity of each drug according to the homeopathic materia medica, they are able to determine the probable reaction and response of the patient to administration of drugs by the homeotherapeutic method. Finally a single drug is prescribed, to be administered in the *minimum* effective dose (keeping in mind, however, that concomitant administration of drugs in physiological or the usual pharmacological dosage may interfere with or negate the therapeutic effectiveness of homeotherapeutics).

Although of limited value for patients receiving physiological medication in minimal or moderate dosage (though compatible with some antibiotics, homeotherapeutic agents are usually rendered ineffective when sulfa drugs, steroids, and other potent pharmacological drugs are administered concomitantly or immediately before homeotherapy), homeotherapeutics has been most effective in treating infants, children, and individuals who have received little or no physiological (allopathic) medication. Moreover, it is the safest therapeutic method for patients who have an allergic diathesis or history of previous drug reactions, whether iatrogenic or toxicological. Wholistic in nature, homeotherapeutics is compatible with most areas of medicine (including obstetrics and surgery), immunotherapy, nutritional therapy (including vitamin supplementation), endocrine therapy (including hormones), psychotherapy, physical therapy, osteopathy, chiropractic, and naturopathy.

When employed precisely in accordance with the Principle of Similars, homeotherapeutics possesses certain definite advantages over many other methods in the control and alleviation of disorders that are amenable to its application. Homeotherapeutic agents can often be prescribed in lieu of antibiotics and toxic therapeutic agents; moreover, they are often effective in disorders for which no specific medication exists. The dosage, as well as expense, is minimal, and sensitivity reactions, toxic manifestations (including poisoning), and severe iatrogenic effects are extremely rare. Once initiated, the process of

---

*Spelled holistic in original text.

recovery is usually progressive, automatic, and simple (though a second or even a third prescription may be called for in the case of complicated or phasic conditions). Relapses are unusual, and suppression of symptoms with subsequent appearance of other illnesses is avoided.

*Note: The word homeopathy/homoeopathy has been spelled according to the preference of the individual organization.*

## Groups and Associations

### (239) LOS ANGELES COUNTY HOMEOPATHIC MEDICAL SOCIETY
c/o G. Brunler, MB, ChB (Edin.), President
435 South Curson, Apt. MJ
Los Angeles, CA 90036

(213) 933-3810

Maintains up-to-date membership list for the Los Angeles area, has speakers' bureau, and provides information on homeopathy for physicians.

### (240) BAY AREA HOMOEOPATHIC STUDY GROUP
c/o Randall Neustaedter
645 62nd Street
Oakland, CA 94609

Conducts laymen's homoeopathic study group.

### (241) INTERNATIONAL HOMEOPATHIC LEAGUE and the SAN FRANSICSO HOMEOPATHIC MEDICAL SOCIETY
c/o Frederic W. Schmid, MD, D-HT
6200 Geary Boulevard
Medical Building at 26th Avenue
San Francisco, CA 94121

(415) 221-4111

Maintains an up-to-date membership list for the San Francisco area, as well as an international list, has a speakers' bureau, and provides information on homeopathy for physicians.

### (242) SANTA CRUZ HOMOEOPATHIC LAY LEAGUE
c/o Lucinda Concannon
131 Sunnyside Avenue
Santa Cruz, CA 95062

Conducts laymen's homoeopathic study group.

### (243) DENVER HOMOEOPATHIC LAYMEN'S LEAGUE
c/o Orville Hudley
229 South Franklin Street
Denver, CO 80209

Conducts laymen's homoeopathic study groups.

### (244) HOMOEOPATHIC STUDY GROUP OF WESTCHESTER AND FAIRFIELD COUNTIES
c/o Phyllis Freeman
27 Spicer Road
Westport, CT 06880

Conducts laymen's homoeopathic study group.

### (245) MICHIGAN HOMEOPATHIC LAYMEN'S SOCIETY
c/o Leonard Lystad
29546 Norma
Warren, MI 48093

Conducts laymen's homeopathic study group.

### (246) HOMOEOPATHIC STUDY GROUP OF ROCHESTER, NY
c/o Jeffrey Van Riper
60 East Avenue
Brockport, NY 14420

(716) 637-6126

Conducts laymen's homoeopathic study group.

### (247) HOMOEOPATHIC LAYMEN'S LEAGUE OF NEW YORK
c/o Mrs. L.C. Becker
90 La Salle Street, Apt. 18-D
New York, NY 10027

Conducts laymen's homoeopathic study group.

### (248) HOMOEOPATHIC LAYMEN'S LEAGUE OF THE NORTHEAST
c/o Lorina Cooper
Hawley Road
North Salem, NY 10560

Conducts laymen's homoeopathic study group.

### (249) L.J. DEWEESE FOUNDATION
c/o Marilyn DeWeese
6280 Garber Road
Dayton, OH 45415

Conducts laymen's homoeopathic study group.

### (250) WOMEN'S NATIONAL HOMEOPATHIC LEAGUE, INC.
1911 Walnut Street
Dover, OH 44622

*Mrs. Horace Reed, Secretary*

Conducts laymen's homoeopathic study group.

### (251) HOMOEOPATHIC LAYMEN'S LEAGUE, MANHEIM, PENNSYLVANIA
c/o David Fidlers
R.D. # 5
Manheim, PA 17545

Conducts laymen's homoeopathic study group.

**(252) LEHIGH VALLEY NATURAL HEALING**
c/o Bill Brodhead
R.D. #1
Box 298A
Northampton, PA 18067

(215) 262-1171

Conducts laymen's homoeopathic study group.

**(253) HOMOEOPATHIC LAYMEN'S LEAGUE, PITTSBURGH, PA.**
c/o Steffne Witney
120 Genessee Road
Pittsburgh, PA 15241

(412) 833-3859

Conducts laymen's homoeopathic study group.

**(254) SALT LAKE CITY HOMOEOPATHIC LEAGUE**
c/o Edith S. Willes
2603 South Eighth Street East
Salt Lake City, UT 84106

(801) 486-8924

Conducts laymen's homoeopathic study group.

**(255) AMERICAN ASSOCIATION OF HOMOEO-PATHIC PHARMACISTS**
6231 Leesburg Pike, Suite 506
Falls Church, VA 22044

(703) 534-4363

Coordinates efforts of American pharmacists who specialize in homoeopathic prescriptions. Assists in the up-dating of the U.S. Homoeopathic Pharmacopoea and in updating research, methodology, and types of medication for homoeopathic practice.

**(256) AMERICAN BOARD OF HOMOEO-THERAPEUTICS**
6231 Leesburg Pike, Suite 506
Falls Church, VA 22044

(703) 534-4363

*Allen C. Neiswander, MD, President*

Diploma granting board for proficiency and accomplishment in homoeopathy.

**(257) THE AMERICAN INSTITUTE OF HOMEOPATHY**
6231 Leesburg Pike, Suite 506
Falls Church, VA 22044

(703) 534-4363

A nonprofit organization of physicians who believe in and use the methodology of homeotherapeutics. The organization works to disseminate information on homeopathy, improving the standards of medical education, and obtaining the general recognition and public acceptance of homeopathy. A reference library and information center are open to the public. Membership is limited to Doctors of Medicine, Osteopathy, or Dentistry who hold a valid license to practice medicine in one of the states of the United States or one of the provinces of Canada, and who shall be prepared to practice homeotherapeutics. Founded 1844.

**(258) AMERICAN FOUNDATION FOR HO-MOEOPATHY**
6231 Leesburg Pike, Suite 506
Falls Church, VA 22044

(703) 534-4363

*Wyrth Post Baker, MD, Trustee*

Fund-raising and grant-in-aid organization for programs in the field of homoeopathy.

**(259) THE NATIONAL CENTER FOR HOMOEOPATHY, INC.**
6231 Leesburg Pike, Suite 506
Falls Church, VA 22044

(703) 534-4363 and 534-4364

*Ralph Packman, Executive Director*

Maintains an educational summer program offering courses in history and philosophy of homoeopathy, therapeutic approach, clinical experience review, and materia medica. Although this program is geared to the health professional, additional educational programs are also offered to laymen in the belief that informed laymen make better patients. A division of research develops research projects relating to homoeopathy, and a division of publications includes an extensive library of classics, working texts, journals, and monographs on homoeopathy. Membership in the national center is open to both individuals and groups, sharing a common interest in the support and perpetuation of homoeopathy and homoeotherapeutics. Founded 1922 as the Postgraduate School in Homoeopathy.

*AFFILIATE AND STATE LAY ASSOCIATIONS*

**SUBURBAN HOMOEOPATHIC LAYMEN'S LEAGUE**
Mary Hunt Steven Chapter
c/o Arthur Drechney
1753 North New England
Chicago, IL 60635

Member of the National Center for Homoeopathy, Inc. Conducts laymen's homoeopathic study groups.

**GLENVIEW HOMOEOPATHIC LAYMEN'S LEAGUE**
c/o Craig H. Swain
1041 North Roselle Road
Hoffman Estates, IL 60195

Member of the National Center for Homoeopathy, Inc. Conducts laymen's homoeopathic study groups.

**HOMOEOPATHIC LAYMEN'S LEAGUE OF KENTUCKY**
c/o Josephine Bryant
418 Chinoe Road
Lexington, KY 40502

Member of the National Center for Homoeopathy, Inc. Conducts laymen's homoeopathic study groups.

**METROPOLITAN DETROIT AREA HOMOEO-PATHIC STUDY GROUP**
c/o Mary L. DeFauw
2013 West Houstonia
Royal Oak, MI 48073

Member of the National Center for Homoeopathy, Inc. Conducts laymen's homoeopathic study groups.

**TWIN CITIES HOMOEOPATHIC ASSOCIATION**
c/o Michael Carlston
434 Fourth Street, N.E.
Minneapolis, MN 55413

Member of the National Center for Homoeopathy, Inc.
Conducts laymen's homoeopathic study groups.

**HOMOEOPATHIC CHAPTER OF SOUTHERN NEW JERSEY**
c/o Diana Gammuto
39 Barnwell Drive
Willingboro, NJ 08046

Member of the National Center for Homoeopathy, Inc.
Conducts laymen's homoeopathic study groups.

**NORTHWEST HOMOEOPATHIC FOUNDATION**
c/o Nancy Kojac
Saugerties Health Food Store
48 Market Street
Saugerties, NY 12477

Member of the National Center for Homoeopathy, Inc.
Conducts laymen's homoeopathic study groups.

**HOMOEOPATHIC LAYMEN'S CHAPTER OF GREATER PHILADELPHIA**
c/o Mrs. Madhupuri Bailey
P.O. Box 26037
Philadelphia, PA 19128

(215) VI8-9654

Member of the National Center for Homoeopathy, Inc.
Conducts laymen's homoeopathic study groups.

**DALLAS CHAPTER OF THE HOMOEOPATHIC LAYMEN'S LEAGUE**
c/o Mary Volz
3227 Rotan Lane
Dallas, TX 75229

(214) 352-2534

Member of the National Center for Homoeopathy, Inc.
Conducts laymen's homoeopathic study groups.

**ROANOKE VALLEY CHAPTER OF THE NATIONAL CENTER FOR HOMOEOPATHY**
c/o Mrs. Lester Greenwalt
Star Route # 1, Box 83B
New Castle, VA 24127

Member of the National Center for Homoeopathy, Inc.
Conducts laymen's homoeopathic study groups.

**HOMOEOPATHIC LAYMEN'S LEAGUE OF WASHINGTON, DC**
c/o Pat Everette
1741 Burning Tree Drive
Vienna, VA 22180

(804) 281-4297

Member of the National Center for Homoeopathy, Inc.
Conducts laymen's homoeopathic study groups.

**NORTHWEST HOMOEOPATHIC FOUNDATION**
c/o Judith Papineau
3918 Pinney Bay Drive
Bremerton, WA 98310

(206) 377-6460

Member of the National Center for Homoeopathy, Inc.
Conducts laymen's homoeopathic study groups.

**PUGET SOUND HOMOEOPATHIC MEDICAL SOCIETY**
c/o John E. Osburn
19522 88th Avenue
Edmonds, WA 98020

Member of the National Center for Homoeopathy, Inc.
Conducts laymen's homoeopathic study groups.

**(260) AUSTRALIAN INSTITUTE OF HOMEOPATHY**
c/o Mrs. G. Reynolds, Secretary
7 Hampden Road
Artarmon 2064, Australia

Association to promote homeopathy. Full member of IFPNT **(72)**

**(261) THE BRITISH HOMOEOPATHIC ASSOCIATION**
43 Russell Square
London WC1, England

Maintains membership list and distributes information. Sponsors lectures and seminars.

**PSIONIC MEDICAL SOCIETY** (dowsing and homeopathy)/Surrey, England **(see 717)**

**(262) HOMÖOPATHISCHER VEREIN E.V.**
2000 Hamburg 20
Eppendorfer Baum 4
West Germany

Association to promote the use of homeopathic methods. Full member of IFPNT **(72)**.

**(263) DEUTSCHER VERBAND FÜR HOMÖOPATHIE UND LEBENSPFLEGE**
7057 Winnenden B. Stuttgart
Ahornweg 7, West Germany

Association of homeopaths and life-care practitioners engaged in various methods of natural and alternative healing. Full member of IFPNT **(72)**.

## Schools, Centers, and Clinics

**BERKELEY HOLISTIC HEALTH CENTER** (educational)/Berkeley, CA **(see 76)**

**(264) HERING FAMILY HEALTH CLINIC**
2340 Ward Street, Suite 107
Berkeley, CA 94705

(415) 548-1992

*Randall Naustaedter, Clinic Coordinator*

Provides family health care including pediatric and gynecological services. Homeopathic medicine is the main form of treatment used. Additional services include nutritional counseling, child care counseling, and social employment counseling. Educational programs in homeopathic theory, homeopathic first-aid, childbirth, and preventive health care are also offered.

**(265) HOMEOPATHIC EDUCATIONAL SERVICES**
1801 Woolsey
Berkeley, CA 94703

(415) 655-3659

*Dana Ullman*

Offers workshops dealing with the homeopathic principle and practice.

**KHALSA MEDICAL AND COUNSELING ASSOCIATES** (multidisciplinary clinic)/Los Angeles, CA **(see 92)**

**WHITE CROSS SOCIETY** (workshops)/Lucerne Valley, CA **(see 93)**

**McCORNACK CENTER FOR THE HEALING ARTS** (wholistic clinic)/Mendocino, CA **(see 95)**

**AGE OF ENLIGHTENMENT CENTER FOR HOLISTIC HEALTH** (trancendental meditation with therapy)/San Diego, CA **(see 104)**

**HOLISTIC LIFE UNIVERSITY** (multidisciplinary workshops)/San Francisco, CA **(see 111)**

**HIMALAYAN INSTITUTE COMBINED THERAPY CENTER** (multidisciplinary, residential center)/Glenview, IL **(see 125)**

**(265.1) U.S. HOMOEOPATHIC RESEARCH, INC.**
Homoeopathic Center
107 East 38th Street
New York, NY 10016

(212) 532-4538

*Bhagat Singh, MD (HOMOEO), President*

A clinic facility where homeopathic treatment is given, USHRI also has available a 10 week introductory course followed by a series of 4 advanced courses in homeopathy. The course is opened to medical doctors as well as the lay public. A computer bank containing a vast amount of information on symptomatic indications for treatment and the homeopathic remedy to be used, is being installed and this service will be made available to physicians and practitioners interested in the use of homeopathic preparations. A newsletter is published from time to time containing news on developments at the center.

**ALTERNATIVE HEALTH EDUCATION CENTER** (wholistic)/Rochester, NY **(see 143)**

**CLYMER HEALTH CLINIC** (multidisciplinary)/Quakertown, PA **(see 150)**

**TYRINGHAM NATUROPATHIC CLINIC** (wholistic spa)/Bucks, England **(see 177)**

**(266) ROYAL LONDON HOMEOPATHIC HOSPITAL**
Great Ormond Street
London, WC1N 3HR
England

Maintains complete homeopathic hospital facilities for public use. A complete line of homeopathic books as well as xeroxed copies of articles that appeared in the *British Homeopathic Journal* are available by writing to the Librarian at the above address.

**SANATORIUM SCHLOSS HAMBORN** (anthroposophical clinic)/West Germany **(see 824)**

## Journals and Publications

**WELL-BEING MAGAZINE** (natural therapies)/San Diego, CA **(see 186)**

**(267) HOMEOTHERAPY**
P.O. Box 31100
San Francisco, CA 94131

(415) 824-7306

*Alain Naude, Editor*

Organ of the Homeopathic Physicians of the Pacific. Contains articles on relevance of homeopathy to medical and psychiatric problems. Published bimonthly by the California State Homeopathic Medical Society. Founded 1975.

**ALTERNATIVES JOURNAL** (multidisciplinary New Age articles)/Miami, FL **(see 193)**

**(268) THE HOMEOPATHIC DIGEST**
Box 667
Ossining, NY 10562

(914) 941-3678

*T.C. Cherian, Editor and Publisher*

Quarterly journal of naturotherapeutics with emphasis on homeopathy. Founded 1976.

**JOURNAL OF THE AMERICAN INSTITUTE FOR HOMEOPATHY**/Falls Church, VA **(see 257)**

**THE LAYMAN SPEAKS** (homoeopathic journal)/Falls Church, VA **(see 259)**

**JOURNAL OF THE RESEARCH SOCIETY FOR NATURAL THERAPEUTICS** (multidisciplinary)/Dorset, England **(see 70)**

**(269) BRITISH HOMEOPATHIC JOURNAL**
Headley Brothers, Ltd.
Invicta Press
Ashford, Kent TN24 8HH
England

Journal of the Faculty of Homeopathy, Royal London Homeopathic Hospital **(266)**.

## Products and Services

**(270) HORTON & CONVERSE**
621 West Pico Boulevard
Los Angeles, CA 90015

(213) 273-0850

Pharmacy stocking homeopathic preparations.

**(271) STANDARD HOMOEOPATHIC COMPANY**
436 West Eighth Avenue
Los Angeles, CA 90014

(213) 627-1555

Manufactures and stocks homeopathic preparations. Regular member of the American Association of Homoeopathic Pharmacists.

**(272) MYLANS HOMEOPATHIC PHARMACY**
222 O'Farrell Street
San Francisco, CA 94102

(415) 781-0053

Pharmacy stocking homeopathic preparations. Associate member of the American Association of Homoeopathic Pharmacists.

**(273) SANTA MONICA DRUG**
1513 Fourth Street
Santa Monica, CA 90401

(213) 395-1131

Pharmacy stocking homeopathic preparations.

**(274) EHRHART & KARL, INC.**
17 North Wabash Avenue
Chicago, IL 60602

(312) 332-1046

Manufactures and stocks homeopathic preparations. Regular member of the American Association of Homoeopathic Pharmacists.

**(275) WASHINGTON HOMOEOPATHIC PHARMACY**
4914 Delray Avenue
Bethesda, MD 20014

Manufactures and stocks homeopathic preparations. Regular member of the American Association of Homoeopathic Pharmacists.

**(276) LUYTIES PHARMACAL COMPANY**
4200 Laclede Avenue
St. Louis, MO 63108

(800) 325-8080

Manufactures and stocks homeopathic preparations. Regular member of the American Association of Homoeopathic Pharmacists.

**(277) HUMPHREYS PHARMACAL COMPANY**
63 Meadow Road
Rutherford, NJ 07070

(201) 933-7744

Manufactures and stocks homeopathic preparations. Regular member of the American Association of Homoeopathic Pharmacists.

**FREEDA PHARMACY** (homeopathic preparations)/New York, NY **(see 530)**

**(278) KIEHL PHARMACY, INC.**
109 Third Avenue
New York, NY 10003

(212) 475-3400

Pharmacy stocking homeopathic preparations. Large and well-known supplier of quality herbs, oils, and perfumes.

**U.S. HOMOEOPATHIC CENTER**/New York, NY **(see 265.1)**

**(279) WELEDA, INC.**
30 South Main Street
Spring Valley, NY 10977

(914) 352-6145

Pharmacy manufacturing and stocking homeopathic and anthroposophic preparations. Associate member of the American Association of Homoeopathic Pharmacists.

**(280) JOHN A. BORNEMAN & SONS**
1208 Amosland Road
Norwood, PA 19074

Manufactures and stocks homeopathic preparations. Regular member of the American Association of Homoeopathic Pharmacists.

**(281) BOERICKE & TAFEL, INC.**
1011 Arch Street
Philadelphia, PA 19107

(215) 922-2967

Manufactures and stocks homeopathic preparations. Regular member of the American Association of Homoeopathic Pharmacists.

**(282) ANNANDALE APOTHECARY**
7023 Little River Turnpike
Annandale, VA 22003

(703) 256-1565

Pharmacy stocking homeopathic preparations.

**HERITAGE STORE** (Cayce)/Virginia Beach, VA **(see 230)**

**(283) SAKTI DISTRIBUTORS**
320 State Street
Madison, WI 53703

(608) 255-5007

Distributor of homeopathic books.

**(284) D.L. THOMPSON HOMEOPATHIC SUPPLIES, INC.**
844 Yonge Street
Toronto 5, Ontario
Canada

Pharmacy stocking homeopathic preparations.

**(285) NELSON'S PHARMACY**
73 Duke Street, Grosvenor Square
London W1, England

Manufacturers and distributors of homeopathic preparations.

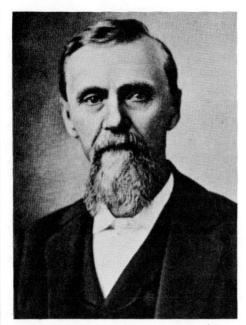

Andrew Taylor Still, discoverer of the principles of osteopathy, born in 1828; courtesy *Osteopathic Physician* magazine.

# Osteopathy

*J. Dudley Chapman, DO, DSc*

Osteopathy is based on the concept that the body has the inherent ability to heal itself if its physical and physiological integrity is intact. The principles of osteopathic medicine were set forth by Andrew Taylor Still (1828–1917). An early abolitionist and supporter of women's suffrage, Still acquired medical skills at the College of Physicians and Surgeons in Kansas City but abhorred the quality and theory (what there was of it) of the medicine of the day. Epidemics of cholera, smallpox, and meningitis were common, and there was no effective treatment: one merely watched the very strong survive and the weak perish. The existing therapies were crude and unscientific; there were as yet no federal agencies to regulate drugs or set standards for medical practice. The prevailing school of thought concentrated on the disease, rather than the body as a functioning unit. Still believed that within "the total man" are the forces or substances necessary for health. Moreover, he felt that progress could be achieved in the study of disease only if a study were first made of health—that is, normalcy. By 1874, he had developed his own system of medicine.

The question of whether illness is the result of outside forces or whether it originates within had been debated for centuries. Still concluded: "It is our natures that are the physicians of our disease." Moreover, he stated, "Order and health are universally one, in union." The dictum of osteopathic medicine is the practical application of these concepts to the treatment of disease.

Still's principles were based on the assumption that within the body there is the capability for health if this capacity is recognized and normalized. Given the opportunity to mobilize its forces, the body will cure itself. One of Still's major points was that "the rule of the artery is supreme"; that is, increased circulation to an affected area—bringing leukocytes, immunological agents, etc.—can determine the course of an illness.

Moreover, Still noted that the body's musculoskeletal system is a structure subject to disorder and when disordered may effect changes in other parts of the body, altering its function, health, and welfare. Thus Still's approach was named osteopathy—"the treatment of bones"—when in fact it emphasizes body structure.

Still observed that the joints of the body, particularly those of the spine, develop unusual manifestations of stress. It seemed these bones joined or articulated in a manner best suited for the horizontal rather than the upright position. The effects of this stress upon the joints he felt, are transmitted through the nervous system and circulatory system, and thus have both local and remote effects.

Still defined these areas of circumscribed change in body tissue as "lesions." A common example of an osteopathic lesion is a sprain. Such a condition means altered motion, pain, and a decrease in function. When motion (normal or accessory) is impeded, the joint no longer responds properly to stresses or demands. Normal motion then becomes a greater stress and source of irritation, and tissue changes result because of limited motion (function); further changes similar to inflammation (primarily a circulatory change) may occur. Lesions cannot be detected by means of xrays or autopsies, any more than a sprained ankle could.

With these principles and concepts in mind, augmented by a careful study of anatomy, Still chartered his first school "to establish a college of osteopathy, the design of which is to improve our present system of surgery, obstetrics and treatment of disease generally." This was the beginning—a certain improvement over the favored practices of the day (leeching, blood-letting, etc.) in the management of the infectious diseases ravaging the country.

Today there are some 14,000 osteopathic physicians and surgeons. The new drugs and technology of standard medical practice have been introduced into osteopathic schools, hospitals, and offices. In fact, today osteopathic medicine so resembles its allopathic cousin, practitioners fear it may eventually be subsumed, incurring the loss of the "whole man" philosophy of practice, as well as the osteopathic structural concept. Manipulation therapy has survived because patients have found it effective; however, it has yet to be subjected to a double-blind study. Osteopathic practitioners hope that, as the merging of schools of thought continues, the scientific standards of the medical mainstream will be applied to the lesion concept, proving its worth.

## Groups and Associations

(286) **NORTH AMERICAN ACADEMY OF MANIPULATIVE THERAPY**
c/o C.R. Hooper, MD, DO
12238 113th Avenue, Suite 106
Youngtown, AZ 85363

(602) 933-8787

Originally organized by a group of Canadian and American physicians, the Society's purpose is to establish, maintain, and conduct a membership organization of doctors to further the knowledge and practice of manipulative medicine. Formed 1965-1966.

(287) **AMERICAN ACADEMY OF OSTEOPATHY**
2630 Airport Road
Colorado Springs, CO 80910

(303) 632-7164

*Louis W. Astell, Executive Director*

Concerned with the development of osteopathic management in total health care. Conducts programs to improve the skills of the individual DO, investigates new methods of manipulation, and develops teaching models for these methods. Also publishes original papers for the Academy membership.

(288) **THE CRANIAL ACADEMY**
c/o Carl H. Rathjen, Secretary-Treasurer
1140 West Eighth Street
Meridian, ID 83642

A component society of the American Academy of Osteopathy, the Cranial Academy represents osteopaths engaged in the field of Cranial Osteopathy.

(289) **AMERICAN ASSOCIATION OF COLLEGES OF OSTEOPATHIC MEDICINE**
5200 South Ellis Avenue
Chicago, IL 60615

(312) 363-6800

*J. Leonard Azneer, DO, President*

Advances and enriches education in osteopathic medicine. Membership limited to osteopathic colleges and nonprofit associations dedicated to the advancement of osteopathic medicine. Publishes bimonthly and weekly newsletters.

(290) **AMERICAN COLLEGE OF OSTEOPATHIC OBSTETRICIANS AND GYNECOLOGISTS**
Box 66
Merrill, MI 48637

(517) 643-5500

*Arthur A. Speir, Executive Director*

Studies and researches all phases of obstetrical and

gynecological practice, emphasizing the application of osteopathic principles and practice. Membership is open to osteopathic Ob-Gyns and to DOs in closely related fields.

(291) **STUDENT OSTEOPATHIC MEDICAL ASSOCIATION**
770 Providence Road, A210
Aldan, PA 19018

Information about osteopathic student activities in the United States.

(292) **AMERICAN OSTEOPATHIC ASSOCIATION**
212 East Ohio Street
Chicago, IL 60611

(312) 944-2713

The national organization of osteopathic physicians. Maintains updated list of state associations as well as individual osteopathic physicians.

*AFFILIATE AND STATE ASSOCIATIONS*

**AMERICAN OSTEOPATHIC FOUNDATION**
212 East Ohio Street
Chicago, IL 60611

(312) 944-2713

Supports research into osteopathic medicine.

**A.T. STILL OSTEOPATHIC FOUNDATION AND RESEARCH INSTITUTE**
212 East Ohio Street
Chicago, IL 60611

(312) 944-2713

Supports research relating to the field of osteopathy.

**AUXILIARY TO THE AMERICAN OSTEOPATHIC ASSOCIATION**
212 East Ohio Street
Chicago, IL 60611

(312) 944-2713

Develops public health and educational activities of the osteopathic profession. Encourages volunteer service associations to be established and continued in osteopathic hospitals, and participates in national and community health endeavors. Membership open to a wife, mother, daughter, sister, or widow of an osteopathic physician.

**NATIONAL OSTEOPATHIC FOUNDATION**
212 East Ohio Street
Chicago, IL 60611

(312) 944-2713

Advances and improves national health care through the extension of osteopathic theory and practice and solicits funds in support of osteopathic education and research.

**OSTEOPATHIC TRUST**
212 East Ohio Street
Chicago, IL 60611

(312) 944-2713

Supports research into the cause, treatment, and prevention of disease, as well as research into osteopathic principles and practice.

**ARIZONA OSTEOPATHIC MEDICAL ASSOCIATION**
5057 East Thomas Road
Phoenix, AZ 85018

(602) 959-0460

**ARKANSAS ASSOCIATION OF OSTEOPATHIC PHYSICIANS AND SURGEONS**
709 Kingwood Road
Little Rock, AR 72207

(501) 666-2445

**OSTEOPATHIC PHYSICIANS AND SURGEONS OF CALIFORNIA**
31582 Coast Highway
Suite C
South Laguna, CA 92677

(714) 499-3435

**COLORADO OSTEOPATHIC ASSOCIATION**
4701 East Ninth Avenue
Denver, CO 80220

(303) 322-1752

**CONNECTICUT SOCIETY OF OSTEOPATHIC PHYSICIANS AND SURGEONS**
Box 124
Roxbury, CT 06783

(203) 354-3398

**DELAWARE STATE OSTEOPATHIC MEDICAL SOCIETY**
P.O. Box 845
Wilmington, DE 19899

(302) 764-6120

**OSTEOPATHIC ASSOCIATION OF THE DISTRICT OF COLUMBIA**
430 "M" Street, S.W.
Washington, DC 20024

(202) 554-4210

**FLORIDA OSTEOPATHIC MEDICAL ASSOCIATION**
P.O. Box 1444
161 North Causeway
New Smyrna Beach, FL 32069

(904) 427-3489

**GEORGIA OSTEOPATHIC MEDICAL ASSOCIATION**
2170 Idlewood Road
Tucker, GA 30084

(404) 934-3434

**HAWAII ASSOCIATION OF OSTEOPATHIC PHYSICIANS AND SURGEONS**
1015 Bishop Street
Honolulu, HI 96813

(808) 531-7966

**IDAHO OSTEOPATHIC MEDICAL ASSOCIATION**
Box 605
Council, ID 83612

(208) 253-4568

**ILLINOIS ASSOCIATION OF OSTEOPATHIC PHYSICIANS AND SURGEONS**
5206 South University Avenue
Chicago, IL 60615

(312) 363-1105

**INDIANA ASSOCIATION OF OSTEOPATHIC PHYSICIANS AND SURGEONS, INC.**
1930 Indiana Tower
Indianapolis, IN 46204

(317) 636-3551

**IOWA SOCIETY OF OSTEOPATHIC PHYSICIANS AND SURGEONS**
827 Insurance Exchange Building
Des Moines, IA 50309

(515) 283-0002

**KANSAS ASSOCIATION OF OSTEOPATHIC MEDICINE**
835 Western
Topeka, KS 66606

(913) 234-5563

**KENTUCKY OSTEOPATHIC MEDICAL ASSOCIATION**
2221 Douglass Boulevard
Louisville, KY 40205

(502) 456-4241

**LOUISIANA ASSOCIATION OF OSTEOPATHIC PHYSICIANS**
614-15 Hibernia Bank Building
New Orleans, LA 70112

(504) 588-9494

**MAINE OSTEOPATHIC ASSOCIATION**
99 Western Avenue
Drawer "M"
Augusta, ME 04330

(207) 623-1101

**MARYLAND STATE OSTEOPATHIC ASSOCIATION, INC.**
1510 Gordon Cove Road
Annapolis, MD 21403

(301) 268-9449

**MASSACHUSETTS OSTEOPATHIC SOCIETY**
343 Washington Street
Newton, MA 02158

(617) 527-1701

**MICHIGAN ASSOCIATION OF OSTEOPATHIC PHYSICIANS AND SURGEONS**
33100 Freedom Road
Farmington, MI 48024

(313) 476-2800

**MINNESOTA STATE OSTEOPATHIC ASSOCIATION**
701 South Main
Park Rapids, MN 56470

(218) 732-5609

**MISSOURI ASSOCIATION OF OSTEOPATHIC PHYSICIANS AND SURGEONS**
P.O. Box 748
325 East McCarty Street
Jefferson City, MO 65101

(314) 634-3415

**MONTANA OSTEOPATHIC ASSOCIATION**
1116 First Avenue North
Great Falls, MT 59401

(406) 452-6353

**NEBRASKA ASSOCIATION OF OSTEOPATHIC PHYSICIANS AND SURGEONS**
1210 Thirteenth Street
Aurora, NE 68818

(402) 694-2525

**NEVADA OSTEOPATHIC MEDICAL ASSOCIATION**
618 South Sixth Street
Las Vegas, NV 89101

(702) 382-5544

**NEW HAMPSHIRE OSTEOPATHIC ASSOCIATION**
29 Green Street
Concord, NH 03301

(603) 224-1242

**AMERICAN OSTEOPATHIC HOSPITAL ASSOCIATION**
John F. Kennedy Memorial Hospital
18 East Laurel Road
Stratford, NJ 08084

(609) 784-4000

*B.A. Zeiher, Chairman of the Board*

Fosters and promotes cooperation between osteopathic hospitals and governmental agencies, and carries out programs to maintain and improve the quality of osteopathic health care delivery. Membership primarily drawn from osteopathic hospitals.

**NEW JERSEY ASSOCIATION OF OSTEOPATHIC PHYSICIANS AND SURGEONS**
1212 Stuyvesant Avenue
Trenton, NJ 08618

(609) 393-8114

**NEW MEXICO OSTEOPATHIC MEDICAL ASSOCIATION**
12517 Prospect, N.E.
Albuquerque, NM 87112

(505) 298-2115

**NEW YORK STATE OSTEOPATHIC SOCIETY**
1973 Morris Gate
Seaford, NY 11783

(516) 826-2212

**NORTH CAROLINA OSTEOPATHIC SOCIETY, INC.**
230 West Pennsylvania Avenue
Southern Pines, NC 28387

(919) 692-8558

**NORTH DAKOTA STATE OSTEOPATHIC ASSOCIATION**
8 South Terrace
Fargo, ND 58102

(701) 235-5923

**OHIO OSTEOPATHIC ASSOCIATION**
53 West Third Avenue
Columbus, OH 43201

(614) 299-2107

**OKLAHOMA OSTEOPATHIC ASSOCIATION**
1310 Citizens Tower Building
Oklahoma City, OK 73106

(405) 528-7095

**OREGON OSTEOPATHIC ASSOCIATION**
15745 Southeast Monner Road
Portland, OR 97236

(503) 658-2032

**PENNSYLVANIA OSTEOPATHIC MEDICAL AS-SOCIATION**
1330 Eisenhower Boulevard
Harrisburg, PA 17111

(717) 939-9318

**RHODE ISLAND SOCIETY OF OSTEOPATHIC PHYSICIANS AND SURGEONS**
1660 Broad Street
Cranston, RI 02905

(401) 781-6870

**SOUTH CAROLINA OSTEOPATHIC ASSOCIATION**
106 West Fifth Street
South Summerville, SC 29483

(803) 871-1242

**SOUTH DAKOTA SOCIETY OF OSTEOPATHIC PHYSICIANS AND SURGEONS**
981 East Main
Sturgis, SD 57785

(605) 347-3616

**TENNESSEE OSTEOPATHIC MEDICAL ASSOCIA-TION**
Box 390
Pikeville, TN 37367

(615) 447-2606

**TEXAS OSTEOPATHIC MEDICAL ASSOCIATION**
512 Bailey
Fort Worth, TX 76107

(817) 336-0549

**UTAH OSTEOPATHIC ASSOCIATION OF MEDICINE AND SURGERY**
10565 South State
Sandy, UT 84070

(801) 571-5601

**VERMONT STATE ASSOCIATION OF OS-TEOPATHIC PHYSICIANS AND SURGEONS**
15 Western Avenue
Brattleboro, VT 05301

(802) 254-2944

**VIRGINIA OSTEOPATHIC MEDICAL ASSOCIA-TION**
1707 Osage Street
Suite 402
Alexandria, VA 22302

(703) 836-2565

**WASHINGTON OSTEOPATHIC MEDICAL AS-SOCIATION**
4210 Southwest Oregon Street
P.O. Box 16309
Seattle, WA 98116

(206) 937-5358

**WEST VIRGINIA SOCIETY OF OSTEOPATHIC MEDICINE**
400 North Lee Street
Lewisburg, WV 24901

(304) 425-2121

**WISCONSIN ASSOCIATION OF OSTEOPATHIC PHYSICIANS AND SURGEONS**
216 Green Bay Road
Thiensville, WI 53092

(414) 242-4650

**WYOMING ASSOCIATION OF OSTEOPATHIC PHYSICIANS AND SURGEONS**
2823 Central Avenue
Cheyenne, WY 82001

(307) 638-3712

**(293) BRITISH COLUMBIA OSTEOPATHIC AS-SOCIATION**
461 Martin Street
Penticton, British Columbia
Canada

Information about osteopathic activities in British Colum-bia.

**(294) CANADIAN OSTEOPATHIC ASSOCIATION**
575 Waterloo Street
London, Ontario
Canada N6B 2R2

Information about osteopathic activities in Canada.

**AUSTRALIAN CHIROPRACTORS, OSTEOPATHS AND NATURAL PHYSICIANS ASSOCIATION/**New South Wales (see 439)

**(295) AUSTRALIAN OSTEOPATHIC ASSOCIATION**
71 Collins Street
Melbourne, Victoria 3191
Australia

Information about osteopathic activities in Australia.

**(296) SOCIETY OF OSTEOPATHS**
c/o Peter K. Blagrave, Hon. Secretary
16 Green Lane
Chislehurst, Kent BR7 5JY
England

Tel: 01-467-3096

Association of osteopathic practitioners. Full member of IFPNT **(72)**.

**BRITISH NATUROPATHIC AND OSTEOPATHIC ASSOCIATION/**London (see 440)

**(297) BRITISH OSTEOPATHIC ASSOCIATION**
24-25 Dorset Square
London, N.W. 1, England

Information about osteopathic activities in Great Britain.

**(298) ASSOCIATION FRANCAISE DE DEFENSE OSTEOPATHIQUE**
c/o F.P. Berthenet, Secrétaire Général
2 Residence des Grilles
14-18, Rue des Grilles
93500 Pantin, France

Organization to promote osteopathic methods in France and legally protect its practitioners. Full member of IFPNT **(72)**.

**NEW ZEALAND ASSN. OF NATUROPATHS & OSTEOPATHS/**Aukland (see 443)

## Osteopathic Hospitals

**(299) EISENHOWER HOSPITAL (Osteopathic)**
33 Barnes Avenue
Colorado Springs, CO 80909

(303) 475-2111

**(300) ROCKY MOUNTAIN OSTEOPATHIC HOSPITAL**
4701 East Ninth Avenue
Denver, CO 80220

(303) 388-5588

**(301) GRAND JUNCTION OSTEOPATHIC HOSPITAL**
Box 220
Grand Junction, CO 81501

(303) 242-0920

**(302) SUN COAST OSTEOPATHIC HOSPITAL**
2025 Indian Rocks Road
Largo, FL 33540

(813) 581-9474

**(303) OSTEOPATHIC GENERAL HOSPITAL**
1750 Northeast 167th Street
North Miami Beach, FL 33162

(305) 949-0211

**(304) TAMPA OSTEOPATHIC HOSPITAL**
4555 South Manhattan Avenue
Tampa, FL 33611

(813) 839-6341

**(305) CHICAGO OSTEOPATHIC HOSPITAL**
5200-5250 South Ellis Avenue
Chicago, IL 60615

(312) 363-6800

**(306) WIRTH OSTEOPATHIC HOSPITAL**
Hwy. 64 West
Oakland City, IN 47560

(812) 749-4017

**(307) SOUTH BEND OSTEOPATHIC HOSPITAL**
2515 East Jefferson Boulevard
South Bend, IN 46615

(219) 288-8311

**(308) DAVENPORT OSTEOPATHIC HOSPITAL**
111 West Kimberly Road
Davenport, IA 52806

(319) 391-2020

**(309) OSTEOPATHIC HOSPITAL OF WICHITA**
2622 West Central Avenue
Wichita, KS 67203

(316) 943-9353

**(310) JAMES A. TAYLOR OSTEOPATHIC HOSPITAL**
268 Stillwater Avenue
Bangor, ME 04401

(207) 942-5286

**(311) OSTEOPATHIC HOSPITAL OF MAINE, INC.**
355 Brighton Avenue
Portland, ME 04102

(207) 774-3921

**(312) WATERVILLE OSTEOPATHIC HOSPITAL**
200 Kennedy Memorial Drive
Waterville, ME 04901

(207) 873-0731

**(313) BAY OSTEOPATHIC HOSPITAL**
3250 East Midland Road
Bay City, MI 48706

(517) 686-2920

**(314) CLARE OSTEOPATHIC HOSPITAL**
104 West Sixth Street
Clare, MI 48617

(517) 386-9951

**(315) DETROIT OSTEOPATHIC HOSPITAL**
12523 Third Avenue
Detroit, MI 48203

(313) 869-1200

**(316) ZIEGER OSTEOPATHIC HOSPITAL**
4244 Livernois Avenue
Detroit, MI 48210

(313) 897-6400

**(317) BOTSFORD GENERAL HOSPITAL (Osteopathic)**
Ziegler Osteopathic Hospitals
28050 Grant River
Farmington Hills, MI 48024

(313) 476-7600

**(318) FLINT OSTEOPATHIC HOSPITAL**
3921 Beecher Road
Flint, MI 48502

(313) 235-8511

**(319) GRAND RAPIDS OSTEOPATHIC HOSPITAL**
1919 Boston Street, S.E.
Grand Rapids, MI 49506

(616) 247-7200

**(320) JACKSON OSTEOPATHIC HOSPITAL**
121 Seymour Avenue
Jackson, MI 49202

(517) 787-1440

**(321) PONTIAC OSTEOPATHIC HOSPITAL**
50 North Perry Avenue
Pontiac, MI 48058

(313) 338-7271

(322) **SAGINAW OSTEOPATHIC HOSPITAL**
515 North Michigan Avenue
Saginaw, MI 48602

(517) 753-7751

(323) **TRAVERSE CITY OSTEOPATHIC HOSPITAL**
550 Munson Avenue
Traverse City, MI 49684

(616) 947-5121

(324) **RIVERSIDE OSTEOPATHIC HOSPITAL**
150 Traux Street
Trenton, MI 48183

(313) 676-4200

(325) **BI-COUNTY COMMUNITY HOSPITAL**
13355 Ten Mile Road
Warren, MI 48089

(313) 758-1800

(326) **WETZELS OSTEOPATHIC HOSPITALS, INC.**
1302-04 North Main
Carrollton, MO 64633

(816) 542-0166

105 East Ohio Street
Clinton, MO 64735

(816) 885-8171

(327) **MINERAL AREA OSTEOPATHIC HOSPITAL**
1212 Weber Road
Farmington, MO 63640

(314) 756-4581

(328) **CHARLES E. STILL OSTEOPATHIC HOSPITAL**
1125 South Madison Street
Jefferson City, MO 65101

(314) 635-7141

(329) **OAK HILL OSTEOPATHIC HOSPITAL**
932 East 34th Street
Joplin, MO 64801

(417) 623-4640

(330) **CENTER FOR HEALTH SCIENCES OF THE KANSAS CITY COLLEGE OF OSTEOPATHIC MEDICINE**
2105 Independence Avenue
Kansas City, MO 64124

(816) 283-2300

(331) **KIRKSVILLE OSTEOPATHIC HOSPITAL**
800 West Jefferson Street
Kirksville, MO 63501

(816) 626-2121

(332) **AXTELL OSTEOPATHIC HOSPITAL**
308 South Broadway
Princeton, MO 64673

(816) 746-3225

(333) **SPRINGFIELD GENERAL OSTEOPATHIC HOSPITAL**
2828 North National Avenue
Springfield, MO 65801

(417) 869-5571

(334) **NORMANDY OSTEOPATHIC HOSPITAL— NORTH**
7840 Natural Bridge Road
St. Louis, MO 63121

(314) 389-0015

(335) **NORMANDY OSTEOPATHIC HOSPITAL— SOUTH**
530 Des Peres Road
St. Louis, MO 63131

(314) 821-3850

(336) **BRADSHAW MEMORIAL OSTEOPATHIC HOSPITAL**
130 "A" Street, S.W.
Miami, OK 74354

(918) 542-3385

(337) **HILLCREST OSTEOPATHIC HOSPITAL**
2129 Southwest 59th Street
Oklahoma City, OK 73119

(405) 685-6671

(338) **MOOTS OSTEOPATHIC HOSPITAL**
8 North Rowe Avenue
Pryor, OK 74361

(918) 825-2155

(339) **OKLAHOMA OSTEOPATHIC HOSPITAL**
Ninth & Jackson Streets
Tulsa, OK 74127

(918) 587-2561

(340) **CRATER OSTEOPATHIC HOSPITAL**
600 South Second Street
Central Point, OR 97501

(503) 664-1205

(341) **EASTMORELAND OSTEOPATHIC HOSPITAL**
2900 Southeast Steele Street
Portland, OR 97202

(503) 234-0411

(342) **ALLENTOWN OSTEOPATHIC HOSPITAL**
1736 Hamilton Street
Allentown, PA 18104

(215) 439-4000

(343) **CLARION OSTEOPATHIC COMMUNITY HOSPITAL**
214 South Seventh Avenue
Clarion, PA 16214

(814) 226-9500

(344) **DOCTORS' OSTEOPATHIC HOSPITAL**
252 West Eleventh Street
Erie, PA 16501

(814) 455-3961

(345) **ERIE OSTEOPATHIC HOSPITAL ASSOCIATION**
5515 Peach Street
Erie, PA 16509

(814) 864-4031

(346) **SHENANGO VALLEY OSTEOPATHIC HOSPITAL**
2200 Memorial Drive Extension
Farrell, PA 16121

(412) 981-3500

(347) **COMMUNITY GENERAL OSTEOPATHIC HOSPITAL**
4300 Londonderry Road
Harrisburg, PA 17109

(717) 652-3000

(348) **HOSPITALS, PHILADELPHIA COLLEGE OF OSTEOPATHIC MEDICINE**
4150 City Avenue
Philadelphia, PA 19131

(215) 878-9400

(349) **MEMORIAL OSTEOPATHIC HOSPITAL**
325 South Belmont Street
York, PA 17403

(717) 843-8623

(350) **SOUTHWEST OSTEOPATHIC HOSPITAL**
2828 Southwest 27th Street
Amarillo, TX 79103

(806) 355-8181

(351) **COMANCHE COMMUNITY OSTEOPATHIC HOSPITAL, INC.**
211 South Austin
Comanche, TX 76442

(915) 356-2012

(352) **CORPUS CHRISTI OSTEOPATHIC HOSPITAL**
1502 Tarlton Street
Corpus Christi, TX 78415

(512) 884-4592

(353) **DALLAS OSTEOPATHIC HOSPITAL**
5003 Ross Avenue
Dallas, TX 75206

(214) 824-3071

(354) **EAST TOWN OSTEOPATHIC HOSPITAL**
7525 Scyene Road
Dallas, TX 75227

(214) 381-7171

(355) **STEVENS PARK OSTEOPATHIC HOSPITAL**
2120 West Colorado Boulevard
Dallas, TX 75211

(214) 943-4631

(356) **DENTON OSTEOPATHIC HOSPITAL**
2026 University Drive West
Denton, TX 76201

(817) 387-6101

(357) **FORT WORTH OSTEOPATHIC HOSPITAL**
1000 Montgomery Street
Fort Worth, TX 76107

(817) 731-4311

(358) **LUBBOCK OSTEOPATHIC HOSPITAL**
5301 University Avenue
Lubbock, TX 79413

(806) 795-9301

(359) **STANDRING MEMORIAL OSTEOPATHIC HOSPITAL**
12845 Twelfth Avenue S.W.
Seattle, WA 98146

(206) 243-1455

(360) **NEW VALLEY OSTEOPATHIC HOSPITAL**
3033 Tieton Drive
Yakima, WA 98902

(509) 453-4704

(361) **WEIRTON OSTEOPATHIC HOSPITAL**
3045 Pennsylvania Avenue
Weirton, WV 26062

(304) 723-1200

(362) **MAIDSTONE OSTEOPATHIC CLINIC**
c/o S.G.J. Wernham, President
30 Tonbridge Road
Maidstone, Kent
England

Provides full osteopathic treatment. Associate member of IFPNT **(72)**.

**BRITISH NATUROPATHIC AND OSTEOPATHIC ASSOCIATION**/London **(see 440)**

## Schools (Colleges)

(363) **THE SUTHERLAND CRANIAL TEACHING FOUNDATION, INC.**
1140 West Eighth Street
Meridian, ID 83642

Professional course and instruction in cranial technique.

(364) **CHICAGO COLLEGE OF OSTEOPATHIC MEDICINE**
1122 East 53rd Street
Chicago, IL 60615

*Thaddeus P. Kawalek, PhD, President*

State accredited institution granting degree of Doctor of Osteopathy.

(365) **COLLEGE OF OSTEOPATHIC MEDICINE AND SURGERY**
3200 Grand Avenue
Des Moines, IA 50312

*J. Leonard Azneer, PhD, President*

State accredited institution granting degree of Doctor of Osteopathy.

**(366) MICHIGAN STATE UNIVERSITY—COLLEGE OF OSTEOPATHIC MEDICINE**
Fee Halls
East Lansing, MI 48824

*Myron S. Magen, DO, Dean*

State accredited institution granting degree of Doctor of Osteopathy.

**(367) KANSAS CITY COLLEGE OF OSTEOPATHIC MEDICINE**
2105 Independence Boulevard
Kansas City, MO 64124

*Rudolph S. Bremen, PhD, President*

State accredited institution granting degree of Doctor of Osteopathy.

**(368) KIRKSVILLE COLLEGE OF OSTEOPATHIC MEDICINE**
204 West Jefferson Street
Kirksville, MO 63501

*H. Charles Moore, PhD, President*

State accredited institution granting degree of Doctor of Osteopathy.

**(369) AMERICAN OSTEOPATHIC COLLEGE OF RHEUMATOLOGY**
Box DOC
Maybrook, NY 12543

(914) 427-2141

*Mrs. Donald I. Phillips, Executive Secretary*

Promotes the study of and research and education in the field of arthritis diagnosis and treatment. Circulates abstracts, reports, and information on seminars, courses, and publications to the membership. Membership limited to physicians interested in the study of rheumatology. A state accredited institution granting degree of Doctor of Osteopathy.

**(370) AMERICAN COLLEGE OF NEURO-PSYCHIATRISTS**
27 East 62nd Street
New York, NY 10021

(212) 980-3318

*Ned Baron, DO, President*

Promotes osteopathy in the fields of neurology and psychiatry, maintains professional standards among osteopathic neurologists and psychiatrists, and stimulates and publishes original research in osteopathic neurology and psychiatry. Membership open both to DOs and non-DOs in related professions.

**(371) OKLAHOMA COLLEGE OF OSTEOPATHIC MEDICINE AND SURGERY**
120 East Ninth Street
Tulsa, OK 74119

*John Barson, EdD, President and Acting Dean*

State accredited institution granting degree of Doctor of Osteopathy.

**(372) PHILADELPHIA COLLEGE OF OS-TEOPATHIC MEDICINE**
4150 City Avenue
Philadelphia, PA 19131

*Thomas M. Rowland, Jr., LLD (Hon), President*

State accredited institution granting degree of Doctor of Osteopathy.

**(373) TEXAS COLLEGE OF OSTEOPATHIC MEDICINE**
3516 Camp Bowie Boulevard
Fort Worth, TX 76107

*C.C. Nolen, LLD, President*

State accredited institution granting degree of Doctor of Osteopathy.

**(374) WEST VIRGINIA SCHOOL OF OS-TEOPATHIC MEDICINE**
400 North Lee Street
Lewisburg, WV 24901

*Roland P. Sharp, DO, President*

State accredited institution granting degree of Doctor of Osteopathy.

## Journals and Publications

**(375) JOURNAL OF THE AMERICAN OS-TEOPATHIC ASSOCIATION**
212 East Ohio Street
Chicago, IL 60611

(312) 944-2713

Official publication of the American Osteopathic Association, publishes various articles and research papers in the field of osteopathic medicine.

**(376) OSTEOPATHIC PHYSICIAN**
O.P. Publications Corporation
733 Third Avenue
New York, NY 10017

(212) 867-7520

*J. Dudley Chapman, DO, Editor*

Independent monthly journal with articles on osteopathy and wholistic medicine. Established 1933.

**JOURNAL OF THE RESEARCH SOCIETY FOR NATURAL THERAPEUTICS** (multidisciplinary)/ Dorset, England **(see 70)**

**(377) JOURNAL OF THE SOCIETY OF OS-TEOPATHS**
28 Tonbridge Road
Maidstone, Kent
England

*Harold S. Klug, DO, Editor*

Published twice yearly (spring and autumn) and issued to members of the Society and circulated to practitioners and others in the field of osteopathy and allied professions.

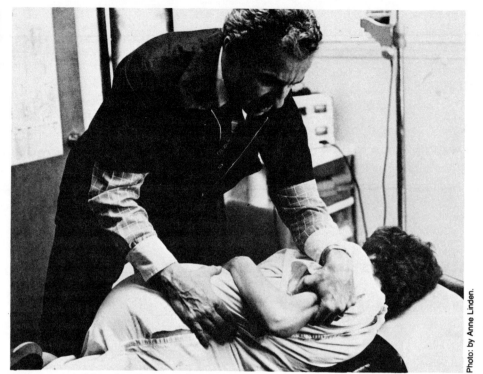

Photo: by Anne Linden.

Adjustment to pelvic region, Paul Muscalino, DC.

# Chiropractic Today

*Julius Dintenfass, DC*

A dramatic change in attitudes toward health and disease was made in 1895 by D. D. Palmer, the discoverer of chiropractic, when he urged that in seeking the causes and cures of disease we must turn to the body itself. From the start chiropractors—convinced that healing is grounded on cooperation with nature—have expounded the natural, healthful living concepts of clean air, pure water, sunshine, and good food, as a necessary adjunct to the chiropractic body of knowledge.

The profession of chiropractic is in a continuous state of evolution. It takes advantage of new research and contemporary breakthroughs to expand further its insights and applications. From the earliest days of the profession, chiropractors have been instrumental in developing innovations in the examination and treatment of the human body which have proved to be important to other branches of the healing arts. Chiropractic offers a biomechanical approach to health which emphasizes the study of body mechanics, applied kinesiology, postural stability, vertebral adjustments, and the dynamic self-regulation control system of the body.

Ever since its inception, the profession of chiropractic, which does not employ drugs or surgery, has maintained a wholistic* approach to patient care. It has steadfastly maintained that healing is the prerogative of the living organism and is brought about by the homeostatic, inherent, curative powers of the body. Chiropractors hold that the human body is the intermediary between the external world and health, and that optimal physiological function is obtained when interference is removed from the communication systems of the body. The nervous system is the primary focus of concern, because it is the master system of the body. It integrates and coordinates all body functions in response to external and internal influences and changes. Its therapeutic goal is to organize the body in such manner as to enable it to utilize its own biological resources for a return to normal function.

Our human body is a highly automated organism, and the basic function of the nervous system is not the

---

*Spelled holistic in original text.*

transformation of energy but rather the processing of information or data. Its effectiveness in processing information to maintain homeostasis for body function is dependent on inputs and outputs. These signals are derived from ingoing nerve impulses and set off by the receptor end organs of the body, which send nerve impulses to important nerve control centers. These centers react to these signals and set off outgoing, or effector, nerve impulses to bring about actions required to establish body equilibrium and homeostasis. If this feedback is disorganized, it can lead to functional disorders and eventual disease.

The doctor of chiropractic examines the patient thoroughly, not only using the standard procedures for making a diagnosis of the ailment, but also making a complex neuromechanical, kinesiological examination of the body to determine the underlying causes of the problem.

Clinical evidence proves that when the underlying cause of a condition is corrected, symptoms will clear up, because they are an intrinsic part of natural processes. Although the chiropractic profession is concerned with structural mechanics as a primary cause of disturbance of the control and communication systems of the body and its correction by manipulative procedures, it does recognize that there may be other factors upsetting body balance—for example, the eating habits typical of our national diet overburdening the digestive system, or the pressures of everyday living causing nervous tension and emotional instability.

Traditionally, the profession has been associated with the diagnosis and correction of disrelated segments of the skeletal system, especially those of the spine and pelvis. Many people, therefore, believe that the doctor of chiropractic is primarily concerned with spinal problems. Although clinical successes with these problems have been excellent, the chiropractor is primarily concerned with the many human ailments precipitated by underlying neurological disturbances. These may cause symptoms in all parts of the body. The following are examples of the major kinds of problems the chiropractic profession has dealt with successfully:

1. *Spinal and pelvic involvements:* e.g., disc syndromes, low back problems, cervical, thoracic, and lumbar strains, sprains and subluxations, migraine headaches having origin in the cervical spine;
2. *Spinosomatic syndromes:* neuralgias arising in the spinal column and the pelvis but radiating into the arms and legs;
3. *General muscular ailments:* e.g., fatigue and postural defects of the body (causing muscle pain in back and neck), sprains and strains of the ribcage, traumatic bursitis or tendonitis of the shoulder or elbow;
4. *Spinal visceral syndromes:* functional disorders of the internal organs and systems that are a consequence of mechanical irritation of nerve pathways.

Some other conditions that have responded very well to chiropractic care are asthmatic syndromes, functional cardiovascular syndromes, high blood pressure associated with peripheral tension, vasomotor spasms, gastrointestinal neuroses, and functional dysmenorrhea.

Since the fundamental principle of chiropractic is the maintenance of the structural and functional integrity of the nervous system it employs as a primary therapeutic agent, manipulation and adjustment of the joints and soft tissues of the body, especially the spine, to restructure nerve communication pathways. Chiropractic research and clinical studies have broadened its approach to treatment so as to include not only the spinal correction but the use of physical modalities and nutrition which may be necessary to stabilize and maintain the structural correction. The doctor of chiropractic follows all of the approved methods of diagnosis to determine, as far as possible, what the nature of the trouble is. The present-day chiropractor is professionally trained in clinical diagnosis, clinical neurology, differential diagnosis, laboratory diagnosis, and the use of special instruments needed for regional diagnoses.

Since structural integrity has been the keystone of chiropractic therapy, it was only natural that the chiropractic profession study the science of kinesiology, which deals with the study of muscle movement, as it relates to nerve and body functions. Certain chiropractic colleges had courses in this subject back in 1950. In the early 1960s a new way of working with muscles was developed by George J. Goodheart, DC, to interpret muscle action. He discovered that it was possible to test the muscles of the body not only to determine strength or weakness, but also as indicators for understanding body language.

Once muscle weakness has been determined, it may be used as an aid to diagnosis, and it presents a number of therapeutic options to treat many conditions. This system of chiropractic kinesiology can determine the muscles and nerves that are not functioning at their optimum levels and bring them back to normal function. This has proved to be most important in the diagnosis and treatment of many conditions of disease. As this new approach of chiropractic kinesiology developed, it has drawn the attention of many practitioners of other health professions such as medicine and dentistry and osteopathy, because of its widespread application in the healing arts.

It is becoming recognized more and more by health authorities that, in the future, the health care professions must emphasize preventive and predictive procedures. These approaches could contribute greatly to the reduction of today's soaring health care costs. Patients with mild or nonspecific complaints are often considered to have problems considered too ''trivial'' to be given much attention. Yet early diagnosis and correction could prevent many of these ailments from blossoming into serious conditions.

The nature of chiropractic practice directed attention to this problem early in its history because it recognized the importance of spinal biomechanics to the body's economy. Studies have established that many disease problems can be prevented from developing by early recognition of the signs of mechanical stress and of disrelationships of the musculoskeletal system. Uncorrected mechanical stress can lead to altered form and function of nerves, bones, joints, and the ligamentous and muscular supporting elements of the body.

Chiropractic care is fast becoming recognized as an indispensable element in the treatment of many diseases and as an active program of health promotion. However, the chiropractic profession continues to recognize the interdependence and complementarity of all branches of the healing arts oriented toward human ecology and the wholistic view of health care.

# The Posture Of A Profession

*Joseph Janse, DC*

Every profession profiles a phylogenesis. No profession begins totally tailor-made. Within all professional disciplines there have to be conjugations and increments. So it has been in chiropractic. Essentially, it began as an emphasis on the idea that there is an intimate relationship between spinal biomechanics and the neurological element. The theory and concept originally advanced by the founder, D. D. Palmer, and his immediate successors, could well have been somewhat "overly conclusive." However, there was the attending emphasis on the fact that once the neurological element was disturbed, dysfunction ensued and could express itself in various ways, not only at the original site of disturbance but also in other structural and functional areas.

Subsequently, the wholistic* concept was expanded through input from several eclectic sources and the thinking of a cadre of leading personalities in the chiropractic profession. The following statements represent the basic indices of the wholistic mosaic of the chiropractic concept:

1. In *Homo sapiens* (the biped), the biomechanical conduct of the spine plays a significant role in conditioning the neurological element from the time of birth to the end of life.
2. The neurological bed, which relates to the arthrological, syndesmological, and myological components of spinal and pelvic segments, comprises the major conditioning, controlling, and beneficial or detrimental influences upon the entire nervous system.
3. These inputs to the nervous system, arising from the articular elements of the motor beds of the spine and the pelvis, often represent either primary, secondary, precipitating, or prolonging factors in health restoration, if positive in quality, or the production of pathophysiological disturbances that lead to disease, if aberrant in quality.
4. Clinical neurophysiologists are encountering the truth of these claims almost constantly as they expand their researches. Such terms as somatovisceral, viscerosomatic, somatocerebral and cerebrosomatic feedback, spinosomatic and spinovisceral syndromes, and pathophysiological spread due to synaptic overlap and contamination have become as common outside chiropractic as within
5. For decades, leading chiropractic educators have emphasized the pathophysiological concept that one thing leads to another and that essentially there is no "localization of effect." Disturbance of the neurological element at one point will eventually project disturbance to other key areas, the nature of which is often determined by the predispositions that exist. Although secondary, these areas may of themselves become primary foci of disturbance and set up a *circulus vitiosus,* a pathophysiological merry-go-round.
6. Essentially, there is but one nervous system, and any classification or segmentation of its components is solely for academic purposes. It is impossible, from a functional standpoint, to isolate one component from the other in aspects of dysfunction, causation, or health-restorative measures. For every somatic neurological experience, there is a visceral, mental, and emotional affectivity. For every visceral, mental, or emotional event, one may encounter a mirroring of it in the somatic structures.
7. It is not to be overlooked that the life process within the organism is the result of stimulation applied to the primary sensoria to include the sensory elements of the cutaneum, the subderma, myofascial planes, the all-important proprioceptive beds of the spinal and pelvic articular complexes, the organs of special sense, as well as the mental and emotional processes. If this is the

---

*Spelled holistic in original text.*

case, it follows that any natural modicum that will provide these sensoria with normal, restorative, and corrective impulsation would constitute good therapy.

It is the purpose of chiropractic education to emphasize the significance of these basic wholistic principles at levels of both basic and clinical sciences. The teaching of anatomy, chemistry, physiology, microbiology, and pathology simply for pedantic purposes would beg the issue. Profound instruction in diagnosis simply for classifying symptoms and memorizing the names of pathological and disease processes is a mere exercise in mental gymnastics. But to know the basic and clinical sciences in order to comprehend all the dimensions of a disease process and the multifaceted ramification of the same, both with respect to causological and radiating affectivities, lends purpose to any of the sciences and demands a wholistic overview of their interrelations. This is a must that confronts all professional education if it is to fulfill purpose and to demonstrate practical clinical meaningfulness. Unfortunately, the educational process in the therapeutic world has too often been a pathology of segmentation, with an overemphasis on so-called specialization. As a result, the art, the science, and the need of general practice at any level have been obscured.

In today's chiropractic education, acceptable standards and procedures are as common as they are to any other primary health deliverers. Preprofessional requirements, as well as a standard curriculum, have been set by the Council on Chiropractic Education. The criteria and procedures for institutional accreditation as established by the Council's Commission on Accreditation have been approved by the United States Office of Education. The educational standards, procedures, and criteria are no longer a question for chiropractic and should no longer be an issue.

Like all other health care and delivery professions, chiropractic insists upon the privilege, the right, and the opportunity of further development, expansion, and the broadening of its base if it can show integrity, competence, and purpose. Chiropractic is most sensitive to its responsibilities and is mindful of its obligations. It also draws pertinent attention to the desperate need for ecumenism among all health care professions. Causeways of dialogue, interchange, and consultation comprise undeniable imperatives. The chiropractic of today fully acknowledges its mishaps, defects, and need for improvement. It calls upon every segment of government and the health care community to proclaim the great need for systems, overviews, and programmings in health care, especially in prevention, restoration, and rehabilitation.

## Groups and Associations

### (380) INTERNATIONAL CHIROPRACTORS' ASSOCIATION OF CALIFORNIA
542 "A" Street
Hayward, CA 94541

(415) 537-2157

*Michael D. Pedigo, DC, President*

Information about chiropractors in California, member of International Chiropractors Association.

### (381) THE WORLDWIDE CHRISTIAN CHIROPRACTIC ASSOCIATION
2224 South College Avenue
Fort Collins, CO 80521

Has wide membership of chiropractic missionaries in various countries, e.g., Indonesia, Peru, Quebec, Bolivia, Ethiopia, and Monaco.

### (382) INTERNATIONAL CHIROPRACTORS ASSOCIATION
741 Brady Street
Davenport, IA 52808

(319) 322-4447

*B.E. Nordstrom, DC, Public Information Director*

Dedicated to the advancement of chiropractic art, science, and philosophy. Maintains listings of State Chiropractic Examining Boards and associations. Founded 1926.

### (383) AMERICAN CHIROPRACTIC ASSOCIATION
2200 Grand Avenue
Des Moines, IA 50312

(515) 243-1121

A national nonprofit professional membership organization, having a working relationship with state chiropractic associations. The ACA is primarily dedicated to establishing and maintaining the standards of education, ethics, and professional competency necessary or desirable to meet the requirements of the profession and the expectations of society. Services of the ACA include professional councils in such areas as diagnosis and internal disorders, mental health, neurology, nutrition, orthopedics, physiotherapy, and women chiropractors; technical assistance within the chiropractic profession and with other professions, organizations, government and insurance agencies; and educational services in the form of printed and audiovisual materials, radio and television public service announcements, public service billboards, workshops, and continuing education, and a "Correct Posture Month" in May and a "Spinal Health Month" in October. The Association also serves as a national resource for current data and state-of-the-art information relative to the profession and its contribution to public health. Publisher of the *Journal of the American Chiropractic Association*.

*AFFILIATE AND STATE ASSOCIATIONS*

**ALABAMA STATE CHIROPRACTIC ASSOCIATION, INC.**
P.O. Box 3335
Montgomery, AL 36109

**ALASKA ASSOCIATION OF CHIROPRACTIC PHYSICIANS**
c/o D.E. Hampton, DC, Secretary-Treasurer
1500 Airport Way
Fairbanks, AK 99701

**ALASKA CHIROPRACTIC SOCIETY**
c/o Donald D. Nickel, DC, Secretary
P.O. Box 2721
Kenai, AK 99611

**ARIZONA CHIROPRACTIC ASSOCIATION**
c/o William B. Risley, DC, Secretary
1125 East Glendale Avenue
Phoenix, AZ 85020

**CHIROPRACTIC PHYSICIANS ASSOCIATION OF ARIZONA INC.**
4747 North Sixteenth Street, Suite B-122
Phoenix, AZ 85016

*Randall Earick, DC, Secretary*

**ARKANSAS CHIROPRACTIC ASSOCIATION**
c/o Felix Cannatella, Jr., DC, Secretary-Treasurer
7410 Base Line Road
Little Rock, AR 72204

**CALIFORNIA CHIROPRACTIC ASSOCIATION**
2201 "Q" Street
Sacramento, CA 95816

*Mr. Charles L. Strauch, Executive Director*

**COLORADO CHIROPRACTIC ASSOCIATION**
8000 East Girard Avenue, Suite 316S
Denver, CO 80231

*Ms. Vera Haney, Executive Secretary*

**CONNECTICUT CHIROPRACTIC ASSOCIATION**
c/o John D. Griswold, Jr., DC, Secretary-Treasurer
1456 North Street
Suffield, CT 06078

(203) 668-5065

**DELAWARE ASSOCIATION OF CHIROPRACTIC PHYSICIANS**
c/o John Paul Feeney, DC, Secretary
183 South DuPont Highway
Midvale, DE 19720

(302) 328-0200

**FLORIDA CHIROPRACTIC ASSOCIATION**
Amherst Building

3203 Lawton Road, Suite 101
Orlando, FL 32803

(305) 896-8561

*Ronald W. Scott, DC, Secretary*

**GEORGIA CHIROPRACTIC ASSOCIATION, INC.**
c/o Hazel C. Cotney, DC, Secretary
308 West Main Street
Thomaston, GA 30286

**HAWAII CHIROPRACTIC ASSOCIATION**
c/o Rex J. Parker, DC, Secretary
1441 Kapiolani Boulevard
Honolulu, HI 96814

**IDAHO ASSOCIATION OF CHIROPRACTIC PHYSICIANS, INC.**
c/o Larry J. Mecham, DC, Secretary
195 South Skyline
Idaho Falls, ID 83401

(208) 524-2834

**ILLINOIS CHIROPRACTIC SOCIETY**
200 East Roosevelt Road
Lombard, IL 60148

(312) 629-0988

*Mr. John P. Quillan, Executive Director*

**INDIANA SOCIETY OF CHIROPRACTIC PHYSICIANS**
c/o Victor K. Fitch, DC, Executive Secretary
6605 East State Boulevard
Ft. Wayne, IN 46805

(219) 486-2147

**INDIANA STATE CHIROPRACTIC ASSOCIATION, INC.**
333 North Penn. Street, Room 918
Indianapolis, IN 46204

(317) 632-9502

*Miss Ann Ajamie, Executive Secretary*

**CHIROPRACTIC SOCIETY OF IOWA**
c/o Russell C. Brown, DC, Secretary-Treasurer
203 Boone National Building
Boone, IA 50036

(515) 432-4201

**IOWA CHIROPRACTIC SOCIETY, INC.**
c/o D.E. McAreavy, DC, Executive Secretary
216 West Platt
Maquoketa, IA 52061

(319) 652-3191

**KANSAS CHIROPRACTIC ASSOCIATION**
3320 Harrison
Topeka, KS 66611

(913) 266-6604

*Milton T. Nida, DC, Secretary-Treasurer*

**KENTUCKY ASSOCIATION OF CHIROPRACTORS, INC.**
c/o Harold W. Evans, DC, Executive Secretary
P.O. Box 1117
Bowling Green, KY 42101

(502) 842-5702

**KENTUCKY CHIROPRACTIC SOCIETY**
c/o Harold Byers, DC, Executive Secretary
105 Lyndon Lane #102
Louisville, KY 40222

(502) 366-1413

**LOUISIANA CHIROPRACTIC SOCIETY, INC.**
c/o Paul J. Adams, DC, Secretary-Treasurer
1101 East Simcoe
Lafayette, LA 70501

(318) 232-6166

**CHIROPRACTIC ASSOCIATION OF LOUISIANA, INC.**
c/o Robert F. Weller, DC, Secretary
214 Cortez Street
Thibodaux, LA 70301

(504) 447-2630

**MAINE CHIROPRACTIC ASSOCIATION**
c/o Roy Slocum, DC, Secretary-Treasurer
30 Bath Street
Brunswick, ME 04011

(207) 725-4222

**MARYLAND CHIROPRACTIC ASSOCIATION**
c/o Harold F. Carbaugh, DC, Secretary-Treasurer
306 North Potomac Street
Hagerstown, MD 21740

(301) 739-1939

**MASSACHUSETTS CHIROPRACTIC SOCIETY, INC.**
c/o Paul M. Hamilton, DC, Secretary-Treasurer
348 Essex Street
Salem, MA 01970

(617) 745-6224

**MICHIGAN CHIROPRACTIC COUNCIL**
c/o James Gregg, DC, Secretary
28252 Ford Road
Garden City, MI 48135

(313) 522-7575

**MICHIGAN STATE CHIROPRACTIC ASSOCIATION**
520 East Michigan Avenue
Lansing, MI 48933

(517) 487-5061

*Richard A. Link, DC, Secretary*

**MINNESOTA CHIROPRACTIC ASSOCIATION**
7300 France Avenue South, Suite 312
Minneapolis, MN 55435

(612) 830-2920

*Donald Saunders, DC, Secretary-Treasurer*

**MISSISSIPPI CHIROPRACTIC ASSOCIATION, INC.**
c/o James L. Ransom, DC, Secretary
406 Garfield Street
Tupelo, MS 38801

(601) 842-4532

**MISSOURI STATE CHIROPRACTORS' ASSOCIATION**
P.O. Box 843
Jefferson City, MO 65101

(314) 636-2553

*Blair S. Alden, DC, Secretary*

**MONTANA CHIROPRACTIC ASSOCIATION**
P.O. Box 593
Helena, MT 59601

(406) 442-1440

*Mr. Alfred F. Dougherty, Executive Secretary*

**NEBRASKA CHIROPRACTIC PHYSICIANS' ASSOCIATION**
c/o Gordon Kuether, DC, Secretary
1454 Colfax Street
Blair, NE 68008

(402) 426-3663

**CHIROPRACTIC ASSOCIATION OF NEVADA**
c/o Lon Harter, DC, Secretary
209 East Corbett
Carson City, NV 89701

(702) 882-0528

**NEW HAMPSHIRE CHIROPRACTIC ASSOCIATION, INC.**
c/o Lorna Fuller, DC, Secretary-Treasurer
Penstock Hill
P.O. Box 510
Hillsboro, NH 03244

(603) 478-5511

**NEW JERSEY CHIROPRACTIC SOCIETY**
c/o Arnold E. Cianciulli, DC, Executive Secretary
940 Avenue "C"
Bayonne, NJ 07002

(201) 339-3186

**NEW MEXICO CHIROPRACTIC ASSOCIATION**
c/o Cathy Riekeman, DC, Secretary
505 San Mateo Boulevard, N.E.
Albuquerque, NM 87110

(505) 255-2466

**NEW YORK STATE CHIROPRACTIC ASSOCIATION**
45 John Street
New York, NY 10038

(212) 571-0910

*Mr. Howard S. Davis, Administrator*

**NORTH CAROLINA CHIROPRACTIC ASSOCIATION, INC.**
5 West Hargett Street, Suite 401
Raleigh, NC 27601

(919) 832-4611

*Mr. Philip R. Smith, Executive Director*

**NORTH DAKOTA CHIROPRACTIC ASSOCIATION**
c/o Roy A. Ottinger, DC, Secretary-Treasurer
Box 1643-1300 Sixth Avenue, N.E.
Jamestown, ND 58401

(701) 252-2424

**OHIO STATE CHIROPRACTIC ASSOCIATION**
c/o Richard H. Arnett, DC, Secretary
7382 East Main Street
Reynoldsburg, OH 43068

(614) 866-5181

**OKLAHOMA CHIROPRACTIC PHYSICIANS' ASSOCIATION**
c/o Rubye Daniel, DC, Secretary
721 Boston
Muskogee, OK 74401

(918) 687-7290

**CHIROPRACTIC ASSOCIATION OF OKLAHOMA**
c/o Robert B. Boese, DC, Secretary
2 North Main
Sapulpa, OK 74066

(918) 224-6363

**OREGON ASSOCIATION OF CHIROPRACTIC PHYSICIANS**
P.O. Box 20455
Portland, OR 97220

(503) 253-3900

*Ms. Betty Tower, Administrative Assistant*

**OREGON CHIROPRACTIC ASSOCIATION**
c/o Daniel E. Beeson, DC, Secretary
7215 Southeast Thirteenth Avenue
Portland, OR 97202

(503) 232-2489

**PENNSYLVANIA CHIROPRACTIC SOCIETY**
1335 North Front Street
Harrisburg, PA 17102

(717) 232-5762

*Mr. Thomas Kepler, Executive Director*

**PENNSYLVANIA ASSOCIATION OF DRUGLESS PHYSICIANS, INC.**
c/o Robert Stippich, Jr., DC, Secretary-Treasurer
446 Rennard Street
Philadelphia, PA 19116

(215) 671-9555

**CHIROPRACTIC SOCIETY OF RHODE ISLAND**
c/o Vincent J. Cavallaro, DC, Secretary
371 Broadway
Providence, RI 02909

(401) 272-1980

**SOUTH CAROLINA CHIROPRACTORS' ASSOCIATION**
c/o Kenneth B. Muckenfuss, Jr., DC, Secretary
1 Yeamans Hall Plaza
Charleston, SC 29406

(803) 747-7986

**SOUTH CAROLINA CHIROPRACTIC SOCIETY**
c/o B.L. Black, DC, Secretary
P.O. Box 536
Mt. Pleasant, SC 29464

(803) 884-3506

**SOUTH DAKOTA CHIROPRACTORS' ASSOCIATION**
c/o Max Winkler, DC, Executive Secretary

108 West Missouri
Pierre, SD 57501

(605) 224-7737

**FEDERATION OF TENNESSEE CHIROPRACTORS**
c/o C.H. Harbrecht, DC, Secretary
105 West End Heights
Lebanon, TN 37087

(615) 444-2245

**TENNESSEE CHIROPRACTIC ASSOCIATION**
c/o Albert W. Horner, Jr., DC, Secretary-Treasurer
418 North Ury Street—P.O. Box 325
Union City, TN 38261

(901) 885-0461

**TEXAS CHIROPRACTIC ASSOCIATION**
303 International Life Building
Austin, TX 78701

(512) 476-1229

*Charles Walker, DC, Executive Director*

**CHIROPRACTIC SOCIETY OF TEXAS**
c/o J.G. Baier, DC, Secretary
6626 Capitol Avenue
Houston, TX 77011

**UTAH CHIROPRACTIC ASSOCIATION, INC.**
c/o C.C. Odden, DC, Secretary
3902 Ogden Avenue
Ogden, UT 84403

(801) 621-1411

**VERMONT CHIROPRACTIC ASSOCIATION, INC.**
c/o James Garand, DC, Secretary
146 Main Street
Montpelier, VT 05602

(802) 223-5677

**VIRGINIA CHIROPRACTORS ASSOCIATION, INC.**
c/o George B. McClelland, Jr., DC, Secretary
131 Huntington Lane
Blacksburg, VA 24060

(804) 951-3424

**CHIROPRACTIC SOCIETY OF VIRGINIA, INC.**
c/o Jerry R. Willis, DC, Secretary
540 East Main Street
Wytheville, VA 24382

(804) 228-3883

**WASHINGTON CHIROPRACTORS ASSOCIATION, INC.**
The Grosvenor House
500 Wall Street, Suite 402
Seattle, WA 98121

(206) 622-8958

*Mrs. LaRhue Eichman, Executive Secretary*

**CHIROPRACTIC SOCIETY OF WASHINGTON**
c/o James Hagen, DC, Secretary
6421 Ash North
Spokane, WA 99208

**ASSOCIATED CHIROPRACTORS OF WASHINGTON**
c/o William F. Wood, DC, Secretary
900 Ferry

Wenatchee, WA 98801

(509) 662-7351

**WEST VIRGINIA CHIROPRACTORS SOCIETY, INC.**
c/o Robert Ballard, DC, Secretary-Treasurer
650 Washington Avenue
Huntington, WV 25701

(304) 522-0061

**WISCONSIN CHIROPRACTIC ASSOCIATION**
22 South Carroll
Madison, WI 53703

(608) 256-7023

*Mr. Del Beno, Executive Director*

**WYOMING CHIROPRACTIC ASSOCIATION**
c/o Lois Foster, DC, Secretary-Treasurer
1229 East Third Street
Casper, WY 82601

(307) 237-7825

**(384) ALBERTA CHIROPRACTIC ASSOCIATION**
F.M. Remedios, DC, Secretary Registrar
203 Royal Alex Place
10106-111 Avenue
Edmonton, Alberta
Canada

Maintains membership list and speakers' bureau, disseminates educational information.

**(385) BRITISH COLUMBIA CHIROPRACTIC ASSOCIATION**
c/o Mr. J.S. Burton, Secretary
535 West Georgia Street
Vancouver 15, British Columbia,
Canada

Maintains membership list and speakers' bureau, provides educational information.

**(386) MANITOBA CHIROPRACTORS' ASSOCIATION**
c/o T.A. Watkins, DC, Registrar
1038 Portage Avenue
Winnipeg, Manitoba
Canada

Maintains membership list and speakers' bureau, provides educational information.

**(387) MARITIME DIVISION (includes)**
New Brunswick Chiropractors' Association
Nova Scotia Chiropractors' Association
Prince Edward Island Chiropractors' Association
c/o Secretary-Treasurer
165 Victoria Street
Amhers, Nova Scotia
Canada

Maintains membership list and speakers' bureau for the area, disseminates educational information.

**(388) CANADIAN CHIROPRACTIC EXAMINING BOARD**
c/o J.A. Langford, DC, Chairman
423 Colborne Street

London, Ontario
Canada

Conducts annual qualifying examinations.

**(389) CANADIAN CHIROPRACTIC ASSOCIATION**
1900 Bayview Avenue
Toronto 17, Ontario
Canada

*D.C. Sutherland, DC, Executive Director*

Maintains membership list and speakers' bureau, provides educational information.

**(390) ONTARIO CHIROPRACTIC ASSOCIATION**
c/o S.W. Stolarski, DC, Executive Director
1900 Bayview Avenue
Toronto 17, Ontario
Canada

Maintains membership list and speakers' bureau, provides educational information.

**(391) ORDER OF QUEBEC CHIROPRACTORS**
c/o Pierre Ste. Marie, DC, Secretary
3980 Sherbrooke Est.
Montreal 36, Quebec
Canada

Services include membership list, speakers' bureau, and educational information.

**(392) CHIROPRACTORS' ASSOCIATION OF SASKATCHEWAN**
c/o B.M. Donbrook, DC, Registrar
305 Sterling Building
Regina, Saskatchewan
Canada

Maintains membership list and speakers' bureau, and disseminates educational information.

**(393) AUSTRALIAN CHIROPRACTOR'S ASSOCIATION**
c/o Mr. Richard K. Deveraux, Executive Director
6 Pound Road
Homsby, New South Wales
Australia

Services include membership list, speakers' bureau, and educational information.

**AUSTRALIAN CHIROPRACTORS, OSTEOPATHS, & NATURAL PHYSICIANS ASSOCIATION**/New South Wales **(see 439)**

**(394) HONG KONG CHIROPRACTORS' ASSOCIATION**
Room 1403
Tak Shing House
20 Des Voeux Road C.
Hong Kong

Services include membership list, speakers' bureau, and educational information.

**(395) JAPANESE CHIROPRACTIC ASSOCIATION**
5-9, 3- Chome Kita-Aoyama
Minato-Ku
Tokyo, Japan

Maintains membership list and speakers' bureau, disseminates educational information.

**(396) NEW ZEALAND CHIROPRACTORS' ASSOCIATION**
P.O. Box 2858
Wellington, New Zealand

Maintains membership list and speakers' bureau, disseminates educational information.

**(397) RHODESIAN CHIROPRACTORS' ASSOCIATION**
P.O. Box 1619
Salisbury, Rhodesia

Services include membership list, speakers' bureau, and educational information.

**(398) THE CHIROPRACTIC ASSOCIATION OF SOUTH AFRICA**
29 Union Club Buildings
69 Joubert Street
Johannesburg, South Africa

Maintains membership list and speakers' bureau, disseminates educational information.

**(399) EUROPEAN PRO CHIROPRACTIC FEDERATION**
CH 4000 Basel,
Gundeldingerstr 139
Switzerland

Tel: 061 341001

Maintains lists of chiropractors and chiropractic organizations throughout Europe, who are members of the European Pro Chiropractic Federation. Contact local associations for information in each country.

*MEMBER ASSOCIATIONS*

**DANISH PRO CHIROPRACTIC ASSOCIATION**
Landsforeningen til Kiropraktikkens Fremme
Øresundsvej 140,
2300 Copenhagen S, Denmark

Tel: 01 5910881

**BRITISH PRO-CHIROPRACTIC ASSOCIATION**
c/o Mr. B. Barraclough-Fell, Hon. Secretary
38 The Island
Thames Ditton, Surrey
England

Tel: 01-398 2098

**THE NETHERLANDS PRO-CHIROPRACTIC ASSOCIATION**
c/o Mr. J. van der Geld, Secretary
Lange Heul 59
Bussum, The Netherlands

Tel: 02159-12531

**NORWEGIAN PRO CHIROPRACTIC ASSOCIATION**
Landsforeningen for Kiropraktikk
c/o Odd Ingebrigtsen, Chairman
Box 333
8001 Bodø, Norway

**SWISS PRO CHIROPRACTIC ASSOCIATION**
c/o Miss Olga Fischer, Secretary
Zelgstr 62
CG 5000 Aarau, Switzerland

Tel: 064 227913

**(400) EUROPEAN CHIROPRACTIC UNION**
Zuchwilerstrasse 10
4500 Solothurn, Switzerland

Tel: 065 29121

Maintains lists of chiropractors and chiropractic organizations throughout Europe, who are members of the European Chiropractic Union. Contact local associations for information in each country.

*MEMBER ASSOCIATIONS*

**EUROPEAN CHIROPRACTIC UNION (BELGIUM)**
c/o J. Gillet, General Secretary
Rue de la Limite 5
1030 Bruxelles, Belgium

Tel: 02 2173219

**DANISH CHIROPRACTIC COUNCIL**
c/o K.E. Nielsen, Secretary
Soendergade 14
8700 Horsens, Denmark

Tel: 05 611415

**EUROPEAN CHIROPRACTIC UNION (DENMARK)**
c/o K.E. Nielsen, Secretary
Soendergade 14
8700 Horsens, Denmark

Tel: 05 611415

**EUROPEAN CHIROPRACTIC UNION (GREAT BRITAIN)**
c/o Jan Hutchinson, Secretary
5, First Avenue
Chelmsford CM1 1RX, England

Tel: 0245 53078

**EUROPEAN CHIROPRACTIC UNION (FINLAND)**
c/o Ragna M.L. Valli
Paanakedonkatu 12
28100 Poro 10, Finland

**EUROPEAN CHIROPRACTIC UNION (FRANCE)**
c/o P. Gruny, DC
8, Chemin de Tison
86000 Poitiers, France

Tel: (49) 41-58-25

**EUROPEAN CHIROPRACTIC UNION (GREECE)**
c/o D.J. Chronis
23 Ivis Street
Old Phaleron
Athens, Greece

**EUROPEAN CHIROPRACTIC UNION (IRELAND)**
c/o F. McCuill
14 Warrington Place
Dublin 2, Ireland

Tel: 6 36 86

**EUROPEAN CHIROPRACTIC UNION (ITALY)**
c/o Thomas E. Rigel, Secretary
Via Emanuele Gianturco, 4
00196 Rome, Italy

Tel: 06 360 58 47

**EUROPEAN CHIROPRACTIC UNION (MONACO)**
St. James
5 Av. Princess Alice
Monte-Carlo, Monaco

Tel: 308725

**EUROPEAN CHIROPRACTIC UNION (NORWAY)**
c/o Kyrre Myhrvold, Secretary
Kirkeveien 59
Oslo 3, Norway

Tel: 02 695192

**EUROPEAN CHIROPRACTIC UNION (SWEDEN)**
c/o Peter W. Lövgren
Birgir Jarlsgatan 106A
114 20 Stockholm, Sweden

Tel: 08 152058

## Schools (Colleges)

**(401) LOS ANGELES COLLEGE OF CHIROPRACTIC**
920 East Broadway
Glendale, CA 91205

(213) 240-7686

State accredited institution granting degree of Doctor of Chiropractic.

**(402) LIFE CHIROPRACTIC COLLEGE**
1269 Barclay Circle
Marietta, GA 30060

(404) 424-0554

State accredited institution granting degree of Doctor of Chiropractic.

**(403) NATIONAL COLLEGE OF CHIROPRACTIC**
200 East Roosevelt
Lombard, IL 60148

(312) 629-2000

State accredited institution granting degree of Doctor of Chiropractic.

**(404) PALMER COLLEGE OF CHIROPRACTIC**
1000 Brady Street
Davenport, IA 52803

(319) 324-1611

State accredited institution granting degree of Doctor of Chiropractic.

**(405) NORTHWESTERN COLLEGE OF CHIROPRACTIC**
2222 Park Avenue
Minneapolis, MN 55404

(612) 871-3001

State accredited institution granting degree of Doctor of Chiropractic.

**(406) LOGAN CHIROPRACTIC COLLEGE**
430 Schoettler Road
P.O. Box 100
Chesterfield, MO 63017

(314) 227-2100

State accredited institution granting degree of Doctor of Chiropractic.

**(407) COLUMBIA INSTITUTE OF CHIROPRACTIC**
P.O. Box 167
Glen Head, NY 11545

(516) 626-2700

State accredited institution granting degree of Doctor of Chiropractic.

**(408) WESTERN STATES COLLEGE OF CHIROPRACTIC**
4525 Southeast 63rd Avenue
Portland, OR 97206

(503) 256-3180

State accredited instituion granting degree of Doctor of Chiropractic.

**(409) SHERMAN COLLEGE OF CHIROPRACTIC**
P.O. Box 5502
Springfield Road
Spartanburg, SC 29301

(803) 585-4372

State accredited institution granting degree of Doctor of Chiropractic.

**(410) TEXAS CHIROPRACTIC COLLEGE**
5912 Spencer Highway
Pasadena, TX 75505

(713) 487-1170

State accredited institution granting degree of Doctor of Chiropractic.

**(411) CANADIAN MEMORIAL CHIROPRACTIC COLLEGE**
1900 Bayview Avenue
Toronto 17
Ontario, Canada

*H.J. Vear, DC, Dean*

Accredited institution granting degree of Doctor of Chiropractic.

**(412) INTERNATIONAL COLLEGE OF CHIROPRACTIC**
Sonora House, First floor
300 Little Collins Street
Melbourne, 3000, Australia

Accredited institution granting degree of Doctor of Chiropractic.

(413) **ANGLO-EUROPEAN COLLEGE OF CHIRO-PRACTIC (AECC)**
2, Cavendish Road
Bournemouth BH IRA
Hampshire, England

Tel: Bournemouth 24777

*K.V. Singarajah, PhD, Dean*

Accredited institution granting degree of Doctor of Chiropractic.

## Journals and Publications

(414) **JOURNALS OF STATE CHIROPRACTIC AS-SOCIATIONS**
For further information regarding the following publications, write to the address of the state association (listed under the American Chriopractic Association **(383)** ).

*The Arizona Chiropractic Association*
*United Chiropractic Journal* (Arizona)
*Pacific Southwest Chiropractic Journal* (California)
*Journal of the Illinois Chiropractic Society*
*The Indiana Journal*
*Journal of the Kansas Chiropractic Association*
*The Louisiana Journal of Chiropractic*
*The Mid-Atlantic Journal of Chiropractic* (Maryland)
*New England Journal of Chiropractic* (Massachusetts)
*Pacific Southwest Chiropractic Journal* (Nevada)
*New Hampshire Chiropractic Journal*
*North Carolina Chiropractic Journal*
*Journal of Ohio State Chiropractic Association*
*Oklahoma Chiropractic Journal*
*The Journal of the Oregon Association of Chiropractic*
*Journal of Pennsylvania Licensed Chiropractic Association*
*New England Journal* (Rhode Island)
*Pacific Southwest Chiropractic Journal* (Utah)
*W.C.A. Journal* (Wisconsin)

(415) **INTERNATIONAL PUBLISHING COMPANY**
Box 2615
Littleton, CO 80122

(303) 333-1581, Ext. 13

*Fern L. Dzaman, Editor*

Publishing a directory of 450 leading chiropractors with biographies, entitled *Who's Who in Chiropractic, International*. Scheduled release: April 1977.

**JOURNAL OF THE AMERICAN CHIROPRACTIC ASSOCIATION**/Des Moines, IA **(see 383)**

(416) **THE DIGEST OF CHIROPRACTIC ECONOMICS**
31393 West Thirteen Mile Road
Farmington Hills, MI 48018

(313) 855-9411

*William L. Luckey, Publisher*

Bimonthly publication "dedicated to the purpose of building and reinforcing professional and economic security through knowledge, information, education and service."

(417) **TEXAS CHIROPRACTIC COLLEGE REVIEW**
5912 Spencer Highway
Pasadena, TX 77505

(713) 487-1170

*William D. Harper, President*

Bimonthly publication of the Texas College of Chiropractic.

(418) **JOURNAL OF THE CANADIAN CHIROPRAC-TIC ASSOCIATION**
1900 Bayview Avenue
Toronto 17
Ontario, Canada

*D.C. Sutherland, DC, Editor*

Official publication of the Canadian Chiropractic Association. Articles deal with all aspects of the field of chiropractic and related subjects.

(419) **PRO CHIROPRAKTIK**
Schweiz. Vereinigung Pro Chiropraktik
Buchdruckerei R. + B. Berthoud
Bümplizstr. 163, 3018 Bern
Switzerland

Tel: 031-56128

Official publication of the Swiss Chiropractic Association.

(420) **ANNALS OF THE SWISS CHIROPRACTORS' ASSOCIATION**
51 av. du Casino
1820 Montreaux
Switzerland

Tel: 021 622680

*E. Valentini, Editor*

Publishes proceedings of the Annual Chiropractic Conference.

## Products and Services

(421) **BIOTRONICS**
7060 Hollywood Boulevard, Suite 601
Hollywood, CA 90028

(213) 466-6157

Distributes the "Lectroflex®" chiropractic adjusting table.

(422) **BAC INDUSTRIES, INC.**
3757 Wilshire Boulevard, Suite 204
Los Angeles, CA 90010

(213) 388-9726

Distributes the "Bac" automatic chiropractic adjustment table.

(473) **ELECTROPEDIC PROFESSIONAL MASSAG-ERS**
3107 Wilshire Boulevard
Los Angeles, CA 90010

(213) 381-2356

Distributes the "Electropedic Massager" massage unit.

**(424) DYNA GYM CORPORATION**
6465 Independence Avenue
Woodland Hills, CA 91367

(213) 348-9260

Distributes the ''Dyna Gym'' exercise slant board.

**(425) MAGUIRE INDUSTRIES**
2112 First Street, West
Bradenton, FL 33505

(813) 746-4443

Distributes the ''Physicare'' gravity traction table.

**(426) ROY CHILDERS ASSOCIATES**
2615 Southeast Fourteenth Street
Ocala, FL 32670

(904) 629-7261

Used chiropractic equipment available at reasonable prices.
Further information available on request.

**(427) WILLIAMS MANUFACTURING CO.**
P.O. Box 104
Elgin, IL 60120

(312) 741-2288

Distributes the ''Zenith-Thompson Pneumatic'' chiropractic
adjustment table.

**(428) THERAPEUTIC SLEEP PRODUCTS, INC.**
1901 Rockdale Road
Dubuque, IA 52001

(319) 556-6733

Distributes the ''Pillo-pedic'' pillow which provides cervical traction during sleep.

**(429) LLOYD TABLE COMPANY**
122 West Main Street
Lisbon, IA 52253

(319) 455-2110

Distributes a full line of chiropractic adjusting tables for all
purposes.

**(430) CONTURPEDIC CORPORATION**
Preston, MN 55965

(507) 765-3881

Distributes the ''Conturpedic Cervical Pillow'' for sleeping.

**(431) POSTUR-PILLO, INC.**
611 Ninth Street
Virginia, MN 55792

(218) 741-5381

Distributes a sculptured contoured pillow for sleeping.

**(432) J.A. PRESTON CORPORATION**
71 Fifth Avenue
New York, NY 10003

(212) 255-8484

Distributes acupressure rotary vibrator massager.

**(433) CAMPILLARY SYSTEMS, INC.**
912 Sunset Avenue
Gettysburg, PA 17325

(717) 334-1478

Distributes the ''Respirizer®'' respirator.

**(434) HILL LABORATORIES COMPANY**
Malvern, PA 19355

(215) 644-2867

Distributes the ''Hill Anatomotor'' chiropractic, massage
and adjustment table.

**GREAT EARTH HEALING, INC.** (ma roller)/East
Montpelier, VT; Montreal, Canada **(see 230.1)**

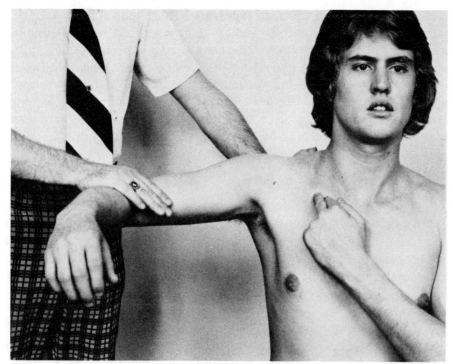

Therapy localization to the sub-clavius muscle (below collar bone) using the deltoid (shoulder muscle) as an indicator muscle. From *Applied Kinesiology* by David S. Walther, DC, published by Systems DC, Pueblo, Colorado.

# Applied Kinesiology

*George J. Goodheart, DC, and*
*Walter H. Schmitt, DC*

The expanding compendium of knowledge called applied kinesiology (AK) stemmed from a simple observation made in early 1964. Most muscle spasm is not primary, but secondary to antagonist muscle weakness. The first applied kinesiology patient was a young man who complained of chronic shoulder pain. Examination revealed the classical signs of a paralyzed serratus anterior muscle, including weakness to standard muscle testing procedures and winging of the scapula. However, palpation of the costal insertions of the involved serratus anterior revealed numerous painful, discrete trigger point-type nodules. After subsequent manipulation with a heavy, rotary pressure, to the doctor's surprise and the patient's delight, the shoulder pain immediately disappeared and function of the serratus anterior completely returned to normal, including full strength to muscle tested.

This incident was the starting point for investigation into the significance of muscle weakness, which in reality represents motorneuron inhibition. The commonly used term "muscle spasm" is not an entity in itself; rather, muscle spasm represents motorneuron facilitation, the reaction to antagonist muscle weakness through reciprocal innervation. Primary muscle spasm occurs so infrequently that it is considered a rarity.

Muscle weakness as it most commonly occurs is a functional rather than pathological reaction of the nervous system. Applied kinesiology has led to the recognition that structural integrity and body function are intimately associated. Virtually any disease state of the body will have a structural manifestation, a specific "body language" pattern, represented by specific muscle weakness patterns. Muscle testing, then, becomes a tool with which to read the body's language, and this tool has opened avenues of investigation that lead into nearly every aspect of the diagnostic and therapeutic modalities available to the present-day wholistic physician.

Much of the early work in applied kinesiology revolved around a correlation of various factors that could cause muscle weakness and the related structural imbalance. The empirical findings of Frank Chapman, DO (neurolymphatic reflexes), Terrence Bennett, DC (neurovascular reflexes), and traditional acupuncture were all related by their discoverers to the body's organ systems. AK investigation showed that each reflex point of each system was also related to a specific muscle weakness. But more importantly, weakness in a specific muscle was found whenever demonstrable dysfunction in a specific organ was identified, and the neurolymphatic, neurovascular, and acupuncture reflex centers for a given organ were all found to be related to this same specific muscle. For example, patients with kidney disease will display concurrent weakness of the psoas muscle; those with gastric disease will show an associated weakness of the pectoralis major, clavicular division, and so on.

These relationships hold true for foot reflexes, hand reflexes, iridology diagnostic areas, cranial reflex centers, etc. Although muscle weakness could be solely of somatic origin, this specific viscerosomatic relationship is an invaluable diagnostic aid. The opportunity to be able to understand and read the body language that a patient presents when his or her structure is faulty is unique; the opportunity to read the structural language is expanded by the relationship that exists between the viscera, which in general are silent, and the muscles that express the language of the viscera.

Experience has shown that not every weak muscle has an associated organ dysfunction, but every organ dysfunction is accompanied by a weak muscle. Therefore, observations of man's structure afford a double diagnostic potential.

Additional advancements in AK revealed that specific nutritional requirements of the body manifest themselves through a specific muscle weakness for each nutrient, and this weakness will be abolished immediately upon ensalivating the appropriate nutritional material. Further, the effectiveness or toxicity of various nutritional products as well as food allergies can be tested by having the patient chew the substance while monitoring the strength of a specific muscle. Obvious food allergens (such as refined sugar to the hyperinsulinism patient) will cause immediate weakening of an associated muscle when the substance is chewed and ensalivated, before any swallowing or usual absorption can take place.

The special importance of spinal integrity, and the widespread effects of pelvic, vertebral, and extremity subluxations are also demonstrated by applied kinesiology methods. Monitoring of muscle strength and weakness as an articulation is moved through specified ranges of motion constitute the "challenge" technique. This procedure permits identification of subluxations and their distant effects, and, more importantly, verification of their correction following adjustment. Similar procedures can be used for the detection and correction of cranial bone articular lesions.

Possibly the most astounding concept in applied kinesiology was the discovery in 1973 of "therapy localization." The acute, kinesthetic sense of the nervous system, particularly the proprioceptive awareness of hand position, can be observed by having the patient place his hands on and off suspected areas of involvement while testing an indicator muscle. When the patient "therapy localizes" to an area of altered function or an irritated "reflex center," the tested muscle will immediately change strength (a weak muscle will strengthen, a strong muscle will weaken). This occurs as long as the patient keeps his hand on the involved area, and the return of the indicator muscle to its previous level of strength occurs instantaneously when the hands are removed. The dramatic impression one receives when first witnessing therapy localization is surpassed only by the response practitioners get when they add the procedure to their diagnostic armamentarium.

Therapy localization, coupled with other applied kinesiology procedures, is capable of identifying virtually all faults and dysfunctions that have an effect on the nervous system. These encompass everything from subluxations of the spine to imbalances in the body's energy fields. Applied kinesiology is based upon the fact that the body language never lies. The opportunity of understanding body language is enhanced by the recognition that the muscles are the mouthpiece of the body's language. The original technique of testing muscles and determining their function, using the method first advocated by Kendall and Kendall, remains the prime diagnostic device. Once muscle weakness has been ascertained, a variety of therapeutic options are available, only a few of which have been mentioned here.

The opportunity to use the body as a laboratory instrument is unparalleled in modern diagnostics because the response of the body is unerring. If physicians approach the problem correctly, using body language as their guide, they will be directed into the correct diagnosis and treatment, and will be rewarded with the deserved satisfactory response, to which the patient is entitled.

The body heals itself; it heals itself in a sure, sensible, practical, reasonable, and observable manner. "The healer within" can be approached from without. Man possesses a potential for recovery through the innate intelligence or the physiological homeostasis of the human structure. This recovery potential with which man is endowed merely awaits the hand and the heart and the mind of a trained individual to bring it to a potential being and allow the recovery which is man's natural heritage to take place.

## Groups and Associations

(434.1) **INTERNATIONAL COLLEGE OF APPLIED KINESIOLOGY**
542 Michigan Building
Detroit, MI 48226

(313) 962-6484

*George Goodheart, DC, Founder*

An association of licensed health professionals who have completed standardized training in kinesiology. The objectives of the organization are to assist in the development of the healing arts through applied kinesiology, to sponsor and promote seminars, to promote research, to disseminate information, and to develop professional standards and ethics for the practice of applied kinesiology.

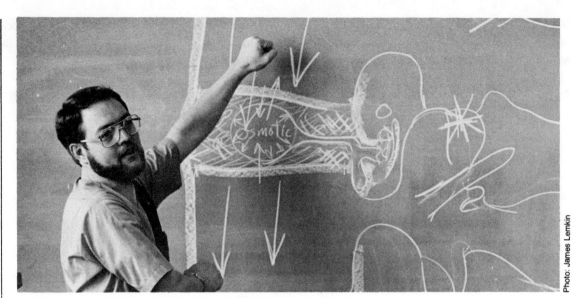

Photo: James Lemkin

An instructor at the National College of Naturopathic Medicine explains the forces at work on the intervertebral disc of the spinal column.

# Naturopathic Medicine: A Separate And Distinct Healing Profession

*Joseph A. Boucher, ND*

*"If I could live my life over again I would devote it to proving that germs seek their natural habitat—diseased tissue—rather than being the cause of diseased tissue; e.g. mosquitos seek the stagnant water, but do not CAUSE the pool to become stagnant."*

*Rudolph Virchow*

In order to fix a time as the starting point of naturopathic medicine one would have to travel well back into antiquity. If it is absolutely necessary to name one person as the founder, we can do no better than to name Hippocrates (ironically dubbed "The Father of Modern Medicine").

However, it is questionable that this modern healing art began with a single individual or even in any particular era; rather, it evolved as civilization evolved. Its history is nothing more than man intelligently observing and applying the laws of nature, as animals do innately. And to the extent and degree that people abided by these laws, to that extent and degree did they enjoy that state we call good health. Conversely, to the extent and degree that they violated the laws, to that extent and degree they gravitated toward the opposite end of that polarity and suffered from disease.

The definition of naturopathy most commonly used and accepted today is that published in the *New Gould Medical Dictionary* (1971): "A therapeutic system embracing a complete physianthropy employing nature's agencies, forces, processes and products, except major surgery." This definition correctly conveys the idea that naturopathic medicine is a separate and distinct healing art. It has features that distinguish it from any other healing arts, such as medicine and surgery, osteopathy, chiropractic, and podiatry. The distinctions are as follows:

1. The naturopathic physician is concerned with the *whole* man rather than with a specific anatomical area. Naturopathic physicians treat people, not conditions.
2. Naturopathic treatment is physiological in nature. Treatment is intended to assist the inherent physiological processes as they relate to healing and normal biochemistry. Any form of treatment that violates natural or physiological law is considered unnatural, especially if such treatment is iatrogenic, causing a new or different illness, or complicating the existing disease process.
3. Naturopathic medicine includes a complete physianthropy, with the emphasis on those methods which evoke a biological response that is therapeutic in nature.

4. Naturopathic physicians are concerned with the immediate *causative* factors of an illness. Equal consideration or treatment is given to the basic, underlying causal factors or circumstances so common in many disorders. Particular emphasis is placed on the maintenance of health (or prevention of disease) through education in nutrition, mental hygiene, physical fitness, and other aspects of bodily care. ("Building health cures disease" is a slogan frequently used in naturopathic literature.)

5. Naturopathic physicians rarely employ a single method or a purely symptomatic approach to bodily disorders; rather, they combine in one well-ordered system of therapeutics the best of all forms of natural healing, by combining multiple methods or approaches best suited to the particular illness being treated.

6. Every naturopathic physician is a true physician in the fullest sense of the dictionary definition ("one who heals") and a true doctor ("a teacher; an instructor"), and a true physician in that patients are instructed what *they* must do to regain and preserve their health.

7. In modern naturopathic colleges, the naturopathic physician is taught all the basic sciences, diagnostic procedures, etc., common to medical doctors in routine office practice.

8. Naturopathic therapeutics involve a multidisciplinary approach to most chronic health problems; e.g., in the treatment of some disorders a botanical or herbal medicine may be used in conjunction with a nutritional or metabolic supplement, diet, diathermy, ultrasound, or spinal manipulations.

9. Naturopathic physicians treat any and all conditions that come within the realm of general practice—cardiovascular, neurological, musculoskeletal, orthopedic, gastrointestinal, genitourinary, pulmonary, dermatological, pediatric, geriatric, etc. Problem cases are frequently referred for specialty care (naturopathic physicians freely cooperate with licensed doctors in the healing professions when such cooperation is in the best interests of the patient).

10. In no way can naturopathic services be considered ancillary in relation to other healing arts or professions. They are, on the contrary, *alternative* in nature.

Naturopathic medicine is very much in favor of all modern, scientific advancement and techniques (many of which, incidentally, verify naturopathic concepts and principles in use for hundreds of years) that extend the life and health of the human body, provided such scientific endeavors do not violate natural or biological principle.

The naturopathic physicians of modern times do not discard a method simply because it is old; neither do they immediately embrace a technique because it is new, popular, and heavily advertised. The methods of naturopathic medicine have been rigidly tested upon the anvil of time and experience.

For this reason, there is today a growing tendency among doctors of other healing professions to employ various aspects of contemporary naturopathic therapeutics.

## Groups and Associations

(435) **AMERICAN ASSOCIATION OF CONSTITUTIONAL MEDICINE**
c/o Kenneth L. Sanders, ND
405 Appleway Avenue
Coeur D'Alene, ID 83814

Information available on the practice and use of Naturopathic Medicine.

(436) **NATIONAL ASSOCIATION OF NATUROPATHIC PHYSICIANS**
Administration Office
609 Sherman Avenue
Coeur D'Alene, ID 83814

(208) 667-0541

*Ronald R. Hoye, Sr., ND, President*

Dedicated to maintaining professional standards, serving as a forum for the exchange of information, and protecting the legal rights of naturopathic physicians to practice. The NANP provides a service whereby a naturopathic physician or patient can become a plaintiff requesting the federal courts to be allowed to practice or receive naturopathic treatment. Activities of the association include national conferences and the publication of the *Journal of Natural Medicine*.

*AFFILIATE AND STATE ASSOCIATIONS*

**ALABAMA ASSOCIATION OF NATUROPATHIC PHYSICIANS**
c/o D.F. Butler, ND
r.O. Box 263
Wetumpka, AL 36092

**THE OKLAHOMA ASSOCIATION & COLLEGE OF NATUROPATH & PHYSIOTHERAPY DOCTORS**
664 West Arbor Vitae Street
Englewood, CA 90301

*Joseph W. Hough, ND*

**FLORIDA ASSOCIATION OF NATUROPATHIC PHYSICIANS**
c/o Charles R. Harvey, ND, President
5508 North Armenia Avenue
Tampa, FL 33603

**FLORIDA ACADEMY OF NATUROPATHIC MEDICINE, INC.**
c/o James C. McKee, ND, BS, President
2125 West Fairbanks Avenue
Winter Park, FL 32789

**IDAHO ASSOCIATION OF NATUROPATHIC PHYSICIANS**
c/o Ronald R. Hoye, ND, President
609 Sherman Avenue
Coeur D'Alene, ID 83814

(208) 667-0541

**THE NATUROPATHIC PHYSICIANS ASSOCIATION OF INDIANA, INC.**
c/o Harry Goble, ND, Secretary-Treasurer
2432 East Lake Shore Drive
Crown Point, ID 46307

**LOUISIANA NATUROPATHIC MEDICAL ASSOCIATION**
c/o T.H. Ketterman, ND, State Board of Examiners
P.O. Box 3806
New Orleans, LA 70177

**MICHIGAN ASSOCIATION OF NATUROPATHIC PHYSICIANS**
c/o William B. Marshall, DC, ND
6399 Sylvania-Petersburg Road
Ottawa Lake, MI 49267

(313) 888-7181

**MONTANA ASSOCIATION OF NATUROPATHIC PHYSICIANS**
c/o Marcel Pitet, ND
423 South 34th Street
Billings, MT 59101

**OHIO ASSOCIATION OF NATUROPATHIC PHYSICIANS**
c/o Earnest D. Boyer, ND
2468 Edsel Avenue
Columbus, OH 43207

**OREGON ASSOCIATION OF NATUROPATHIC PHYSICIANS**
c/o R.M. Finley, ND, Secretary
820 Southwest Tenth Avenue
Portland, OR 97205

**TEXAS ASSOCIATION OF NATUROPATHIC PHYSICIANS**
c/o Richard Earl Watkins, ND
4101 Clemson Drive
Garland, TX 75042

**UTAH ASSOCIATION OF NATUROPATHIC PHYSICIANS**
c/o Jonathan G. Rand, ND, President
90 South 150 East
Orem, UT 84057

(801) 224-3311

**WASHINGTON ASSOCIATION OF NATUROPATHIC PHYSICIANS**
c/o William Bresnan, ND
735 Tenth East
Seattle, WA 98102

**(437) ONTARIO NATUROPATHIC ASSOCIATION**
R.R. 2
Aurora, Ontario
Canada L4G 3G8

*Norah Stewart, ND, Secretary-Treasurer*

Maintains membership list and speakers' bureau, disseminates educational information.

**(438) SASKATCHEWAN ASSOCIATION OF NATUROPATHIC PHYSICIANS**
Corner Board & 15th
Regina, Saskatchewan
Canada

*V.B. Norman, ND, President and Provincial Licensing Examiner*

Services include membership list, speakers' bureau, and educational information.

**(439) AUSTRALIAN CHIROPRACTORS, OSTEOPATHS AND NATURAL PHYSICIANS ASSOCIATION**
c/o Mrs. A. Downer, Secretary
6 /102, Kirribilli Avenue
Kirribilli, New South Wales
Australia

Association of qualified practitioners in chiropractic, osteopathic, and various other forms of alternative healing. Full member of IFPNT (**72**).

**RESEARCH SOCIETY FOR NATURAL THERAPEUTICS** (multidisciplinary professional membership assoc.) /Dorset, England (**see 70**)

**(440) BRITISH NATUROPATHIC AND OSTEOPATHIC ASSOCIATION**
Frazer House,
6 Netherhall Gardens
London NW3 5RR
England

Tel: 01-435 8728

Established to advance the professions of naturopathy and osteopathy in the United Kingdom. Operates a four-year educational program, The British College of Naturopathy and Osteopathy, for training qualified naturopaths and osteopaths. A naturopathic clinic is operated in conjunction with this college. A complete directory of members of the Association is available from the above address.

**(441) INCORPORATED SOCIETY OF REGISTERED NATUROPATHS**
1 Albemarle Road
The Mount
York YO2 1EN, England

Representative body of incorporated Naturopathic Physicians.

**(442) ISRAEL NATUROPATHIC ASSOCIATION**
c/o Alex Hary, Secretary
Shoshanim Street 4
Kiriat-Tivon-36000
Israel

Association of Naturopaths and other qualified practitioners of drugless medicine. Full member of IFPNT **(72)**.

**(443) NEW ZEALAND ASSOCIATION OF NATUROPATHS AND OSTEOPATHS**
c/o E. Cheal, Secretary
P.O. Box 26, 068
Aukland 3, New Zealand

Promotes the use of naturopathic and osteopathic modes of healing and protects the rights of their practitioners. A full member of the IFPNT **(72)**.

## Schools, Centers, and Clinics

**LUKATS' PREVENTION REGENERATION RESORT**/Safford, AZ **(see 164)**

**CHRISTOS SCHOOL OF NATURAL HEALING/**
Taos, NM **(see 135)**

**(444) NATIONAL COLLEGE OF NATUROPATHIC MEDICINE**
510 Southwest Third Avenue, Room 415
Portland, OR 97204

(503) 226-3717

*Brian L. MacCoy, ND, Dean*

3100 McCormick Avenue
Wichita, KS 67213

(316) 942-8662

A four-year medical program leading to a degree in Naturopathic Medicine (ND). The first two years are in basic science, whereas the clinical work in the last two years is basically comprised of related classroom therapeutic subjects. Emphasis on botanical medicine, homeotherapeutics, physiotherapy, natural childbirth, minor surgery, manipulation, and preventative medicine. Candidates must have completed two years of college and coursework in organic chemistry, biology, English, mathematics, and psychology. Founded 1956.

**NATUROPATHIC BIRTH CENTER**/Winston, OR **(see 23)**

**CLYMER HEALTH CLINIC** (multidisciplinary clinic)/
Quakertown, PA **(see 150)**

**TYRINGHAM NATUROPATHIC CLINIC** (wholistic spa)/Bucks, England **(see 177)**

**SHALIMAR HEALTH HOME** (education and rejuvenation resort)/Essex, England **(see 178)**

**BRITISH NATUROPATHIC AND OSTEOPATHIC ASSOCIATION** (4 yr educational program)/London **(see 440)**

**(445) PORT OF HEALTH INTERNATIONAL NATUROPATHIC HEALTHATARIUM**
Apdo. 5-46
Guadalajara 5
Jalisco, Mexico

Tel: 15-30-13

*Dr. Eduard L. Carl, ND, Director*

Center with luxury accommodations for extended nature cure programs. Therapies include colon irrigation, supervised fasting, laetrile, herbs, chelation, deep nerve massage, chiropractic, physiotherapy, hyperbaric oxygen, Koch therapy, and acupuncture.

**(446) NEDERLANDSE COLLEGE VOOR NATUROPATHIE**
van Lenneplaan 16
Hilversum, The Netherlands

College to train naturopaths. Associate member of IFPNT **(72)**.

**BIRCHER-BENNER PRIVATKLINIK** (wholistic clinic)/Zürich, Switzerland **(see 180)**

## Journals and Publications

**(447) JOURNAL OF NATURAL MEDICINE**
1134 North Orchard
Suite 19
Boise, ID 83704

(208) 376-1581

*Louise F. Davis, Managing Editor*

Biannual journal of the National Association of Naturopathic Physicians **(436)**. Articles on natural treatment of specific diseases, homeopathy, herbs, acupuncture, and other naturopathic practices. Founded 1977.

**JOURNAL OF THE RESEARCH SOCIETY FOR NATURAL THERAPEUTICS**/Dorset, England **(see 70)**

**IFPNT NEWSLETTER** (natural healing) /London, England **(see 72)**

## Products and Services

**HEALTH RESEARCH** (books) /Mokelumne Hill, CA **(see 209)**

**W.G. BAZAN** (books) /O'Fallon, MO **(see 224)**

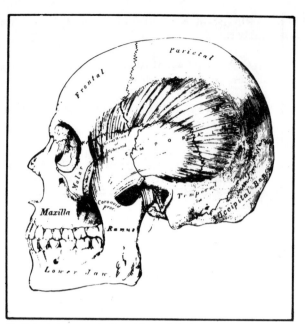

Skull depicting areas indicated in cranial adjustment

# Cranial Technique
*Major B. DeJarnette, DC, DO*

Craniofacial lesions exist in all humanity and most of them go uncorrected, adding pain and disease to one's life.

The cranium is basically a component of eight bones shaped in the approximate form of a ball. Inside that ball will be found depressions for the various parts of the brain. Surrounding those depressions and the brain proper will be found membranes which extend the full length of the spinal cord and house the message transmission system of man, known as the nervous system.

To help manage all of this, and to maintain some semblance of order, there is suspended from the temporal fossa what is known as the mandible, or the lower jaw. This is truly a mechanism of great magnitude for it not only furnishes sockets for our teeth, but also a nerve and blood and lymph supply to nourish them.

In every facial movement, the mandible moves much of man's face and skull. The miracle of the mandible is its ability to compensate for every cranial and facial fault that it cannot correct.

Man's skull and face are held together by toothlike projections which we call sutures (sutures refer to something sewn together). The only suture in the skull and face which is not toothlike is the squamosal, which holds the temporal bone in position in relationship to the frontal, sphenoidal, parietal and occipital bones.

Fully 96 per cent of all humanity has a misalignment of the mandible; consequently, that same percentage has misalignments of the cranial and facial sutures. Few persons escape without some minor warning of a craniofacial fault as, for instance, with sinus problems. Toothache is often due to simple misalignments in which pressure upon a tooth changes from normal to abnormal, causing that tooth to rotate and press upon nerves or blood vessels. A quick glance at the people around you will reveal a number of them to have one eye smaller than the other, another piece of evidence that the total skull and face are misaligned. Headaches, migraine attacks and facial neuralgias are but a sampling of the effects of such cranial or facial faults.

There is only one solution to this burden so many people unnecessarily bear—health practitioners, including dentists, must be trained to recognize and help correct existing craniofaults.

We know that man must have a nervous system capable of instant response if he is to survive in a state of health. We know that the spinal cord has the ability to monitor many of man's needs, but it is only the brain which is capable of transmitting the power to run man's visceral systems and his circulatory, excretory and secretory systems.

To appreciate the need for Cranial Technique, one has but to consider the composition of the right parietal bone for a few minutes to recognize a vital fact about misalignment. That bone can have over one hundred sutural fingers, each being so important that should only two of them twist a piece of membrane between them, it can disturb man's ability to motivate or articulate, focus his hands upon a task, or survive the extreme pressure of vascular excitement.

All of man's cranium does not have to be misaligned to create a problem. A tiny focus of the misalignment can upset the total system. There isn't any question but that man's sight can be preserved longer if one can contain the cranial vault within certain limits. Problems involving man's hearing are widespread with serious consequences not only in sound management, but in body movement management as well.

Every practitioner should be capable of performing a cranial examination to ascertain if faults are present and in need of correction. If correction is needed and not given, no system of healing can progress that patient past those cranial faults. Therefore, further study and consideration of this technique should be encouraged as a necessary adjunct to a total health approach.

## Groups

(447.1) **SACRO OCCIPITAL RESEARCH SOCIETY INTERNATIONAL (SORSI)**
P.O. Box 338
Nebraska City, NB 68410

(402) 873-6769

*M.B. DeJarnette, DC, DO, Founder*

Maintains a four-year cranial training and certification program, which is available to qualified practitioners of chiropractic, orthodontics, and allied fields. Holds annual conference; a major part of the agenda consists of the presentation of current research findings in the field of cranial technique.

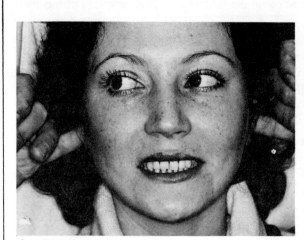
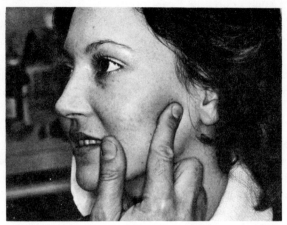

Some TMJ testing techniques
Palpation of condyles through external auditory meatuses.

Palpation of the masseter muscle courtesy, Harold Gelb, DMD.

# The Position Of The Mandible (Lower Jaw) As It Relates To Stress In The Human System
*Willie B. May, BS, DDS*

All therapy is directed toward reduction of stress. Dentistry, through oral orthopedics, reduces stress on the total person. By controlling the functional position of the mandible, it is earning a place in the wholistic concept of health care. Observations begun in 1950 suggest that up to 50 percent of the stress load on the individual can be reduced by maintaining proper functional position of the mandible.

The chewing mechanism can be a source of uninterrupted stress of great magnitude. This continuous stress load is often more pronounced during rest or sleep periods. Thus, it is a two-edged sword: it both adds to the work load and hampers the ability to rest or recover from work.

The natural result of this continuous overload of stress is chronic symptoms of all types and of varying degrees of severity. Besides speeding up the aging process, improper mandibular function affects every facet of life. The symptoms involved often defy all treatment methods, simply because the cause is not removed. Even if a treatment does give the expected results, its effectiveness is reduced. This dental stress, unrecognized until recent years, is capable of overshadowing all therapies.

The treatment available today, pivotal mandibular equilibration, represents a continaul refinement and improvement of procedures that began with papers published independently in the early 1930s by J. B. Costen, MD, and D. J. Goodfriend, DDS. Costen, an EENT physician, had noticed that certain ear symptoms were associated with conditions in the mouth and often were the result of improper functioning of the temporomandibular joint (TMJ). The numerous symptoms he observed accompanying these problems (occlusions, missing teeth, etc.) became known as Costen's syndrome, and the list increased with each report.

At this stage the major question being asked was, can occlusal problems and improper TMJ function be a factor in loss of hearing? There was little concern for the other symptoms that Costen listed in his papers. The focus was broadened in the midforties when Victor H. Sears, DDS, came upon a principle of simple mechanics to improve the stability of complete dentures and at the same time to slow the destructive forces of dentures on the edentulous dental ridges. Sears termed his method, which accomplishes mandibular equilibration, "occlusal pivots."

Denture patients treated with this method consistently reported a lessening of chronic-type symptoms throughout the body. The improvements were often so dramatic that they could not be passed over as coincidental. The treatment for denture patients was modified to apply to persons with natural teeth, and the result was often a complete turnaround of chronic conditions. Sears was then faced with the problem of how to communicate this fact to other dentists—a problem because it went against many principles on which the mechanics of dentistry were firmly established.

Sears soon spread his concept of treatment sufficiently to create the need for a clearinghouse of observations related to TMJ function. The American Equilibration Society, a group of physicians and dentists dedicated to observing, sorting, and reporting data and making their findings available to the dental profession, was founded in 1955. (The American Academy of Craniomandibular Oral Orthopedics, founded later, is also concerned with TMJ therapies.)

The primary objective of the AES was to make all dental colleges of the world aware that this new treatment was available and to encourage them to reorganize their curricula to include this new subject. After 20 years this goal has nearly been accomplished.

In the method of treatment begun by Sears the greatest attention is given to the function of the muscles and their controlling nerves (in other methods, the teeth are the center of attention). Basic principles of orthopedics are observed. In working with edentulous cases, Sears noted that he could easily modify the skeletal support, chin to nose distance, by modifying the denture. This made it possible to provide skeletal support for the chewing muscles. Herein lies the important difference between pivotal mandibular equilibration and other methods. As the muscles are relieved of the need to compensate, they are able to coordinate better with the other muscles in this area. Their action becomes milder or softer and reduces the destructive forces keeping the ridges tender and causing them to continue to shrink.

When this method is adapted to persons with natural teeth, the head skeleton, forehead to chin vertical dimension, is often shorter than the relaxed head muscle(s). This problem is met in the same way that a short leg is treated, with a manmade support to supplement the short skeletal dimension. Once the mandible seems to be stabilized in its corrected neuromuscular-controlled position, rather than the tooth-oriented position, the course of treatment is decided. The alternatives are to keep the patient on the splint to maintain the improved neuromuscular function or to reconstruct the mouth at this corrected position (if the latter course is selected, care should be taken to use materials acceptable to the person's nervous system; this can be done by using applied kinesiology).

Ideally, it is best to establish treatment in early childhood, so that the short dimension in the head skeleton has a chance to correct itself. Also, since children have not been exposed to stress for long, they have a greater potential for response.

The patient should be alerted to watch for return of any symptoms relieved during the treatment. This warning should be in effect even if there are other circumstances that could contribute to the symptoms. For example, a patient who had been relieved of severe neck, shoulder, and back pain through proper mandibular support underwent a radical mastectomy. Some months later the neck, shoulder, and back pains returned. After many tests over an extended period of time, all with negative results, the patient returned for a check of the mandibular position. One simple adjustment of the mandibular support stopped all the pain. Even if correcting the mandibular position does not relieve pain, clearing this stress will permit diagnostic tests to give truer results, and treatment will be more rewarding.

One of the early studies established that all medicinal dosages could be reduced 35 to 65 percent once the dental stress is reduced—with no reduction in results. A broken femur that failed to heal after 7 months and two surgical procedures healed in a few weeks once the mandible was given proper support. Similar results are commonplace in offices using this improved treatment method.

The method can easily be added to any treatment or research program. The only requirements are a staff of two, even part-time, and a very limited space. A single treatment unit of this type could serve many studies in a research and teaching environment.

The explosion of knowledge in the field increases the urgency of comparing results and selecting the methods that have the most benefits for the patients treated for TMJ problems. The observations of all wholistic therapists would greatly contribute to further this knowledge. We can look forward to the day when all initial patient interviews, regardless of the mode of therapy, will include the question, ''Has there been any change in your occlusal pattern or mandibular position?'' Already many therapists are observing, ''I wish all of my patients could be freed of stress in their chewing mechanisms before I begin treatment.''

# Temporomandibular Joint Technique

*Harold T. Perry, DDS, PhD*

The temporomandibular joints are located at the cranial end of the mandible. Their fossae are formed by the base of the temporal bone. The components of the temporomandibular joints are similar to those of all other joints. Foremost are the ligaments, capsule, disc, synovial fluid, muscle, nerve, and blood vessels. The body surfaces of the temporomandibular joints are unlike those of other joints in that they are covered by fibrocartilage. The joints have a possible gliding or hinge movement; a variety of movements are possible when the two joints are acting in concert. Dislocations, dysfunction, and disease will take their toll on this joint, as on any other. However, this joint is distinguished by its close association with the dental apparatus, as well as the totality of the stomatognathic system.

Beginning in 1918, dentists observed that a number of symptoms were directly related to the temporomandibular joints. In 1934 an otolaryngologist, J. B. Costen, grouped these symptoms under the name Costen's syndrome, including (a) pain of the head and neck, about the ears and jaws; (b) otological changes such as tinnitus, deafness; (c) joint tenderness, vertigo, and assorted other oral symptoms. He believed that all these symptoms were due to overclosure of the bite. For many years all disturbances of the temporomandibular joint remained grouped into Costen's syndrome.

In 1957 A. S. Freese reclassified the symptoms with a more logical and acceptable explanation. He also described a conservative treatment regime for the patient possessing the symptoms. Several other investigators and clinicians have since proposed classifications and descriptions that, when taken in toto and reviewed, present a series of signs and symptoms that have been related to the arrangement of the teeth of the mandible to the maxilla, microtrauma, macrotrauma, mental stress, dental procedures, pathology, etc. The following divisions represent the major schools of thought relative to the cause of dysfunction and treatment:

1. *Emotional Stress:* The advocates of stress being a primary cause of temporomandibular joint pain-dysfunction are legion in the healing arts. In the past few years D. M. Laskin and his group at the University of Illinois Dental School have done extensive testing of hundreds of patients with the temporomandibular joint dysfunction symptom. Their studies and reports point to the need for a complete diagnosis in the treatment of these patients. Their work emphasizes the contribution of emotional overtones that may create, contribute to, or complicate the disturbance. This school of thought believes that psychiatric counseling, muscle relaxants, and tranquilizers, in conjunction with muscle exercise, will do much to relieve the disturbance. Their personality analysis of these patients and their treatment regime are keyed to a psychological, rather than a physical or pathological, problem.

2. *Dental Malocclusion:* This school believes that the occurrence of teeth that are out of balance with their counterparts in the opposite jaw initiate neural reflexes that cause a jaw shift. This results, in time, in muscle spasms of certain craniofacial and cervical muscles and a segment of the associated pain dysfunction pattern.

Followers of this school believe it essential to "balance the bite" by means of dental restoration, tooth grinding (occlusal equilibration), or by means of placing a removable denture-like appliance. The latter is designed to disarticulate the teeth of the mandible and maxilla, and thus interrupt the neurogenic reflexes that prompted the jaw shift and myospasm. This group stresses the importance of sound dental procedures and the physiological construction of removable dental appliances.

3. *Neuromuscular:* That this category is recognized distinctly does not imply that the neuromuscular system is not an integral part of the other groups. The separation of this group is intended merely to acknowledge the fact that many practitioners who deal with temporomandibular joint dysfunction may at some junction apply therapy directed solely toward the nerves and muscles. Those individuals who approach the problem as a neuromuscular one believe that spasms of the voluntary

muscles that elevate and move the jaw indicate a shift of the jaw, which in turn alters the relation of the teeth of the maxilla and mandible. Lazlo Schwartz recommended moist heat packs to the involved muscles, muscle relaxants, and even local anesthetic injection into the involved muscles; this treatment is aimed at relieving the spasm to permit the jaw to return to its more normal, balanced posture. H. I. Magoun has cited a possible role of the cranial articulations, fascia, and musculature in his mode of treatment.

4. *Osteoarthritic Pathology:* This particular entity does not eclipse the importance of the preceding, but at all times must be considered as a possible cause of dysfunction and pain in and about the temporomandibular joint.

Clearly, temporomandibular joint dysfunction problems are complex. Though the rationales of treatment among the various groups of practitioners overlap to a certain degree, the universal application of a single procedure to a variety of patients is bound to fail in a number of cases; thus, the mode of treatment chosen must be in accord with the diagnosed cause.

## Groups and Associations

(447.2) **AMERICAN EQUILIBRATION SOCIETY**
School of Dental Medicine
Southern Illinois University
Edwardsville, IL 62025

*Atten: Richard E. Coy, DDS, Secretary*

(618) 692-2000

Organized for the study of lesions in the TMJ (temporal mandibular joint) and related structures.

(447.3) **AMERICAN ACADEMY OF CRANIO-MANDIBULAR ORTHOPEDICS**
Macomb Professional Building
11885 East Twelve Mile Road
Warren, MI 48093

(313) 573-0030

*Stuart Davidson, DDS, Secretary*

Dedicated to elucidating modes of treatment and diagnosis for the syndrome of craniomandibular dysfunction, and to educate the medical-dental profession as to the occurrence of this syndrome. Toward this end the Academy holds monthly regional groups, meetings and workshops, encourages schools and hospitals to establish C.M. dysfunction clinics, supports a journal on the subject, and establishes an international professional meeting ground. A speakers' bureau is available for the dissemination of pertinent information.

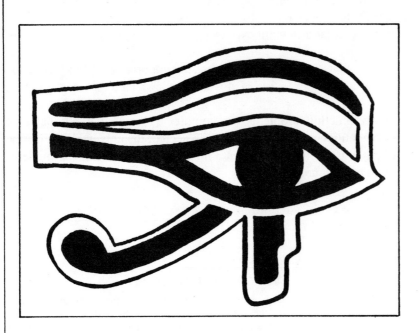

# Developmental Vision Therapy
*Raymond L. Gottlieb, OD*

*"The history of the living world can be summarized as the elaboration of ever more perfect eyes within a cosmos in which there is always something more to see.*

*Teilhard de Chardin*

The importance of vision in our daily lives can hardly be overstated. How well we see and remember has an obvious impact on us as we develop. This is true not only in terms of academic and professional achievement, but in regard to social and personal adjustment and self-esteem as well. If people can be taught to see twice as fast, remember twice as much and with less effort, profound change is bound to occur in the quality and consciousness of their lives. They become more powerful and vital human beings. If the quality of perceptual skills can be improved in children, the benefit to their lives may be immeasurable.

Developmental visual training is designed to do just that. It was originally conceived as a result of the observation that some people are unskilled at some basic visual abilities, such as the ability to aim the eyes precisely, to move the eyes from point to point, to follow a moving object, to use the two eyes together. Clearly, once learned and integrated, this coordination could lead to profound and surprising changes in a patient's whole life.

Two facts soon became evident: that vision is a learned and therefore trainable process; and that the way people use their visual system is a measure of the way they use their brain and thus is, to some extent, an analog of their consciousness and system of reality.

"The prison house is the world of sight," stated Plato over two millennia ago. History is filled with ideas about vision and its relation to health and consciousness. Developmental vision therapy has emerged over the past 70 years as a growing optometric specialty. Like so many other evolving forms of therapies which deal with human potential, its model is diversified and increasingly wholistic.*

---

*Spelled holistic in original text.*

The therapy is itself usually highly individualized, depending on the needs and circumstances of the patient. Approaches include techniques involving optical devices such as stereoscopes; movement, using balancing and trampoline devices; lenses and prisms, as training devices; flashing light sources; specific color therapy, to stimulate and balance the sensory systems and the body; biofeedback; hypnotism; posture and body work; and nutrition. Most practitioners use a variety of approaches. All, however, observe some common principles, such as staying very sensitive to the functioning process that a patient displays as a new goal or skill is learned and integrated. Such behavioral characteristics as attention span, frustration level, coordination, efforting, avoidance of dependency behavior, and figure-ground, central-peripheral, temporal and multisensory organization and flexibility are important for developing useful and integrated visual perception and human potential.

## Groups and Associations

(448) INTERNATIONAL ORTHOKERTOLOGY SECTION OF THE NATIONAL EYE RESEARCH FOUNDATION
18 South Michigan Avenue
Chicago, IL 60603

(312) 726-7866

Represents individual optometrists engaged in the field of orthokertology. "Orthokertology is that procedure designed to effect the reduction or elimination of refractive anomalies and binocular dysfunctions by the programmed application of contact lenses." Publishes the *Journal of Orthokertology*.

(449) ACADEMY OF CORRECTIVE OPTOMETRY
6320 Rockhill Road
Kansas City, MO 64131

*Cecil Henry, OD, Secretary-Treasurer*

607 North High Street
California, MO 65018

(314) 396-2222

Promulgates two forms of corrective visual therapy, syntonic optometry and photoretinology. "Photoretinology is the method of bringing the corticovisual system into balance by use of quantum energies of the visual spectrum. These energies incident into the eye increase the efficiency of both the sensory and motor visual pathways. This method improves visual perception, reception and projection to and from the brain, thus resulting in space being perceived as a whole rather than vision becoming a hole in space; the latter being the case when the peripheral fields are constricted." Photoretinology is recommended for patients with slow reading ability, perceptual problems and dyslexia.

(450) THE AMERICAN OPTOMETRIC ASSOCIATION
7000 Chippewa Street
St. Louis, MO 63119

(314) 832-5770

The AOA is a national organization composed of 51 affiliate organizations representing doctors of optometry in the U.S. The Association works toward furthering the quality of vision care provided by its members. Included in its services are programs relating to vision development and its relationship to the total health of the person. The Association publishes the *Journal of the American Optometric Association*, which is concerned with disseminating new and technical information as well as historical and other educational writing in the field of optometry.

(451) THE OPTOMETRIC EXTENSION PROGRAM FOUNDATION, INC.
Duncan, OK 73533

(405) 277-2230

A continuing education program providing optometrists with monthly courses, regional seminars, and information about local study groups. Reprints of research studies also available.

## Schools, Centers, and Clinics

(452) CENTER FOR THE CORBETT-BATES METHOD
17200 Ventura Boulevard, Suite 305
Encino, CA 91316

(213) 986-0886

*Janet Goodrich, PhD*

Offers group classes, private lessons, out-of-town workshops, and a teacher training program in the Corbett-Bates Method of vision improvement. The lessons retrain the mind and eye to see clearly through techniques of movement, relaxation, centralization, imagination, and visual memory. The central premise of the method is that many eye problems are a by-product of tension.

(453) LIBRA CENTER FOR EYES AND VISION (at Wellness Resource Center)
42 Miller Avenue
Mill Valley, CA 94941

(415) 383-3806

*Kenneth Maue, PhD, Director*

A holistic treatment program for nearsighted, farsighted, and astigmatic persons. Uses the Bates Method and centering techniques, as well as "Info-Flow" learning games that put vision in the context of activity.

SAN ANDREAS HEALTH CENTER (multidisciplinary)
/Palo Alto, CA (see 101)

**SAN DIEGO NATURAL HEALTH CLINIC** (holistic clinic)/San Diego, CA **(see 108)**

**CORNUCOPIA CENTERS** (educational) /Miami, FL **(see 124)**

**RAMANA HEALTH CENTRE** (wholistic hospital) / Hants, England **(see 161)**

**(454) PSYCHOSENSORIAL TRAINING** (applied neurophysiology)
10, Boulevard Princess Charlotte
Bloc 1
Monte Carlo, Monaco

Tel: 301067

*Marguerite Quertant, Director*

The purpose of psychosensorial training (PST) is to eliminate functional disorders using an educational method of applied neurophysiology. The Quertant method consists of two parts: examination to determine the presence of the functional disorder which determines the second part, the educational or training phase. PST uses the eye-optic nerve unit (1) to gain access to the regulatory nerve centers in the base of the brain, (2) to examine their functional efficiency, and (3) to educate gymnastically these same nerve centers to eliminate the disorder. This method is effective in sensory disorders (color blindness, nystagmus, deafness), drug addiction, neurosis and depression, nervous fatigue, severe dyslexia, epilepsy, migraine, psychomotor instability, skin allergies, hypermotivity, and many other disorders. Plans include setting up an international training center and further research. Additional information on request.

## Schools (Colleges and Universities)

**(455) UNIVERSITY OF ALABAMA IN BIRMINGHAM**
School of Optometry/Medical Center
University Station
Birmingham, AL 35294

(205) 934-4011

Offers degree program in vision development therapy training.

**(456) UNIVERSITY OF CALIFORNIA, BERKELEY**
School of Optometry
101 Optometry Building
Berkeley, CA 94720

(415) 642-3303

Offers degree program in vision development therapy training.

**(457) COLLEGE OF OPTOMETRISTS IN VISION DEVELOPMENT**
P.O. Box 285
Chula Vista, CA 92012

(714) 420-3010

Certifying body for optometrists in vision therapy, as it relates to strabismus (cross-eyed), amblyopia (lazy-eyed) and binocular (coordination problems). Publishes quarterly journal providing information in the field.

**(458) SOUTHERN CALIFORNIA COLLEGE OF OPTOMETRY**
2001 Associated Road
Fullerton, CA 92631

(714) 870-7226

Offers degree program in vision development therapy training.

**(459) ILLINOIS COLLEGE OF OPTOMETRY**
3241 South Michigan Avenue
Chicago, IL 60616

(312) 225-1700

Offers degree program in vision development therapy training.

**(460) INDIANA UNIVERSITY**
School of Optometry
Bloomington, IN 47401

(812) 337-4447

Offers degree program in vision development therapy training.

**(461) NEW ENGLAND COLLEGE OF OPTOMETRY**
424 Beacon Street
Boston, MA 02115

(617) 261-3430

Offers degree program in vision development therapy training.

**(462) FERRIS STATE COLLEGE**
College of Optometry
Big Rapids, MI 49307

(616) 796-9971

Offers degree program in vision development therapy training.

**(463) STATE UNIVERSITY OF NEW YORK**
State College of Optometry
100 East 24th Street
New York, NY 10010

(212) 477-7900

Offers degree program in vision development therapy training.

**(464) THE OHIO STATE UNIVERSITY**
College of Optometry
338 West Tenth Avenue
Columbus, OH 43210

(614) 422-2647

Offers degree program in vision development therapy training.

**(465) PACIFIC UNIVERSITY**
College of Optometry
Forest Grove, OR 97116

(503) 357-6151

Offers degree program in vision development therapy training.

(466) **PENNSYLVANIA COLLEGE OF OPTOMETRY**
1200 West Godfrey
Philadelphia, PA 19141

(215) 424-5900

Offers degree program in vision development therapy training.

(467) **SOUTHERN COLLEGE OF OPTOMETRY**
1245 Madison Avenue
Memphis, TN 38104

(901) 725-0180

Offers degree program in vision development therapy training.

(468) **UNIVERSITY OF HOUSTON**
College of Optometry
3801 Cullen Boulevard
Houston, TX 77004

(713) 749-3124

Offers degree program in vision development therapy training.

(469) **SCHOOL OF OPTOMETRY**
Montreal University
3333 Queen Mary Road—350
Montreal, PQ, Canada

Offers degree program in vision development therapy training.

(470) **UNIVERSITY OF WATERLOO**
School of Optometry
Faculty of Science
Waterloo, Ontario, Canada

(519) 885-1211

Offers degree program in vision development therapy training.

## Journals and Publications

**JOURNAL OF THE AMERICAN OPTOMETRIC ASSOCIATION**/St. Louis, MO (see 450)

# III
# NUTRITION AND HERBS

---

Preventive Nutrition And Health Maintenance

Macrobiotics And Oriental Medicine

Pharmacognosy In Wholistic Medicine

Parts Or Wholes: An Introduction To The Use Of
Whole Plant Substances In Healing

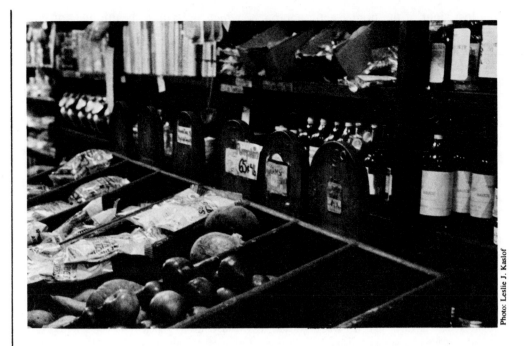

Photo: Leslie J. Kaslof

# Preventive Nutrition And Health Maintenance

*Richard O. Brennan, DO*

*"Living under conditions of modern life, it is important to bear in mind that the preparation and refinement of food products either entirely eliminates or in part destroys the vital elements in the original material."*

United States Government
Dept. of Agriculture

Ancient physicians believed in wholistic* medicine. The early Greek physicians strove to direct the patient's mind and habits into wholesome patterns; thus, they taught their patients to select their foods carefully and to eat less. Hippocrates (460-377 B.C.) taught that the primary treatment of a patient should be based on proper food, rest, fresh air, water, and sunshine. This approach was called *vis medicatrix naturae*, "the healing power of nature," which cures from within.

The advent and the acceptance of the germ theory of disease suddenly rendered the wholistic approach to the treatment and prevention of the chronic degenerative diseases passé. Specificity of the causation of diseases assumed the dominant role in medicine. Medical specialties, based on a disease entity or various body systems, evolved and flourished.

When the "wonder drugs" came into general use, they brought the acute infectious diseases under control. Subsequent advances in medicine consisted of increasingly sophisticated use of antibiotics. New drugs were developed for each disease. Advertising slogans and campaigns touted quick and simple relief from symptoms. The dominance of the drug and chemical industry became a potent force in displacing the ancient idea that medicine should treat the whole person and his or her environment.

Probably the most damaging and stunning blow to the practice and the philosophy of wholistic medicine was dealt by the emergence of the tranquilizer and antidepressant drugs, which can cover up and mask the symptoms of many nutritional-deficiency diseases. Though these symptoms may be alleviated or palliated by such drugs, the patient is not being treated as a whole person and the condition will persist.

We have become far too overeducated and oversophisticated about the details of our metabolic

---

*Spelled holistic in original text.

95

processes. We have lost sight of the homeostatic approach, which is basic to health and, of course, to disease.

Walter B. Cannon, MD, wrote in *The Wisdom of the Body* (W. W. Norton, 1926):

The constant conditions which are maintained in the body might be termed "equilibria." That word, however, has come to have fairly exact meaning as applied to relatively simple physical chemical states, in closed systems, where known forces are balanced . . . . The coordinated physiological processes which maintain most of the steady states in the organism are so complex and so peculiar to living beings—involving, as they may, the brain, nerves, the heart, lungs, kidneys, and spleen, all working cooperatively—that I have suggested a special designation for these states, "homeostates." . . . The word does not imply something set and immobile, as stagnation. It means a condition, a condition which may vary but is relatively constant.

In 1885, the Belgian philosopher Leon Frederick stated:

The living being is an agency of such sorts that each disturbing influence induces by itself the calling forth of compensatory activity to neutralize or repair the disturbance. The higher in the scale of living things, the more numerous, the more perfect, and the more complicated, these regulatory agencies become. They tend to free the organism completely from the unfavorable influences and changes occurring in the environment.

In 1900, Charles Richet, the French philosopher, wrote:

The living being is stable. It must be so, in order not to be destroyed, dissolved, or disintegrated by the colossal forces, often adverse, which surround it. By an apparent contradiction it maintains its stability only if it is excitable and capable of modifying itself according to external stimuli and adjusting its response to the stimulation. In a sense it is stable because it is modifiable—the slight instability is the necessary condition for the true stability of the organism.

The isolation of individual nutrients, initiated in 1911 by the epoch-making discoveries of Casimir Funk, a Polish biochemist, led to our present understanding of the nutrients he called *vitamine*. Clinical observations suggested a connection between isolated and individual nutrients and certain deficiency diseases. Thus, the concept of deficiency disease is relatively modern and is still not sufficiently understood or applied.

The vast amount of research that has been done on the food factors that we call "nutrients" has led to a rapidly expanding recognition of the value of applied nutrition. We understand that these nutrients are necessary to health—indeed, to life—and that inadequate consumption of these nutrients results in disease. However, we often overlook that many deficiency states are attributable to widespread subclinical deficiencies and a lack of essential substances; the idea of minute deficiences is only beginning to gain acceptance.

Many clinicians today are recognizing that the incidence of mild, latent, or "subclinical" deficiencies is much greater than they generally supposed. These deficiencies, rather than the more advanced cases, require our attention if we are to prevent the escalating incidence of chronic degenerative diseases. Clinical deficiences are difficult to detect; they affect great numbers of people and are apt to pass unnoticed and untreated. Since characteristic individual nutrient disease conditions are not prevalent, the patient's general health and efficiency are affected only indirectly.

Two important factors are generally overlooked: (1) many deficiencies are induced by the development of other diseases, without which they would not occur; and (2) nutritional deficiencies may affect other diseases, such as infections. Though some deficiencies may seem to be caused by individual nutrient factors, resulting in a distinctive disease pattern, that does not mean that only those particular diseased tissues are affected—they are interrelated with the other parts of the body.

Nutrients are clearly basic factors in the activities of living cells, though they cannot be made or synthesized by the body. Moreover, nutrients show a consistent lack of toxicity, or potentiality for harm, to the body's basic metabolic processes. While the cells of the body may still function, suboptimally, with an occasional inadequate supply of nutrients, optimal supply favors optimal growth and functions, and an excess has no effect; it is eliminated without injury to the cells and their processes.

Laboratory research projects and the major clinics have concentrated primarily on the effects of the minimum amounts of the nutrient factors (that is, the focus has been mainly on the appearance of frank deficiency disease). Almost no research has been done to determine the optimum amount of essential nutrients and their effect on health. A so-called state of health, in which detectable disease is absent, is insufficient; as far as nutrition is concerned, we need to find out the amounts of nutrients "that would provide the utmost in health." And another subject we need to study is the interrelationships of optimum amounts of nutrients.

One dictionary definition of food is: "What is eaten, or taken into the body, for nourishment, more broadly, whatever supplies nourishment to organic bodies . . . . Nutriment, that on which anything subsists . . . something that sustains." "Sustains" is an excellent word; however, most of our food in America today will support life, but it won't sustain health.

Unfortunately, clinicians wait until deficiency diseases are fully developed and obvious before they think to diagnose nutritional deficiency and institute treatment. Generally speaking, there are four things that should be considered in diagnosing dietary deficiencies. They are (1) an analytical evaluation of the dietary intake, (2) the signs and symptoms of a possible deficiency state, as determined by history and physical examination, (3) laboratory test, and (4) a clinical trial of the "therapeutic augmentation of concentrated nutrients."

To treat the ill, the modern system of specialized medicine today looks first to the alleviation and palliation of symptoms, then to surgery. The basic processes of healing and restoring function, which should be considered an integral part of medicine, have been neglected or, too often, recommended by persons lacking in source material and background to give proper counseling. Modern medicine needs to rediscover the aphorisms of ancient medicine. The world is crying out for wholistic preventive medical health care.

## Groups and Associations

(471) INTERNATIONAL ACADEMY OF BIOLOGICAL MEDICINE, INC.
P.O. Box 31313
Phoenix, AZ 85046

*Paavo O. Airola, PhD, ND, President*

Equips participating physicians with theoretical and practical knowledge on effective nutritional and other biological alternatives to conventional therapies and drugs.

(472) CALIFORNIA ORTHOMOLECULAR MEDICAL SOCIETY
2340 Parker Street
Berkeley, CA 94704

(415) 848-8595

*Michael Lesser, MD, President*

Areas of interest include role of vitamins in the prevention and treatment of disease, air ionization, chelation therapy, hair analysis, acupuncture, and kinesiology. An annual meeting is held in which original research is presented.

(473) THE NATIONAL HEALTH FEDERATION
212 West Foothill Boulevard
Monrovia, CA 91016

(213) 358-1155

A national, consumer rights organization that educates legislators, health planners, and other concerned groups about the role of alternative medical practices in the overall health care system of the nation. Also involved in legislative action to minimize harassment of such movements. Indi-

viduals and groups are invited to join, and receive a subscription to the Federation's newsletter. There is also an associated NHF library for legal briefs and information on practice and philosophy of various therapeutic disciplines.

(474) AMERICAN ACADEMY OF MEDICAL PREVENTICS
11311 Camarillo Street
North Hollywood, CA 91602

(213) 878-1234

*Garry F. Gordon, MD, President*

Provides educational programs and conferences for physicians and the lay public in nutrition, megavitamins, and chelation therapy. Also maintains a referral service of physicians knowledgeable in chelation therapy, and a reference library on chelation therapy and related subjects. Founded 1973.

CENTER FOR INTEGRAL MEDICINE (educational)
/Pacific Palisades, CA (see 57)

(475) INTERNATIONAL ACADEMY OF METABOLOGY, INC.
1000 East Walnut Street, Suite 247
Pasadena, CA 91106

(213) 795-7772

*Gerard E. Stavish, PhD (Cand.), Executive Director*

Nonprofit organization of dentists, nutritionists, physicians, biologists, biochemists, and other scientists with a special interest and knowledge in the field of metabolic diseases. Develops educational programs, clinical approaches, and research projects in metabology. Cassette tape recordings of workshops and conferences are available from the Academy. Publishes a bimonthly newsletter with research notes on vitàmins, endocrinology, allergy and food science.

**(476) THE ACOS FOUNDATION**
649 Irving Street
San Francisco, CA 94122

(415) 664-1464

*Jimmy Scott, PhD, Executive Director*

A nonprofit education and research foundation sponsoring workshops and symposia in nutrition, with special reference to its role in psychophysiology. In planning is a Community Health and Nutrition Center which will include a shop that will sell vitamins, minerals, books, and other health items, a lending library, and support groups for fasting, exercise, and other health activities.

**(477) SAN FRANCISCO VEGETARIAN SOCIETY**
1450 Broadway, #4
San Francisco, CA 94109

*Alexander Everett, Vice President*

A nonprofit organization which holds seminars and lectures on vegetarianism and nutrition. Publishes a newsletter, *Veg News.*

**(478) THE HEALTH CORPS**
P.O. Box 333
Venice, CA 90291

(213) 275-3314

*Joan Simmons, Director*

Disseminates information on nutrition and natural treatment for metabolic disorders such as hypoglycemia. A practical health care system, Inner Ecology, is the mainstay of the Corps and involves attention to food groups, vitamins, and minerals. The Corps will send free to any interested party a copy of a diagnostic "Health Indicator Test," designed for patients with blood sugar disorders. Exercise, meditation, and other healing methods are taught through written and taped lessons, a monthly health bulletin and a bimonthly newsletter. Founded 1976.

**(479) NATIONAL NUTRITIONAL FOODS ASSOCIATION**
7727 South Painter Avenue
Whittier, CA 90602

(213) 945-2669

Membership organization seeking to improve products and to disseminate information in the nutritional field. Holds annual conference spotlighting various issues and speakers in the field.

**(480) HUXLEY INSTITUTE FOR BIOSOCIAL RESEARCH**
Green Farms, CT 06436

(203) 259-2191

*Anne Crellin Seggerman, President and Founder*

Provides information on treatment for a variety of disorders which include alcoholism, anorexia nervosa, autism, drug addiction, hyperactivity, learning disabilities, memory loss, retardation, schizophrenia, and senility. This information is available to professionals, government, and the public. The Institute believes in individualized treatment through nutrition and vitamins. Services include speakers' bureau, newsletter, professional referral service, and a library (for members).

**(481) THE AMERICAN NATURAL HYGIENE SOCIETY, INC.**
National Headquarters
1920 Irving Park Road
Chicago, IL 60613

(312) 929-7420

Coordinates local chapters throughout the U.S., Canada, England, and Australia. Natural Hygiene is a system of living, emphasizing the value of unadulterated, vegetarian foods, and fasting. A wide range of books on the subject are available from the Natural Hygiene Press, at the above address. Has list available of professional hygienists and fasting retreats around the country.

**(482) FOUNDATION FOR NUTRITIONAL RESEARCH**
1 North LaSalle Street
Chicago, IL 60602

A nonprofit, public service institution, chartered to investigate and disseminate nutritional information. A special focus of the Foundation is the development of dietary regimes for diabetes and hypoglycaemia.

**SOCIETY FOR THE PROTECTION OF THE UNBORN THROUGH NUTRITION**/Chicago, IL **(see 4)**

**(483) SOCIETY OF BIOLOGICAL PSYCHIATRY**
Tulane Medical Center
1415 Tulane Avenue
New Orleans, LA 70112

(504) 588-5231

*Arthur W. Epstein, MD, Secretary-Treasurer*

A group of research oriented scientists and clinicians interested in the biological nature of psychiatry. The disciplines of various members include neurology, psychology, neurophysiology, neuroanatomy, and neurochemistry. Founded 1945. Incorporated 1949.

**(484) ECOLOGOS**
80 Martin Road
Milton, MA 02186

(617) 698-9161

An intentional community and research organization dedicated to maximizing the world's food supply and human health through return to a diet of raw fruits, green leafy vegetables, and nuts. Toward this end, Ecologos is in the process of establishing healing clinics emphasizing raw food diet, fasting and hygiene, planting organic orchards of fruit and nut trees, training teachers of natural healing and ecologically harmonious lifestyle, and establishing research stations for study of the optimum relationship between human life and other natural processes.

**(485) NUTRITIONAL RESEARCH ASSOCIATION**
610 Third Avenue
Bradley Beach, NJ 07720

A fraternal organization whose main objective is to restore, maintain, and improve the physical and spiritual health of the United States by educating its members about food and nutrition, exercise and natural living, and spiritual advancement, and by compiling and disseminating nutritional research information. Membership available; contact the Association for further information.

**(486) THE AMERICAN VEGAN SOCIETY**
Box H
Malaga, NJ 08328

(609) 694-2887

Nonprofit, nonsectarian organization advocating abstinence from all animal products (including both foods and products such as cosmetics) and the doctrine of Ahimsa (nonslaughter, nonviolence, harmlessness). The Society is involved in researching alternative sources for animal products currently used (e.g., milk, honey, wool, fur, leather), and conducting educational programs on the virtues of Ahimsa. The society publishes a bimonthly magazine, *Ahimsa*. Books and literature on veganism are also available by mail.

**(487) NORTH AMERICAN VEGETARIAN SOCIETY**
501 Old Harding Highway
Malaga, NJ 08328

(609) 694-2887

Nonprofit, nonsectarian educational organization involved in coordinating the vegetarian movement in the USA and Canada. Organizes national and international vegetarian congresses, establishes centers for educational vegetarian work, and promotes research into the scientific, ethical, and other aspects of vegetarianism. The Society also disseminates information on these subjects, and publishes a bimonthly magazine, *Vegetarian Voice*. Membership is open both to vegetarians and nonvegetarians with an interest in the movement.

**(488) HEALTH ASSOCIATES**
2910 Grand Concourse, #3B
Bronx, NY 10458

(212) 298-1295

*Lewis Harrison, BA, AA, Director*

Has available information on the importance of good nutrition in maintaining health.

**JEWISH VEGETARIAN SOCIETY**/Forest Hills, NY **(see 494)**

**(489) ACADEMY OF ORTHOMOLECULAR PSYCHIATRY**
1691 Northern Boulevard
Manhasset, NY 11030

(516) 627-7260

*Allan Cott, MD, President*

Disseminates scientific information in the field of orthomolecular psychiatry and serves as a meeting ground for professionals to extend their knowledge in the field. Also coordinates training in orthomolecular psychiatry. Professional membership is limited to those practicing orthomolecular psychiatry or to those who have made some original contribution to the field. Members receive the *Journal of Orthomolecular Medicine*. Founded 1971.

**(490) INTERNATIONAL ACADEMY OF PREVENTIVE MEDICINE**
10409 Town & Country Way, Suite 200
Houston, TX 77024

(713) 468-7851

*Joseph A. Nowell, Executive Director*

Nonprofit educational society for health care professionals interested in the prevention of disease and the applications of medical nutrition in health maintenance. The Academy sponsors conferences and seminars for health care professionals and publishes proceedings books, a journal, and a newsletter for members. A directory of members is available from IAPM for $3.50, postage paid, to assist in locating healthcare professionals interested in preventive medicine.

**(491) CANADIAN ASSOCIATION FOR PREVENTIVE AND ORTHOMOLECULAR MEDICINE**
2177 Park Crescent
Coquitlam, British Columbia
Canada V3J 6T1

(604) 461-9383

*Loyd Wisheart, President*

Organization of physicians, nonmedical healers, and lay persons dedicated to promoting and developing orthomolecular medicine, encouraging the improvement of food quality and elimination of additives and adulterants, and disseminating information in these areas through meetings, seminars, lectures, and the publication of literature. Founded 1975.

**(492) CANADIAN HEALTH FOOD ASSOCIATION**
c/o Mrs. Florence Hogg
20440 Douglas Crescent
Langley, British Columbia
Canada V3A 4B4

Represents the cause of natural therapeutics to the legislative bodies of British Columbia and Canada.

**(493) CONSUMER HEALTH ORGANIZATION OF CANADA**
108 Willowdale Avenue
Willowdale, Ontario M2N 4X9
Canada

(416) 222-3083

*L. Shelly, Director*

An affiliate of the National Health Federation, the CHOC holds seminars and symposia concerned with all aspects of health and nutrition.

**(494) THE JEWISH VEGETARIAN SOCIETY**
855 Finchley Road
London NW11 8LX
England

Tel: 01-455 0692

*Philip L. Pick, FFS, President*

American Secretariat
c/o Judah Grosberg
63-38 Yellowstone Boulevard
Forest Hills, NY 11375

(212) 459-1014

Through educational programs and a journal *(Bet Teva)* the Society encourages vegetarianism on an interantional level as a solution to the world's food problems. Emphasis is on making known the Jewish teachings concerning vegetarianism as a way of life.

(495) **THE HOWEY FOUNDATION**
2a Lebanon Road
Croydon
Surrey, CRO 6UR
England

Tel: 01-654 5817

*W. Gummer, General Secretary*

An independent, nonsectarian, nonprofit organization dedicated to developing solutions to the ecological problems of modern society. It concerns itself with such issues as pollution, artificial additives, meat eating and vegetarianism, organic agriculture, and husbandry. The Foundation relies entirely on donations and is a registered charity.

## Schools, Centers, and Clinics

**HEALTH AWARENESS INSTITUTE** (clinic) /Phoenix, AZ **(see 74)**

**BERKELEY HOLISTIC HEALTH CENTER** (educational) /Berkeley, CA **(see 76)**

**PSYCHOSOMATIC MEDICINE CLINIC** (holistic therapy) /Berkeley, CA **(see 78)**

**CENTER FOR FAMILY GROWTH** (birth) /Cotati, CA **(see 8)**

**BIOLOGY OF THE MIND/BODY** (workshop)/Davis, CA **(see 80)**

**NATIONAL ARTHRITIS MEDICAL CLINIC**/Desert Hot Springs, CA **(see 81)**

**WHOLISTIC MEDICINE AND PERSONAL GROWTH CENTER**/Hawthorne, CA **(see 84)**

**ISLA VISTA OPEN DOOR MEDICAL CLINIC**/Isla Vista, CA **(see 85)**

(496) **INTERNATIONAL COLLEGE OF APPLIED NUTRITION**
Box 386
La Habra, CA 90631

Nonprofit organization disseminating scientific information in the field of nutrition. Publishes the *Journal of Applied Nutrition.*

**BARAKA** (holistic center) /Los Angeles, CA **(see 87)**

**HOLISTIC HEALTH CENTER** (educational center) /Los Angeles, CA **(see 90)**

**INSTITUTE OF REALITY AWARENESS** (health counseling) /Los Angeles, CA **(see 91)**

**KHALSA MEDICAL AND COUNSELING ASSOCIATES** (multidisciplinary clinic) /Los Angeles, CA **(see 92)**

**WHITE CROSS SOCIETY** (workshops) /Lucerne Valley, CA **(see 93)**

**McCORNACK CENTER FOR THE HEALING ARTS** (multidisciplinary clinic) /Mendocino, CA **(see 95)**

**LOMI SCHOOL** (body work) /Mill Valley, CA **(see 835)**

**WELLNESS RESOURCE CENTER** (preventive therapy center) /Mill Valley, CA **(see 96)**

**WHOLISTIC HEALTH AND NUTRITION INSTITUTE** (educational) /Mill Valley, CA **(see 97)**

**AUTOGENIC HEALTH CENTER** /Oakland, CA **(see 98)**

**GEORGE OHSAWA MACROBIOTIC FOUNDATION**/Oroville, CA **(see 535)**

**SAN ANDREAS HEALTH CENTER** (multidisciplinary)/Palo Alto, CA **(see 101)**

**LIFE AND HEALTH MEDICAL GROUP** (clinic) / Redlands, CA **(see 102)**

**SACRAMENTO MEDICAL PREVENTICS CLINIC** (holistic clinic) /Sacramento, CA **(see 103)**

**AGE OF ENLIGHTENMENT CENTER FOR HOLISTIC HEALTH** (Transcendental Meditation and health) /San Diego, CA **(see 104)**

**SAN DIEGO NATURAL HEALTH CLINIC** (holistic clinic) /San Diego, CA **(see 108)**

**EAST-WEST ACADEMY OF HEALING ARTS** (educational) /San Francisco, CA **(see 110)**

**NURSE CONSULTANTS AND HEALTH COUNSELORS** (educational) /San Francisco, CA **(see 112)**

**ASSOCIATED PSYCHOLOGISTS OF SANTA CLARA**/Santa Clara, CA **(see 114)**

**FAMILY PRACTICE CENTER** (clinic) /Santa Rosa, CA **(see 116)**

**INTEGRAL HEALTH SERVICES** (multidisciplinary clinic) /Putnam, CT **(see 120)**

**STAMFORD CENTER FOR THE HEALING ARTS** (wholistic clinic in a church) /Stamford, CT **(see 121)**

**INSTITUTE OF PNEUMOLOGY** (acupuncture) / Washington, DC **(see 638)**

**MANKIND RESEARCH FOUNDATION** (heuristic research) /Washington, DC (see 122)

**CORNUCOPIA CENTERS** (educational center) /Miami, FL (see 124)

**(497) HUMAN LIFE STYLING**
Box 3405
Seminole, FL 33542

(813) 894-4151

*John McCamy, MD, Chairman*

Maximizing of health level through nutrition, movement, and stress reduction. Serves as consultants to industry and offers workshops in the design of preventive health care systems.

**(498) HUMAN ECOLOGY RESEARCH FOUNDATION**
505 North Lake Shore Drive
Chicago, IL 60611

(312) 828-9480

*Theron G. Randolph, MD, Director*

Attempts to demonstrate nutritional/environmental causes of heretofore unexplained diseases. Patients first fast in an environmentally controlled "ecology unit," and are then fed single food meals. Patients are observed after they return to home and work, and correlations are made between specific foods and somatic imbalance.

**FOUNDATION OF TRUTH** (spiritual growth) / Indianapolis, IN, also Essex, England (see 62)

**CENTERS FOR HEALTH AND LIFE** (education and treatment) /Des Moines, IA (see 126)

**MARTIN BUBER INSTITUTE** (educational wholistic center) /Columbia, MD (see 127)

**INSTITUTE FOR HUMANISTIC AND TRANSPERSONAL EDUCATION**/Amherst, MA (see 1147)

**EAST WEST FOUNDATION** (macrobiotics) /Boston, MA (see 536)

**(499) HIPPOCRATES HEALTH INSTITUTE**
25 Exeter Street
Boston, MA 02116

(617) 267-9525

*Ann Wigmore, DD, Director*

Provides a residential center for education and body cleansing. The method includes a raw food diet primarily consisting of sprouted seeds and the use of a high-chlorophyll, wheat-grass extract. The Institute has claimed the program to be efficacious in treating a wide gamut of maladies, including cancer. Educational programs include classes in polarity massage, organic gardening indoors, and reflexology. Founded 1963.

**ACUPUNCTURE CENTER OF MASSACHUSETTS**/ Newton, MA (see 130)

**(500) AMERICAN ACADEMY OF NUTRITIONAL CONSULTANTS**
500 Dorian Road
Westfield, NJ 07090

(201) 233-5858

*Arnold J. Susser, President*

Sponsors 20 seminars per year on nutrition and related fields. Membership open to any health care professional who attends at least ten of these.

**DESERT LIGHT FOUNDATION** (educational clinic) / Albuquerque, NM (see 134)

**(501) SCHOOL OF SCIENTIFIC NUTRITION, INC.**
1605 Coal Avenue, S.E.
Albuquerque, NM 87106

(505) 243-6749

*Hazel R. Parcells, PhD, Founder*

Offers classes in beginning and advanced radiesthesia and nutrition.

**(502) NATIONAL NUTRITION WORKSHOP CENTERS, INC.**
99 Railroad Station Plaza
Hicksville, NY 11801

(516) 931-1575

Holds workshops in the New York-Long Island area on nutrition and publishes a newsletter, *Nutrition Naturally.*

**HEALTHORIUM** (nutritional information) /Lawrence, NY (see 20)

**INSTITUTE FOR SELF DEVELOPMENT** (educational) /Manhasset, NY (see 137)

**ARTHRITIS MEDICAL CENTER** /New York, NY (see 138)

**(503) NUTRITION INSTITUTE OF AMERICA**
200 West 86th Street, Suite 17-A
New York, NY 10024

(212) 595-9256

*Gary Null, Director*

Nonprofit research, evaluation, and referral center in the fields of nutrition, psychology, environmental studies, chemistry, and paranormal healing. Maintains a large comprehensive research laboratory, library, and research files, all open to the serious investigator. Publishes a monthly consumer magazine, *Caveat Emptor.*

**TREE OF LIFE** (educational center) /New York, NY (see 142)

**(504) NUTRITION EDUCATION CENTER, INC.**
P.O. Box 303
Oyster Bay, NY 11771

(516) 692-5150

*Eleanor Krinsky, Executive Director*

Serves as a centralized clearing house for information on all aspects of nutrition and related fields. Sponsors lectures, workshops, and structured courses in nutrition, and publishes a newsletter, *Nutrition in Life*, which condenses important research and articles in the field.

**ALTERNATIVE HEALTH EDUCATION CENTER** (educational) /Rochester, NY **(see 143)**

**PSI CENTER** (educational and clinic facilities) / Cincinnati, OH **(see 145)**

**EUGENE CENTER FOR THE HEALING ARTS** (educational) /Eugene, OR **(see 148)**

**(505) GREAT OAKS SCHOOL OF HEALTH**
82644 North Howe Lane
Creswell, OR 97426

(503) 895-4967

*Isabelle Moser, RN, PhD, and Douglas Moser, PhD, Directors*

Provides supervision for fasting, and educational programs in megavitamins, nutrition, yoga, meditation, and alternative healing methods. Also offers marriage and family counseling, and testing for allergy.

**INSTITUTE OF PREVENTIVE MEDICINE** (medical counseling) /Portland, OR **(see 149)**

**NATUROPATHIC BIRTH CENTER**/Winston, OR **(see 23)**

**(506) AMERICAN MEDICAL SYMPOSIA** (a trust)
7616 LBJ Freeway, Suite 229
Dallas, TX 75251

(214) 233-8039

*Don Cerveny, Director*

Offers monthly "electromedical therapeutic teaching seminars" plus an annual midwinter conference with emphasis on nutrition, preventive health care, and holistic concepts.

**(507) DR. SHELTON'S HEALTH SCHOOL**
P.O. Box 1277
San Antonio, TX 78295

(512) 497-3613

*Herbert M. Shelton, PhD, Director*

Dedicated to teaching a "hygienic way of life," through fasting, organic foods, exercise, sunbathing, and "right living."

**HOME CENTER** (medical educational center) /Virginia Beach, VA **(see 155)**

**PREVENTIVE MEDICINE CLINIC**/Bellevue, WA **(see 156)**

**COLD MOUNTAIN INSTITUTE** (educational) / Vancouver, B.C., Canada **(see 1130)**

**SERENITY HEALTH EDUCATION CENTRE** (educational) /Vancouver, B.C., Canada **(see 159)**

**DIAT- UND KNIEPP-SANATORIUM DR. FELBER-MAYER** (clinic) /Austria **(see 812)**

**LATIN AMERICAN MISSION PROGRAM, INSTITUTO NATURISTA ADVENTISTA** (wholistic clinic) /Guatemala, Central America **(see 160)**

**3-L BHAVAN** (herbs) /Hull, England **(see 162)**

**ITA-WEGMAN-KLINIK** (anthroposophical clinic) / Arlesheim, Switzerland **(see 813)**

**LUKAS KLINIK** (anthroposophical clinic) /West Germany **(see 814)**

**OTTO BUCHINGER CLINIC** (wholistic) /West Germany **(see 181)**

**PARACELSUS-KRANKENHAUS** (anthroposophical rest home) /West Germany **(see 822)**

**SANATORIUM SCHLOSS HAMBORN** (anthroposophical clinic) /West Germany **(see 824)**

## Resorts

**LUKATS' PREVENTION REGENERATION RESORT**/Safford, AZ **(see 164)**

**HIDDEN VALLEY HEALTH RANCH** (fasting and rest home) /Escondido, CA **(see 166)**

**MEADOWLARK** (holistic resort) /Hemet, CA **(see 167)**

**ORR SPRINGS ASSOCIATION** (retreat)/Ukiah, CA **(see 170)**

**(508) PAWLING HEALTH MANOR**
Box 401
Hyde Park, NY 12538

(914) 889-4141

*Robert R. Gross, Director*

A resort atmosphere. Encourages fresh air, exercise, natural foods, and rational fasting. No medical advice is given. Founded 1959.

**NEW AGE HEALTH FARM** (resort) /Neversink, NY **(see 172)**

**(509) VEGETARIAN HOTEL**
Woodridge, NY 12789

(914) 434-4455

A health-camp resort, featuring vegetarian meals. Open May 28 through September. Founded 1920.

**TYRINGHAM NATUROPATHIC CLINIC** (wholistic spa) /Bucks, England **(see 177)**

**(510) VILLA VEGETARIANA HEALTH SPA**
Box 1228
Cuernavaca, Mexico

Tel: 3-10-44

*David and Marlene Stry*

Rejuvenation resort specializing in fasting and nutritional education. Founded 1966.

**RIO CALIENTE S.A.** (rest resort) /Guadalajara, Mexico **(see 179)**

## Journals and Publications

**(511) JOURNAL OF APPLIED NUTRITION**
Box 386
La Habra, CA 90631

Published by the International College of Applied Nutrition **(496)**. Contains scientific articles, editorials, abstracts, and book reviews in the field.

**(512) CANCER CONTROL JOURNAL**
2043 North Berendo
Los Angeles, CA 90027

(213) 663-7801

The journal of the Cancer Control Society, which emphasizes the therapeutic uses of Vitamin B17 (found in apricot kernels), as well as other alternative approaches to the treatment of malignancy.

**(513) LET'S LIVE**
444 North Larchmont Boulevard
Los Angeles, CA 90004

(213) 469-3901

*James F. Scheer, Editor*

Monthly magazine with articles on biological medicine, nutrition, natural cosmetics, organic gardening, and natural health.

**NHF NEWSLETTER** (National Health Federation) / Monrovia, CA **(see 473)**

**THE MACROBIOTIC** (journal) /Oroville, CA **(see 535)**

**(514) WHEN** (World Health and Ecology News)
Box Number One
Palm Springs, CA 92262

Newspaper containing articles on nutrition and related subjects.

**INTERNATIONAL ACADEMY OF METABOLOGY NEWSLETTER** (nutrition) /Pasadena, CA **(see 475)**

**COMMON GROUND** (multidisciplinary directory San Francisco Bay Area) /San Francisco, CA **(see 187)**

**LEAVES OF HEALING** (health newsletter) /Santa Monica, CA **(see 189)**

**(515) CNI WEEKLY REPORT**
1910 "K" Street, N.W.
Washington, DC 20006

(202) 833-1730

Newsletter of the Community Nutrition Institute. Articles on federal issues such as welfare, food stamps, and food supplements.

**(516) HEALTHLINE MAGAZINE**
P.O. Drawer 24200
Southwest Station
Washington, DC 20024

(202) 554-2292

*Kern Smith, Publisher*

Articles on nutrition, preventive medicine, and new developments in medicine. Founded 1975.

**(517) NUTRITION ACTION**
Center for Science in the Public Interest
1779 Church Street, N.W.
Washington, DC 20036

(202) 332-4250

Politically oriented newsletter reporting on various situations affecting legislation dealing with nutrition. Ralph Nader affiliate organization.

**ALTERNATIVES JOURNAL** (multidisciplinary new age articles)/Miami, FL **(see 193)**

**SUNSPARK PRESS** (directory of publications) /St. Petersburg, FL **(see 194)**

**ORDER OF THE UNIVERSE** (and other publications of the East West Foundation) (macrobiotic publication) Boston, MA **(see 537)**

**EAST WEST JOURNAL** (multidisciplinary new age articles) /Brookline, MA **(see 195)**

**NEW AGE JOURNAL** (multidisciplinary) /Brookline, MA **(see 196)**

**(518) ACRES U.S.A.**
Box 9547
Raytown, MO 64133

(816) 837-0064

Monthly publication dealing with organic growing methods, nutrition, and environmental science.

**AHIMSA** (journal-vegetarian) /Malaga, NJ **(see 486)**

**JOURNAL OF ORTHOMOLECULAR MEDICINE**/Manhasset, NY (see Academy of Orthomolecular Psychiatry, **498**)

**SEEKER** (multidisciplinary newsletter directory NY area) /New York, NY **(see 202)**

**(519) NATURAL HEALTH BULLETIN**
c/o Parker Publishing Co.
West Nyack, NY 10994

*Carlson Wade, Editor*

Contains articles on herbs, health foods, healing techniques, and various aspects of natural therapeutics and nutrition.

**(520) PLAY 'N TALK BULLETIN**
P.O. Box 18804
Oklahoma City, OK 73118

*Marie A. LeDoux, President*

Newsletter with articles on nutrition, cooking, and vitamins.

**PREVENTION MAGAZINE** (natural health) /Emmaus, PA **(see 205)**

**(521) NATURAL FOOD NEWS**
P.O. Box 210
Atlanta, TX 75551

*Tom Lavin, Editor*

Published monthly by the Natural Food Associates. Makes available information and news in the natural food industry. Also publishes the *Natural Food and Farming* magazine.

**JOURNAL OF THE INTERNATIONAL ACADEMY OF PREVENTIVE MEDICINE** (nutrition) /Houston, TX **(see 490)**

**(522) DR. SHELTON'S HYGIENIC REVIEW**
P.O. Box 1277
San Antonio, TX 78295

(512) 438-9293

*Herbert M. Shelton, PhD, Editor and Publisher*

Monthly magazine with articles on nutrition, fasting, and natural hygiene.

**HEALTHVIEW NEWSLETTER**/Charlottsville, VA **(see 198)**

**(523) PROVOKER PRESS**
St. Catharines, Ontario
Canada L2R 7C9

*John Tobe, Publisher*

Publishes *The Provoker*, a bimonthly, and *Live to Be 100 Newsletter*, both dealing with nutritional concerns.

**BET TEVA** (Jewish vegetarian journal) /London, England **(see 494)**

## Products and Services

**(524) HEALTH EVALUATIONS, INC.**
P.O. Box 187
Hayward, CA 94543

(415) 582-0286

*Victoria D. Bonnington, Vice President*

A nonprofit corporation dedicated to developing services and disseminating information on a health optimization system. Services include low-cost nutritional evaluation; computerized dietary analysis; hair analysis for nutritional minerals and for toxic environmental metals; referral service to nutritionally oriented physicians; and a health books mail order service. Health Evaluations also sponsors a comprehensive series of nutrition-oriented workshops.

**HEALTH RESEARCH** (books) /Mokelumne Hill, CA **(see 209)**

**AURORA BOOKS** (health) /Denver, CO **(see 217)**

**NUTRI-BOOKS** (health) /Denver, CO **(see 218)**

**(525) ELMET DIVISION ELECTRO-METALS, INC.**
13 Summit Street
East Hampton, CT 06424

(203) 267-4200

Distributor of "Purette" water filter.

**(526) SUPER DISTILLERS, INC.**
c/o Rosemary Piccolo
57 Trumbull Street
New Haven, CT 06510

(203) 469-5185

Distributor of the Jack Ellis Super Water Distiller.

**(527) LEWIS LABORATORIES INTERNATIONAL, LTD.**
P.O. Box 2081
Belden Station
Norwalk, CT 06852

(203) 226-7529

Distributor of "Staminex," a food supplement.

**(527.1) THE NUTRITIONAL ACADEMY**
P.O. Box 345
Des Plaines, IL 60016

(312) 298-7270

The purpose of the Academy is to develop an effective, individualized system of nutritional programming to balance body chemistry; a system that can be used in the physician's office without additional personnel; a biochemical upgrading program that restores the patient's basic functional health and reserve level; and a system of continual upgrading of nutritional programs in line with current advances in the field of biochemical and nutritional research. Use of the Academy's facilities is available to clinicians who wish to restore the balance necessary to maintain successful, gratifying clinical practice. The clinicians of the Academy, with their expanded understanding of cellular biochemistry, are returning to standard medical laboratory procedures to subject them to review. It is the purpose of the research projects now underway to make those tests available to the medical community. As these tests are used to extend the physician's biochemical awareness, preventive medicine as well as the wholesome health of the individual patient, will have made great advancement. Further information regarding activities and computer bank service may be obtained by writing to the Academy.

**(528) CLEAN WATER SOCIETY**
22707 Dequinder Road
Hazel Park, MI 48030

(313) 399-1460

Distributors of two stage water distillers.

**SUN PUBLISHING COMPANY** (books) /Albuquerque, NM **(see 225)**

**(529) CENTER FOR HEALTHFUL LIVING**
275 Central Park West, Suite 1C
New York, NY 10024

(212) 864-3229

*Michael Riciardi, Director*

Diet and nutrition counseling, nutrition information and referral service, water analysis, health evaluation testing. Products available: food supplements, water distillers, fruit and vegetable juicers, home colonic equipment, home exercisers, books, biorhythm charting. Services and products available by appointment only.

**(530) FREEDA PHARMACY**
110 East 41st Street
New York, NY 10017

(212) 685-4980

Distributor of Kosher natural vitamins, homeopathic medication, and herbal medicinal preparations.

**(531) MIRACLE EXCLUSIVES, INC.**
16 West 40th Street
New York, NY 10018

(212) 398-0880

Distributors of juicers, extractors, sprouters, grain mills, and other nutritional aids.

**(532) SUNDANCE INDUSTRIES**
28 Vermont Avenue
White Plains, NY 10606

(914) 946-9340

Distributes "Wheateena" electric (wheatgrass) juicers.

**(533) DENNISON DISTILLATOR** ™
440 Centenary Avenue
Cleveland, TN 37311

Distributor of the "Dennison (water) Distillator."

**(534) ALBION LABORATORIES, INC.**
P.O. Box E
Clearfield, UT 84015

Offers a diet analysis based on a carefully kept record of all foods eaten by a person in a 5-day period. The nutritive content of the diet is then correlated with urine, hair, and saliva analysis to determine what the body "has absorbed or rejected after the food was swallowed." The results have been useful in diagnosis, treatment, and prevention of specific mineral related disorders.

**HERITAGE STORE** (Cayce)/Virginia Beach, VA **(see 230)**

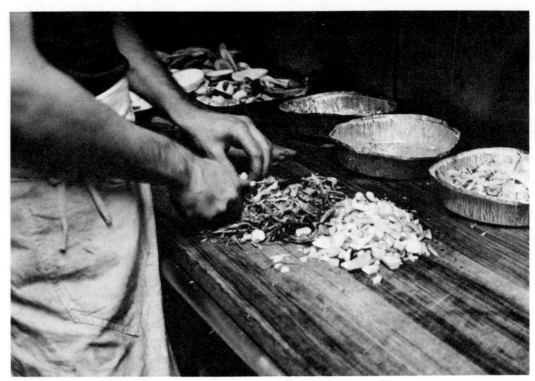

Photo: Leslie J. Kaslof

Caldron Restaurant, New York City;

# Macrobiotics And Oriental Medicine
*Michio Kushi*

More than forty years ago, Dr. Alexis Carrel, a Nobel Prize-winning physiologist at the Rockefeller Institute in New York, wrote a book entitled *Man the Unknown*. In this work, Dr. Carrel called attention to the rising incidence of worldwide individual and social decline confronting man in the twentieth century and pointed toward the increasingly urgent need for a synthesis of all past medical, scientific, and philosophical knowledge into a comprehensive understanding of man, nature, and the universe. Dr. Carrel felt that only with the development of such a wholistic approach could our modern crisis be solved.

At about the same time, thousands of miles away in Japan, Nyoichi Sakurazawa, known in the West as George Ohsawa, had arrived at a similar conclusion, based on his own experience of having cured himself of what was considered a terminal case of tuberculosis many years earlier.

After being abandoned by modern medicine, Ohsawa investigated the approach of traditional Eastern medicine, in particular the application of the ancient dialectical philosophy of *yin* and *yang* to diet, and it was through this application that he was able to cure himself.

Through continued study and experience, Ohsawa began to realize that by applying this traditional philosophy biologically to the selection and manner of preparing food, it was possible to relieve not only physical illness but also psychological, spiritual, and even social malaise. Ohsawa then dedicated his life to spreading the understanding of this philosophy and way of life (later named ''macrobiotics,'' from the Greek *macro,* ''large'' or ''great,'' and *bios,* ''life'') to many thousands of people throughout the world.

I first met George Ohsawa in Japan not long after the end of the Second World War, surprisingly enough through my interest in world peace through world government. At that time, Ohsawa asked me a question, ''Have you ever thought of the dialectic application of diet for world peace?'' Of course, I had never considered a solution as simple as this, but after coming to America soon afterwards, I began to understand the importance of food in determining our individual physiological, psychological, and spiritual conditions, and hence the condition of our society and the world at large.

To illustrate how the Order of the Universe, or yin and yang, operates, let us consider several basic examples. Within our bodies, we are continuously maintaining a dynamic balance between the centripetal tendency of contraction and the centrifugal tendency of expansion, or the forces of yin and yang. We can see this basic polarity in our bodies in things like the rhythmic expansion and contraction of the heart and lungs in circulation and respiration, and in the stomach and intestines during the digestion and absorbtion of food. Also, this relationship exists chemically in the complementary and antagonistic balance between sodium and potassium in the human body, as well as in the nervous system between the orthosympathetic and parasympathetic branches of the autonomic nervous system.

In fact, when we view the body as a whole, we discover countless complementary and antagonstic, or yin and yang, relationships. For example, such a relationship exists between the compacted yang head and the expanded yin torso. This becomes particularly apparent when we consider the relationship between the brain, which represents the major organ of the head, and the intestines, which are its complement in the torso.

We can consider that the spinal cord and the brain were created originally in the form of a spiral beginning at the region where the spinal cord begins and terminating with the brain, specifically the region of the midbrain. This compacted, or yang, system continually attracts and processes a more yin form of our surrounding environment in the form of waves or vibration, such as light, sound, image, dream, and memory. We can also view the intestines and digestive vessel as a spiral. This more yin, or expanded, spiral begins at the region known in the Orient as *hara*, which is located in the small intestine, three fingers below the navel. We can see that the intestines and digestive tract are hollow and expanded in comparison to the brain and spinal cord, which are more tightly compacted. This more yin system therefore attracts and processes a complemental form of the surrounding environment, which is the more yang, physicalized food which we eat every day.

This complemental and antagonistic relationship was well understood in traditional Oriental medicine, which viewed the smooth coordination of these two major systems as vital to our health and well-being. Along this line, it was not unusual for a traditional doctor to consider psychological or emotional problems as having their root cause in some dysfunction in the intestines or digestive system. More often than not, their recommendations for correcting these types of problems were directed toward reestablishing a smooth functioning in the intestinal region through adjustments in the patient's diet.

In traditional Oriental medicine, the recognition of complementary and antagonistic relationships in the body was extended to the major organs. For example, the *Nei-Ching*, or *Yellow Emperor's Classic of Internal Medicine*, composed several thousand years ago in China, divides the major organs into two groups: the yang, compacted, or solid organs; and the yin, hollow or expanded organs. Also, each organ was grouped with its complementary partner, showing the interrelationship between the compacted organs and their expanded counterparts.

Traditional Oriental medicine classifies the major organs as follows:

| Yang | Yin |
|---|---|
| Lungs | Large intestine |
| Heart | Small intestine |
| Kidneys | Bladder |
| Spleen and pancreas | Stomach |
| Liver | Gall bladder |

This classification is the basis of the entire realm of Oriental medicine, which includes the practice of acupuncture, moxibustion, shiatsu, herb medicine, palm healing, and dietary adjustment. Fundamental to the practice of these forms of treatment is the understanding of *ki* (in China called *chri*, in Korea *gee*), which can be translated as "electromagnetic energy." Ancient people viewed all material phenomena as a manifestation of ki. They also saw the human body in this light, and understood that this energy coursed through the body along certain pathways, or meridians, corresponding to the organs. Each organ was a manifestation of ki, which flowed continuously to the organ from the surrounding environment through its corresponding meridian and also continually discharged through this same passageway. They understood that sickness was primarily an imbalance or blockage of this energy, either within the organ or along the corresponding meridian. Therefore, in Oriental medicine treatments aim at reestablishing energy balance or releasing stagnation by stimulating certain points along these meridians, with needles (as in acupuncture), finger pressure (as in shiatsu), or heat (as in moxibustion).

We can clearly understand the principle of yin and yang when we consider the genesis and development of various disease conditions. Let us take as an example a condition such as leukemia. Within the bloodstream we generally have two different types of cells: more yang, or compacted, red cells and more yin, or expanded, white cells. In the same way, we can divide all of our food substances into these same general categories. Foods such as meat, eggs, salt, and other animal products exert a more constrictive effect and are therefore yang, whereas sugar, fruits, liquid, and most chemicals create an expansive effect and are therefore yin. Generally speaking, leukemia results from the proliferation of the yin white blood cells as the yang red blood cells decrease. This condition is simply the result of an overconsumption of yin foods such as sugar, dairy products (e.g., ice cream), soft drinks, fruit juices, and chemicals.

To relieve this condition, one should stop ingesting the excessively yin foods just mentioned, as well as animal foods such as meat and eggs. Yang attracts yin, so if one's diet is based on animal products, then sugar, fruits, alcohol, etc. are needed to create balance. Instead of an extreme balance such as this, a diet based on whole cereal grains, cooked vegetables, beans, seaweed, and soup is more advisable. (Soup made from traditionally fermented soybean products such as miso and tamari is recommended.) People with leukemia should observe a more careful way of eating until their condition improves, at which time they may add other foods such as an occasional salad, cooked seasonal fruit, and some animal food, preferably in the form of fish. A slightly more yang method of selecting and preparing food is advisable to offset leukemia, which is a yin condition. Among vegetables, yang root vegetables such as carrots and burdock should be emphasized, and a person with this condition should eat only cooked foods until the blood condition becomes stabilized.

The above illness is just an example of how we can understand all sickness in terms of yin and yang. We can also understand that the most direct way of approaching any illness is to discover its origin or cause, which inevitably leads us to an individual's way of eating. By correcting this fundamental point, we are able to eliminate the cause of sickness, permitting the body to reestablish natural balance with the environment. This condition, called "health," can be maintained continuously through balanced and orderly eating.

The goal of macrobiotics is the application of the Order of the Universe, or yin and yang, to our biological and physiological foundation through our daily food. When practiced by individuals, this way of life can lead to health, happiness, and freedom. When understood and practiced by society, it can lead to an age of endless human development towards love, justice, and peace.

## Centers

**(535) GEORGE OHSAWA MACROBIOTIC FOUND-
ATION**
1544 Oak Street
Oroville, CA 95965

(916) 533-7702

*Herman Aihara, President*

Center for the dissemination of the teachings of George Ohsawa. Seminars, cooking classes, workshops in such areas as nutrition, herbs, healing, acupuncture, shiatsu, and do-in. Annual weekend and summer retreats are held on the Foundation's land in Northern California. Pamphlets, books, and a monthly publication, *Macrobiotic*, are published including the topics mentioned above.

**(536) THE EAST WEST FOUNDATION**
359 Boylston Street
Boston, MA 02116

*Michio Kushi, President*

Presents regular monthly seminars and study programs covering many aspects of Oriental medicine, philosophy, and culture, and is presently publishing periodicals and books which deal with these same areas. Specific subjects studied in the Foundation's seminars include shiatsu (acupressure), massage, Oriental visual diagnosis, palm healing, moxibustion, acupuncture, meditation and spiritual practices, and psychology and consciousness. Recently, the East West Foundation participated with Harvard University School of Medicine in research which demonstrated cholesterol levels and blood pressure lower than the American norm in individuals adhering to a macrobiotic-style diet. In addition, the Foundation is engaged in educational and research programs studying the role of diet in the prevention and treatment of cancer. A list of national and international centers connected with East West Foundation is available on request.

## Journals and Publications

**HAPPINESS PRESS** (do-in books) /Magdia, CA **(see 847)**

**(537) Periodicals of the EAST WEST FOUNDATION**
359 Boylston Street
Boston, MA 02116

*One Peaceful World*, quarterly newsletter of Foundation activities.

*Michio Kushi Seminar Reports*, monthly, direct transcriptions of the ongoing seminars of Michio Kushi.

*Case History Reports*, a quarterly with personal accounts of experiences with macrobiotic curing, including such illnesses as cancer, heart disease, and allergies.

*Order of the Universe Magazine*, quarterly magazine featuring articles based on the seminars of Michio Kushi.

**EAST WEST JOURNAL** (multidisciplinary new age articles) /Brookline, MA **(see 195)**

**SWAN HOUSE PUBLISHING COMPANY** (macrobiotic books) /Brooklyn, NY **(see 226)**

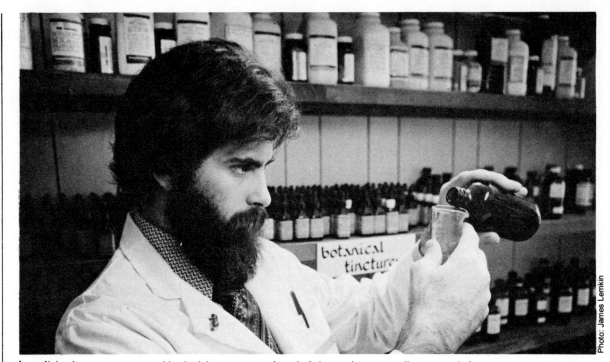

In a clinic pharmacy, a naturopathic physician measures a botanical tincture in compounding a prescription.

# Pharmacognosy In Wholistic Medicine
*Norman R. Farnsworth, PhD*

Pharmacognosy is a multifaceted discipline concerned with the study of drugs, potential drugs, and other economic products derivable from plants and animals. Its history parallels that of humanity; its unwritten history may greatly exceed the recorded portion. Since much of our knowledge in this field has been passed from generation to generation by word of mouth, undoubtedly becoming distorted along the way, such information is referred to as "folklore." However, when such information has been documented in an acceptable way, it is perhaps better to refer to it as "ethnomedicine."

There are many disciplines within pharmacognosy; those most pertinent to wholistic medicine are the study of ethnomedicine, the laboratory verification of biological activity in ethnomedically authenticated plants and animals, and the isolation and structure-elucidation of biologically active plant and animal constituents.

There is perhaps no subject more poorly understood than the importance and role of botanical extracts and their active principles in current medical practice. A few statistics can be cited to clarify this situation. During the period 1959-74, roughly 25 percent of all prescriptions dispensed from community pharmacies in the United States contained one or more plant principles or plant extracts as their active ingredient (in 1974 alone, the American consumer spent about $3 billion on such prescriptions). Microbial prescription products (chiefly antibiotics) accounted for an additional 13.3 percent of all prescriptions that year, and animal-derived prescriptions about 2.7 percent of the total. Thus, in 1974, about 41.2 percent of all prescriptions dispensed in the U.S. were derived from natural products.

Most of these prescriptions contained pure plant principles as their active ingredients, extracted, for the most part, from plants that once were used in the form of extracts. However, a large number of prescriptions are still composed entirely or partially of crude botanical products. Table 1 presents some interesting figures:

Table 1. Plant Extracts Used in Prescriptions in the U.S.A. (1973)

| Plant Name | Common Name | Pharmacological Category | Percent of Category |
|---|---|---|---|
| *Rauvolfia serpentina* | Rauwolfia | Cardiovascular drugs | 16.51 |
| *Veratrum album* | Veratrum | Cardiovascular drugs | 4.62 |
| *Veratrum viride* | Veratrum | Cardiovascular drugs | 0.14 |
| *Digitalis purpurea* | Foxglove | Miscellaneous cardiovascular drugs | 10.34 |
| *Papaver somniferum* | Opium | Analgesics | 0.16 |
| *Cephaelis ipecacuanha* | Ipecac | Antitussive and decongestants | 8.72 |
| *Atropa belladonna* | Belladonna | Antispasmodics | 9.59 |
| *Papaver somniferum* | Opium | Antidiarrheals | 13.32 |
| *Malus sylvestris* | Pectin | Antidiarrheals | 34.28 |
| *Plantago ovata* | Psyllium | Laxatives | 16.67 |
| *Rhamnus purshiana* | Cascara | Laxatives | 12.08 |

These figures do not, of course, include plant preparations sold over the counter or prescription drugs used widely outside of the U.S.A. An extract of *Silybum marianum* (Silybin), for example, is used widely in West Germany, as well as in other European countries, for the treatment of liver ailments; extracts of *Ginkgo biloba* are used for treating hearing disorders. The list of drugs used on a wide scale outside the U.S.A. is almost endless.

Why have synthetic drugs and pure active constituents of plant and animal drugs gained such a foothold as to be the basis of the therapeutic armamentarium of the modern physician? This question has been debated at length (but not in print). Surely one major factor in the diminishing use of extracts by physicians is the fact that medical students are not exposed to the advantages (or disadvantages) of any alternatives to "single-chemical" therapy. Those physicians who do treat congestive heart failure with whole-leaf *Digitalis purpurea*, rather than purified cardiac glycoside digitoxin (or digoxin from *D. lanata*), cite a more easily reproducible activity, better stability, and greater ease in controlling blood levels. However, such subtle differences are difficult to measure; therefore, comparative studies in the published literature are rare. The benefits of using substances in their natural form have not yet been adequately explored.

Anyone who has recently visited the People's Republic of China cannot fail to be impressed with the widespread use of herbal preparations in its health care system. The flora of the P.R.C. comprises some 30,000 species; about 3,000 are used either in the organized system of medicine or as home remedies. Little attempt is being made to isolate and characterize the "active" principles; rather, these days the major effort seems to be directed toward making herbal preparations more stable, palatable, and convenient for home use (refrigeration is virtually nonexistent in China, and the principal dosage form to date has been an aqueous decoction, which is subject to microbial decomposition). The herbal pharmacology delegation from the U.S. that visited the P.R.C. in 1974 concurred that medical care in China is equal to, if not better than, that offered in the U.S.

Thus, although it would be difficult to prove at this point that the use of herbal preparations in a galenical form could be an acceptable adjunct to modern medicine, it is apparent that the people today using this form of drug therapy outnumber those using synthetic or pure natural constituents, or both. The growing movement of persons interested in using herbal preparations as one aspect of wholistic medical practice will create an increasing need for information concerning the efficacy, advantages, and disadvantages of herbal drugs. We hope that pharmacognosy will be able to provide such information in a rational, scientific, and assimilable manner.

# Parts Or Wholes: An Introduction To The Use Of Whole Plant Substances In Healing

*Leslie J. Kaslof*

From the earliest times, humanity has sought to understand the deeper nature of plants. Over the years many elements believed to represent this nature have been identified within plants and grouped according to their properties and effects on living organisms. Some of these elements have been designated vitamins, minerals, proteins, or enzymes; some of those used in medicine have been termed alkaloids, glycocides, and steroids. *However, no characterization or separation of parts can be a substitute for understanding or utilizing plants as whole entities.*

This confusion between parts and wholes is symptomatic of modern science in general, and can be well illustrated by developments in the field of nutrition.

In the past 50 years, because of the depletion in the nutritional values of our food (brought on by certain technological "advances"), the need for a sound, concentrated form of nourishment has clearly emerged. Consequently, millions of persons have embraced the wholesale assortment of food supplements which recently have appeared on the commercial market as the answer to this dilemma. Let us examine this situation more closely:

In the Soviet Union, a country that has recently become quite sophisticated in its use of megavitamins, many physicians have instituted nutritional programs that prescribe periods of high vitamin dosages alternating with periods of no vitamin intake. For example, a person takes a regimen of vitamin supplements for two weeks. Then, for four weeks, s/he takes no vitamin supplements. Although no official explanation has been given for this practice, one can easily extrapolate the reasoning behind it —large doses of these elements weaken the body's ability to extract these same elements from food, and eventually a dependency is created.

This same reasoning can be applied to the use of drugs that have been separated and isolated (S&I) from their whole substance. In addition to these so-called "active ingredients" (the isolated modern drugs), there exist within whole plant substances inactive ingredients and unique organizing principles, many of which have yet to be recognized. Though some of these may, in time, be revealed with the development of more sophisticated analysis and technology, others may never be discovered.

These subtle elements, while not having the dramatic effects of the "active ingredients," are in fact important in catalyzing or balancing the effect of the active principle in the living system. In this sense, whole plant substances have a definite remedial advantage over their isolated constituents.

Nutritional supplementation, or the attempt to restore health through the use of S&I elements, both represents and perpetuates a basic misconception ingrained in our society, which focuses on goals, and pays little attention to the processes through which those goals are attained. Those who favor supplementation assume that once a needed element has been supplied, deficiencies will disappear. However, in many instances, nutritional deficiency is brought on not so much by the unavailability of certain elements as by the body's inability to assimilate them. Even assuming that in some miraculous way an S&I element has all the properties necessary to produce the desired effect in the human system, one cannot simply replace an element *considered* deficient with an S&I approximation. It would still lack the ability to stimulate the vital process of extrapolating elements from the food we eat, a function equally as important as obtaining the elements themselves.

Whole plant substances not only stimulate this exercise of function but also make available, in concentrated form, a vital force—activity sufficient to catalyze a revitalizing biochemical response. The fact that plants both catalyze a healing response in our own systems and also represent that which facilitates the connections between the animal world and terrestrial, solar, and more subtle forces is in itself wholistic. The nature of plants has a direct affinity with our own: we share life in a dynamic process of mutual support. Through plants we reestablish our connection with the environment. Ingested, plants touch and awaken aspects of our nature we may have only dreamed existed. Using whole plant substances is like praying—on a biochemical level.

## Groups and Associations

**(538) SOCIETY FOR ECONOMIC BOTANY, INC.**
Department of Pharmacognosy and Pharmacology
College of Pharmacy
University of Illinois
833 South Wood Street
Chicago, IL 60612

(312) 996-7240

*Edward S. Mika, PhD, Chairman, Membership Committee*

An international scientific organization whose members from many disciplines share a common interest in plants and plant products useful to man. Members receive the quarterly journal, *Economic Botany*, which contains scientific articles on medicinal, industrial, and agricultural uses of plants. Symposia on specific topics are held at annual meetings. Founded 1960.

**(539) INTERNATIONAL INSTITUTE FOR BIOLOGICAL AND BOTANICAL RESEARCH LTD.**
P.O. Box 912
Brooklyn, NY 11202

(212) 638-4141

*L.J. Kaslof, Founder*

A New York State nonprofit scientific and educational foundation, which bridges the gap between the professional plant sciences (researchers and groups engaged in current as well as potential use of plant substances within the field of medicine) and practicing members of the medical and healing arts.

## Schools, Centers, and Clinics

**BERKELEY COMMUNITY HEALTH PROJECT** (free clinic) /Berkeley, CA **(see 75)**

**BERKELEY HOLISTIC HEALTH CENTER** (educational workshops) /Berkeley, CA **(see 76)**

**BERKELEY WOMEN'S HEALTH COLLECTIVE** (educational) /Berkeley, CA **(see 77)**

**CENTER FOR FAMILY GROWTH** (birth) /Cotati, CA **(see 8)**

**NATIONAL ARTHRITIS MEDICAL CLINIC** /Desert Hot Springs, CA **(see 81)**

**(540) ROSEMARY'S GARDEN**
P.O. Box 442
Guerneville, CA 95446

(707) 869-9919

*Rosemary Gladstar, Director*

An herb store that sponsors weekly classes on herbal heal-

ing, gardening, and field identification walks. Retreats are sponsored to provide an opportunity for healers and students to share and teach each other in an informal atmosphere.

**(541) MEDICINE WHEEL**
P.O. Box 1121
Idyllwild, CA 92349

(714) 659-4310

A nonprofit collective dedicated to learning, teaching, and practicing herbology, and other natural healing arts. Interested in facilitating the development of a nationwide alternative herbal and natural healing collective. Distributes medicinal herbs, spices, oils, and miscellaneous earth products through mail order and affiliated Southern California stores.

**ISLA VISTA OPEN DOOR MEDICAL CLINIC** (holistic) /Isla Vista, CA **(see 85)**

**BARAKA** (holistic center and clinic) /Los Angeles, CA **(see 87)**

**WHITE CROSS SOCIETY** (holistic workshops) / Lucerne Valley, CA **(see 93)**

**McCORNACK CENTER FOR THE HEALING ARTS** (multidisciplinary clinic) /Mendocino, CA **(see 95)**

**WHOLISTIC HEALTH AND NUTRITION INSTITUTE** (educational and clinic) /Mill Valley, CA **(see 97)**

**ACUPUNCTURE WHOLISTIC CLINIC**/Monterey Park, CA **(see 635)**

**SACRAMENTO MEDICAL PREVENTICS CLINIC**/ Sacramento, CA **(see 103)**

**ACUPUNCTURE AND HERBS RESEARCH**/San Diego, CA **(see 636)**

**SAN DIEGO NATURAL HEALTH CLINIC** (holistic) /San Diego, CA **(see 108)**

**EAST-WEST ACADEMY OF HEALING ARTS** (educational) /San Francisco, CA **(see 110)**

**(542) NEW AGE CREATIONS-HERBAL COSMETICS**
219 Carl Street
San Francisco, CA 94117

(415) 564-6785

*Jeanne Rose, President*

Classes and workshops on medicinal herbs, herbal first-aid, and culinary herbs. Sells a full line of specially formulated herbal cosmetics and other herbal products.

**ASSOCIATED PSYCHOLOGISTS OF SANTA CLARA**/Santa Clara, CA **(see 114)**

**(543) GARDEN OF SANJIVANI (School of Herbs and Spiritual Healing)**
2083 Ocean Street, Ext.
Santa Cruz, CA 95060

(408) 425-0597

*Michael Tierra, Director*

Offers a three-month residential program in herbology and spiritual healing. Special courses are offered in shiatsu, polarity, and reflexology massage, iridology, acupuncture, the Bach flower remedies, homeopathy, yoga, nutrition, anatomy, and physiology. The program is under the auspices of the Hanuman Fellowship, a California nonprofit corporation. Founded 1976.

**ORR SPRINGS ASSOCIATION** (retreat) /Ukiah, CA **(see 170)**

**COMMUNITY FREE SCHOOL** (education and workshops) /Boulder, CO **(see 119)**

**STAMFORD CENTER FOR THE HEALING ARTS** (wholistic clinic in a church) /Stamford, CT **(see 121)**

**HIMALAYAN INSTITUTE COMBINED THERAPY CENTER** (wholistic resort) /Glenview, IL **(see 125)**

**(544) BOTANICAL MUSEUM**
Harvard University
Oxford Street
Cambridge, MA 02138

(617) 495-2326

*Richard E. Schultes, PhD, Director*

Home of the famous Harvard University Glass Flower exhibit. The museum is open to the public and students, has displays on many interesting aspects of plants. Maintains a herbarium and a library facility for researchers and students of the university.

**(545) ETHNOBOTANICAL LABORATORIES**
Museum of Anthropology
University of Michigan
Ann Arbor, MI 48104

(313) 764-1817

*Richard Ford, PhD, Director*

Maintains a plant identification service, herbarium, and laboratory for the analysis of plant material.

**DESERT LIGHT FOUNDATION** (holistic center and school) /Albuquerque, NM **(see 134)**

**CHRISTOS SCHOOL OF NATURAL HEALING**/ Taos, NM **(see 135)**

**(546) NEW YORK BOTANICAL GARDENS**
Bronx, NY 10458

(212) 220-8777

Maintains a library facility, herbarium, plant information service, (horticultural) gardens and beautifully kept grounds. Membership is available to the public and entitles one to use all the facilities of the Gardens. List of abstracts and publications available for a nominal fee.

**(547) TRAILSIDE NATURE MUSEUM**
Cross River, NY 10518

(914) 763-3993

*Nicholas A. Shoumatoff, Curator*

Specializes in Delaware Indian herblore, the museum sponsors programs and field trips as well as maintaining a library and herbarium facility. Open 9am to 5pm, Wednesday-Sunday.

**SWEDISH INSTITUTE** (massage and herbs) /New York, NY **(see 863)**

**TREE OF LIFE** (educational center) /New York, NY **(see 142)**

**ALTERNATIVE HEALTH EDUCATION CENTER**/ Rochester, NY **(see 143)**

**(548) LLOYD LIBRARY AND MUSEUM**
917 Plum Street
Cincinnati, OH 45202
Atten: Librarian

(513) 721-3707

Founded by John Uri Lloyd, the library and museum represent an internationally famous collection of literature in the natural sciences, with preeminence in the fields of the pharmaceutical sciences, eclectic medicine, botany, and chemistry. A photostat service is available.

**PSI CENTER** (clinical and educational) /Cincinnati, OH **(see 145)**

**INSTITUTE OF PREVENTIVE MEDICINE**/Portland, OR **(see 149)**

**NATUROPATHIC BIRTH CENTER**/Winston, OR **(see 23)**

**CLYMER HEALTH CLINIC** (wholistic) /Quakertown, PA **(see 150)**

**(549) NEBO BEHAVIOR RESEARCH CENTER (NBRC)**
P.O. Box 116
Provo, UT 84663

*Daniel Mowrey, PhD, Director*

Uses standard experimental pharmacological techniques in the study of medicinal, psychotropic, and nutritional herbs. Seeks to publish work in reputable scientific journals, in the belief that good defense against skeptics, cynics, and anti-herbal legislation can only be achieved through rigorous scientific evaluation and verification. Founded 1975.

**THE COMMUNITY HEALTH CENTER** (clinic) / Burlington, VT **(see 152)**

**HOME CENTER** (wholistic center and workshops) / Virginia Beach, VA **(see 155)**

**RADIANCE—HERBS AND MASSAGE**/Olympia, WA **(see 864)**

**SUNSHINE MEDICAL SHOW** (clinic) /Seattle, WA **(see 156.1)**

**(550) DOMINION HERBAL COLLEGE**
7527 Kingsway
Burnaby 3
British Columbia, Canada

*Ella Birzneck, MH, President*

Offers a correspondence course in herbology and basic anatomy and physiology. On graduation, the student is awarded the certificate as ''chartered herbalist,'' and becomes eligible for membership in the Canadian Herbalist Association of British Columbia. Founded 1926.

**(551) EMERSON COLLEGE OF HERBOLOGY, LTD.**
815 Bancroft Street
Pointe Claire, Quebec
Canada H9R 4L6

*Jack Thuna, ND, President*

Offers a certificate and correspondence course in herbal medicine.

**SERENITY HEALTH EDUCATION CENTRE** (multidisciplinary) /Vancouver, BC, Canada **(see 159)**

**(552) EDWARD BACH HEALING CENTRE**
Mount Vernon, Sotwell
Wallingford
Berkshire, England

Disseminates information on the theory and practical application of the Bach Flower Remedies.

**TYRINGHAM NATUROPATHIC CLINIC** (clinic-spa) /Bucks, England **(see 177)**

**RAMANA HEALTH CENTRE** (wholistic hospital) / Hants, England **(see 161)**

**3-L BHAVAN** (yoga and herbs) /Hull, England **(see 162)**

**(553) NATIONAL INSTITUTE OF MEDICAL HERBALISTS**
Registrar
68 London Road
Leicester LE2 OQD
England

Offers a four-year program in herbal medicine, including most of the traditional courses of medical school with emphasis on herbs and natural treatment. Also maintains an active Research Department engaged in the establishment of standards for the herbs used in medicine and the investigation of their therapeutic activity. Founded 1864.

**(554) SWEDISH HERBAL INSTITUTE**
Artillerigatan 25
Gothenburg, Sweden 41502

Tel: 031-252310

*George Wikman, President*

Evaluates traditional medical herbs used in native cultures, from Africa, Asia, and South America. Also markets various herbal products which include Russian root (*Eleutherococcus senticosis*), Ginseng, *Harpago procumbens*, Kava-Kava, Kan Jang, and Tibetan herbal prepara-

tions. The Institute is also engaged in research on the therapeutic effects of negative air ions, bioelectric and electromagnetic therapies, and the use of biofeedback and electroacupuncture.

**SANATORIUM SONNENECK** (anthroposophical clinic) /Badenweiler, Switzerland **(see 815)**

**BIRCHER-BENNER PRIVATKLINIK** (spa-clinic)/ Zürich, Switzerland **(see 180)**

**FILDERKLINIK** (anthroposophical hospital) /West Germany **(see 816)**

**GEMEINNÜTZIGES GEMEINSCHAFTSKRANKENHAUS HERDECKE** (anthroposophical hospital) / West Germany **(see 818)**

**PARACELSUS-KRANKENHAUS** (anthroposophical rest home) /West Germany **(see 822)**

**SANATORIUM FÜR DYNAMISCHE THERAPIE STUDENHOF** (anthroposophical clinic) /West Germany **(see 823)**

# Journals and Publications

**COUNTRY LADY'S DAYBOOK** (birth) /Oakland, CA **(see 43)**

**WELL-BEING MAGAZINE** (natural healing) /San Diego, CA **(see 186)**

**HARTLEY FILM PRODUCTIONS** (multidisciplinary audiovisuals) /Cos Cob, CT **(see 219)**

**ALTERNATIVES JOURNAL** (multidisciplinary new age articles) /Miami, FL **(see 193)**

**SUNSPARK PRESS** (directory of alternative publications) /St. Petersburg, FL **(see 194)**

**(555) FOXFIRE**
Rabun Gap, GA 30568

(404) 746-2561

Quarterly magazine with articles on the mountain culture of southern Appalachia. Includes folklore related to herbs and healing.

**EAST WEST JOURNAL** (multidisciplinary magazine) / Brookline, MA **(see 195)**

**NEW AGE JOURNAL** (multidisciplinary magazine) / Brookline, MA **(see 196)**

**(556) ECONOMIC BOTANY**
Publications Office
New York Botanical Gardens
Bronx, NY 10458

*Richard E. Schultes, PhD, Editor*

A scientific quarterly journal devoted to all aspects of plant uses by man.

**(557) LLOYDIA**
P.O. Box 484
Cincinnati, OH 45201

*Arthur E. Schwarting, PhD, Editor*

Publication of the American Society of Pharmacognosy. Technical information on all aspects of the pharmacological use of plants.

**(558) THE HERBALIST**
224 Draper Lane
P.O. Box 62
Provo, UT 84601

(801) 374-1180

*Bud Clegg, Managing Editor*

Monthly magazine with articles on herbs and herbal therapeutics.

**(559) HEALING YOURSELF**
402 Fifteenth Avenue East
Seattle, WA 98112

(206) 332-6698

*Joyce Prensky, Editor*

A regularly revised manual with information on self-help, herbal remedies, pregnancy and childbirth, diseases and imbalances, and vitamins and nutrition. Provides practical information for home and self-treatment.

**(560) QUARTERLY JOURNAL OF CRUDE DRUG RESEARCH**
Swets Publishing Service
Swets and Zeitlinger B.V.
Heereweg 347 B
Lisse, The Netherlands

*Dr. George M. Hocking, Editor-in-Chief*

Devoted to recording the history, taxonomy, ecology, geographical distribution, morphology, histology, chemistry, methods of identification and determination, pharmacology, and local popular uses of plant and animal crude drugs and their derivatives. Experimental studies and reviews of less well-known drugs of the vegetable and animal kingdoms are also featured.

## Products and Services

**(561) OAK VALLEY HERB FARM**
Star Route
Camptonville, CA 95922

(916) 288-3505

Distributes herbal cosmetics, herbal books, and some dried herbs and tinctures.

**MEDICINE WHEEL** (herbal distributor) /Idyllwild, CA **(see 541)**

**(562) D'FRANSSIA CORPORATION**
4505 West First Street
Los Angeles, CA 90004

(213) 461-3444

Complete line of herbs geared to a Spanish-speaking market.

**HEALTH RESEARCH** (books) /Mokelumne Hill, CA **(see 209)**

**(563) TAYLOR'S HERB GARDEN, INC.**
2649 Stingle Avenue
Rosemead, CA 91770

(213) 280-4639

Box 150C
Cave Creek Stage
Phoenix, AZ 85020

(602) 992-7967

1535 Lone Oak Road
Vista, CA 92083

(714) 727-3485

Distributor of dried herbs and live plants, grown in the three locations.

**(564) NATURE'S HERB COMPANY**
281 Ellis Street
San Francisco, CA 94102

(415) 474-2756

Distributes a full line of dried herbs and a variety of fine quality oils and herbal preparations.

**NEW AGE CREATIONS-HERBAL COSMETICS**/San Francisco, CA **(see 542)**

**RAINBOW BRIDGE** (new age books and records) /San Francisco, CA **(see 213)**

**ACUPUNCTURE AND HERBS RESEARCH**/San Diego, CA **(see 636)**

**(565) HERB TRADE ASSOCIATION**
P.O. Box 409
Santa Cruz, CA 95016

(408) 423-7923

*Paul A. Lee, PhD, Executive Director*

Represents many of the large botanical supply companies in the U.S. Has list of local herb outlets. Presently negotiating with FDA setting standards for botanical material in commercial distribution.

**(566) HOUSE OF QUALITY HERBS**
P.O. Box 14
Woodland Hills, CA 91365

(213) 884-4440

Distributor of herbal preparations, pills, syrups and balms.

**(567) HERBARIUM**
U.S. National Arboretum
Washington, DC 20250

(202) 399-5400

Will identify specimens of plants sent to them. The instructions for obtaining such information are as follows:

1. Send a portion of the plant that is large enough to show leaves, flowers, and fruits.
2. Dry the specimens before sending by placing them over heat, between folds of newspaper and separators, weighted down with a heavy object, tightly bound to ensure flat specimens.

3. Tie the dried specimens (still in newspaper) between two pieces of cardboard; wrap and box for shipping.
4. Attach to each specimen a label containing the following information:
   a. The origin or source of the plant to be identified.
   b. The approximate size of the plant in question, and whether it is an herb, a shrub, tree or vine.
   c. When collected and by whom collected and any other pertinent data, such as flower color, habitat, growth form, etc.
5. Be sure that the address of the sender appears both on the package and in the letter.

### (568) INDIANA BOTANIC GARDENS
P.O. Box 5
Hammond, IN 60473

(219) 931-2480

Packaged herbs and herbal preparations.

### (569) MEER CORPORATION
9500 Railroad Avenue
North Bergen, NJ 07047

(201) 861-9500

Wholesale bulk supplier of raw and processed botanicals.

### (570) VERA PRODUCTS
P.O. Box 1863
Taos, NM 87571

(505) 758-4416

Distributes Lily of the Desert aloe vera products, as well as live aloe plants for planting or potting.

### SWAN HOUSE PUBLISHING COMPANY (macrobiotics and herb books) /Brooklyn, NY (see 226)

### (571) BIO-BOTANICA
2 Willow Park Center
Farmingdale, NY 11735

(516) 752-1583

Manufacturer of a complete line of botanical extracts.

### (572) APHRODISIA
28 Carmine Street
New York, NY 10014

(212) 989-6440

Wholesale and retail distributor of dried herbs and herbal preparations. One of the very few companies that is a supply link between large foreign and domestic suppliers and the small distributor and retail store.

### (573) H.P. KRAUS
16 East 46th Street
New York, NY 10017

(212) 687-4808

Specializes in old and rare herbals, fine flower paintings, gardening, and botanical illustrations.

### KIEHL PHARMACY (herbal preparations and dry herbs) /New York, NY (see 278)

### SERENITY (herb shop) /New York, NY (see 159)

### (574) THE THREE SHEAVES CO.
100 Varick Street
New York, NY 10013

(212) 962-4495

Wholesale, retail, and mail order outlet for imported herbal teas and food supplements. Major distributor of a large line of imported clays for healing as well as cosmetic purposes.

### (575) UNITED COMMUNICATIONS
P.O. Box 320
Woodmere, NY 11598

(516) 374-0943

Distributes the *Herb and Ailment Cross Reference Chart*, as well as a full line of fully illustrated color plant identification charts.

### (576) GARDENS OF THE BLUE RIDGE
P.O. Box 10
Pineola, NC 28662

(704) 756-4339

Distributes live wild flowers, trees, shrubs, plants, and bulbs.

### (577) WESTERN COMFREY, INC.
P.O. Box 45
Canby, OR 97013

(503) 266-3788

Distributes comfrey products.

### (578) TRANSMUTATIONS, INC.
P.O. Box 12673
Philadelphia, PA 19129

Distributes herbal mixtures and pillows. Founded 1976.

### (579) PARK LABORATORIES, INC.
114 Blue Star Street
San Antonio, TX 78204

(512) 224-6977

Distributes salves, oils, and liniments.

### (580) THE HERB SHOP—CHRISTOPHER'S DISTRIBUTING CO.
P.O. Box 352
Provo, UT 84601

(801) 225-7259

Distributes teas, herbs, oils, tinctures, syrups, and ointments.

### (581) NATURE'S MEDICINE CHEST
c/o The Gluten Co., Inc.
P.O. Box 482
Provo, UT 84601

Publishes and distributes a useful set of full color 4 x 6 card photos (field identification cards) of medicinal, edible, and poisonous herbs. Information regarding harvesting, use, and preparation also provided.

### (582) THE APOTHECARY SHOP
Shelburne Museum
Shelburne, VT 05482

(802) 985-3344

This 19th century-style apothecary shop is one of the thirty-five exhibit buildings at the Shelburne Museum. The interior is divided into two sections: a main room stocking drugs, medicines, patent medicines, herbs, and bottles of oils, tinctures, and chemicals; and a compounding room with a brick hearth and copper utensils. Outside the shop is an herb garden containing many of the specialties used by the apothecary. Open from mid-May to mid-October.

**HERITAGE STORE** (Cayce) /Virginia Beach, VA **(see 230)**

**(583) NORTH CENTRAL COMFREY PRODUCERS**
P.O. Box 195
Glidden, WI 54527

(715) 264-2083

Distributes live comfrey plants as well as dried leaves and roots.

**(584) POTTERS (Herbal Supply) LTD.**
Douglas Works, Leyland, Mill Lane
Wigan Lancashire, England

Has available a complete line of herbal extracts and preparations. Catalog available.

**SWEDISH HERBAL INSTITUTE** (herb products) /
Gothenburg, Sweden **(see 554)**

# IV
# HEURISTIC DIRECTIONS IN DIAGNOSIS AND TREATMENT

---

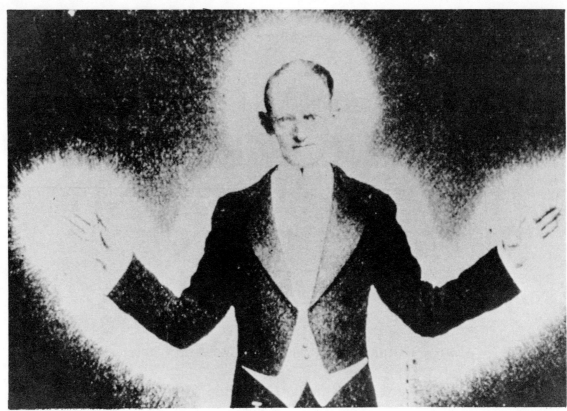

Dr. Strong standing in a 5,000,000 cycle electro-magnetic field as photographed in 1917; courtesy of Earl Lane from *Electrophotography*. By Earl Lane, Berkeley; And Or Press, 1975.

# Introduction To Heuristic Groups And Centers

*Philip Lansky*

*"Cease not to think of the Universe as one living Being, possessed of a single Substance and a single Soul; and how all things trace back to its single sentience; and how it does all things by a single impulse; and how all existing things are joint causes of all things that come into existence; and how intertwined in the fabric is the thread and how closely woven the web."*

*Marcus Aurelius*

Heuristic (from the Greek *heuriskein*: to invent or discover) is defined by Webster as "helping to discover or learn; specifically, designating a method of education or of computer programming in which the pupil or machine proceeds along empirical lines, using rules of thumb to find solutions or answers." It is through a systematic study of the empirical findings described in this section that we sense the imminence of important new "solutions and answers" for the practice of medicine and the living of life.

At our present level of understanding, medicine is conceived and practiced almost entirely at the level of the observable physical body. Though we have learned to use technology to extend our senses (through microscopes and other sensory amplifiers) we still limit our study to observable physical phenomena. Occasionally we may acknowledge a "psychosomatic" dimension, but this seldom goes further than ancillary psychological counseling or as an explanation for diagnostic mysteries.

True wholistic medicine must begin to consider the human organism not as an isolated entity, a "whole" solely unto itself, but rather as a dynamic manifestation of a much greater, infinite whole. In such an expanded view, we do not treat or examine an isolated individual, but rather work to establish balance in the total psychosomatic sphere of which each individual forms his/her own center.

It is my belief that the empirical observations described in this section will, when systematically studied, yield a totally new understanding of the body of man; in this sense they are truly heuristic.

The articles on aeroiontherapy and the effects of light on health are examples of the relationship between physiological events inside the skin and physical events outside the skin. The wholistic physician must know how to bring both into balance.

The sections on acupuncture and Kirlian photography suggest that the energy forces of the individual body extend beyond the traditional limits, and can be observed for purposes of diagnosis (Kirlian) and re-focused for purposes of treatment (acupuncture).

Biorhythms and medical astrology begin to give us a sense of the cyclical changes which influence physiological function. Biorhythms are based on endocrine (hormonal) cycles believed to originate in the body's interior, while astrological movement of the planets occurs on the "exterior." Both, however, are important and perhaps are parts of more universal psychophysical cycles.

Iridology is representative of those sciences which claim that many indices of the body's health can be found through a study of subtle changes in the body's morphology. Related diagnostic sciences might include medical palmistry and physiognomy.

Finally, the sections on fields of life, radionics, and radiesthesia point to the existence of forms of energy more subtle than what we usually regard as physical. In fact, these energies may provide the missing link through which consciousness interacts with the physiology. As is the case with many psychic healers, the diagnostician practicing radionics or radiesthesia need not necessarily be in close proximity to his patient.

To the skeptical among us, these "heuristic directions" may appear to be beyond the pale of rational consideration. However, we should keep in mind that this is always the case with new discoveries in science which threaten to upset existing scientific models. It is my feeling that underlying these heuristic phenomena is a latent revolution in medical thinking as important (and as difficult) for our time as the revolutions of Galen, Pasteur and Darwin were for theirs.

## Groups and Associations

(585) **FLOAT (Association for Research and Communication)**
Big Sur, CA 93920

(408) 667-2194

*Francis J. Busco, Director*

Sponsors seminars, tutorials, and symposia in the scientific study of consciousness.

**NURSE CONSULTANTS AND HEALTH COUNSELORS** (educational) /San Francisco, CA **(see 112)**

(586) **BORDERLAND SCIENCES RESEARCH FOUNDATION**
P.O. Box 548
Vista, CA 92083

(714) 724-2043

*Riley Hansard Crabb, Director*

A nonprofit organization of people with an "active interest in unusual happenings along the borderland between the visible and invisible worlds." Specific areas of interest include psychic phenomena, radiesthesia, Kirlian photography, and UFOs. Offers consultation for individuals with "borderland problems" and spiritual healing through prayer. Publishes the bimonthly *Journal of Borderland Research*. Founded 1951.

**AMERICAN SOCIETY FOR PSYCHICAL RESEARCH**/New York, NY **(see 771)**

## Schools, Centers, and Clinics

**INSTITUTE FOR RESEARCH INTO WHOLISTIC THERAPEUTIC ENERGIES** (radiesthesia) /Boulder Creek, CA **(see 79)**

**NATIONAL ARTHRITIS MEDICAL CLINIC**/Desert Hot Springs, CA **(see 81)**

(587) **PAUL DE SAINTE COLOMBE CENTER**
6230 Mulholland Highway
Hollywood, CA 90068

(213) 467-7058

*Kathi de Sainte Colombe, Director*

Practices a unique science known as "graphotherapy." The prime assumption is that just as changes in the unconscious mind affect the handwriting, so also can intentional changes in the handwriting affect the unconscious mind. The Center has evolved an entire system of psychotherapy based on first analyzing the client's character from his/her handwriting, and then prescribing specific penmanship exercises designed to change the handwriting, and ultimately the personality. The Center has reported success with this approach in treating emotional instability, acute introversion, timidity, learning difficulty, depression, stuttering, juvenile delinquency, sexual aberrations, neurosis, alcoholism and smoking. A text describing the work, entitled *Graphotherapeutics*, by Paul de Sainte Colombe (1966) is available from the center. In bulk quantities, it may be ordered from De Vorss & Co., Box 550, Manna del Rey, CA 90291.

**(588) HUMAN DIMENSIONS INSTITUTE—WEST**
P.O. Box 5037
Ojai, CA 93023

(805) 646-8343

*Luke Gatto*

Dedicated to research into consciousness, parapsychology, and healing science. Areas of investigation either planned or in progress include nutrition and herbology, radiesthesia and medical dowsing, color therapy and radionics, acupressure and massage, and development of a bioshelter experimenting with the recycling of power and energy. Formerly The Institute for Fundamental Studies.

**CHURCH OF GENTLE BROTHERS AND SISTERS** (holistic workshops) /San Francisco, CA **(see 109)**

**(589) INTROSPECTIVE TECHNOLOGY SERVICES (ITS)**
2172 Green Street
San Francisco, CA 94123

(415) 921-3875

To achieve "self-harmony and greater self-realization," ITS uses the Computerized Voice Analyzer which measures minute changes in the voice pattern. The computer is said to "pinpoint the client's positive and negative traits." The client receives a detailed list and description of his/her "unique strengths and weaknesses plus suggestions for improving weaker areas."

**(590) PHYSICS/CONSCIOUSNESS RESEARCH GROUP, INC.**
2 Whiting Street
San Francisco, CA 94133

(415) 441-8720

*Jack Sarfatti, PhD, Director*

Offers personalized tutorial instruction in quantum physics, molecular quantum biophysics, and mathematical models of information processing in the nervous system. Also offered is a seminar in the mind/body problem and the relationship of quantum physics to models of consciousness. Quantum physics is taught in the seminars as a holistic science, with important applications in medical research. Founded 1975.

**THETA SEMINARS** (rebirthing) /San Francisco, CA (also Pacific Palisades and Truckee, CA; Boulder, CO; Miami and Tampa, FL; Honolulu, HI; Arlington, MA) **(see 1064)**

**UNIVERSITY OF CALIFORNIA EXTENSION** (workshops) /Santa Cruz, CA **(see 115)**

**(591) HUNA INTERNATIONAL**
2617 Lincoln Boulevard
Santa Monica, CA 90405

(213) 392-2794

*Sage King, Founder*

Offers courses in psychic development, spiritual healing, and many aspects of parapsychology. Additional work is offered in pyramid energy, astrology, nutrition, color and sound, dreams, radionics, reincarnation, and related subjects. The teachings are strongly influenced by the ancient knowledge of the Polynesian Kahunas.

**(592) THE RADIX INSTITUTE**
225 Santa Monica Boulevard, 6th floor
P.O. Box 3218
Santa Monica, CA 90403

(213) 395-1555

*Charles R. Kelley, PhD, Director*

160 Besant Road
P.O. Box 97
Ojai, CA 93023

(805) 649-8555

Dedicated to "studying the creative process in nature as that process was described by Wilhelm Reich." Offers classes, workshops, and individual sessions in improvement of feeling capacity, self-direction, and visual perception. Workshops are given throughout the U.S. and in Europe. Indepth training is available either in Santa Monica or by extension.

**(593) ADVENTURE TRAILS RESEARCH AND DEVELOPMENT LABORATORIES, INC.**
Laughing Coyote Mountain
Black Hawk, CO 80422

*T.D. Lingo, Director*

Maintains the assumption that 90% of the human brain, especially in the frontal lobes, is dormant. Researching and teaching methods of "brain self-control" to unleash human potential and self-cure neurosis within a year. "The technique of brain self-control is merely to learn the mechanics of brain parts and to harmonize willed behavior with the genetic code encouraging the individual into unlimited growth." Founded 1957.

**COMMUNITY FREE SCHOOL** (educational workshops) /Boulder, CO **(see 119)**

**SHORELINE TRAINING AND EMPLOYMENT SERVICES** (horticultural therapy) /Guilford, CT **(see 1076)**

**YES EDUCATIONAL SOCIETY** (educational) / Washington, DC **(see 123)**

**(594) PSYCHOPHYSICS FOUNDATION, INC.**
347 Northeast 36th Street
Miami, FL 33137

(305) 576-0840

Dedicated to promulgating the science of psychophysics, defined by Dr. Gustav Theodor Fechner in 1861 as "the scientific study of the relation between mental and physical processes." The Foundation is devoted to help those in need of physical and mental assistance by improving the relationship between body and mind. Offers lectures and classes and training programs; maintains a research and reference library of books and tapes on relaxation, self-hypnosis, biofeedback, and parapsychology; provides biofeedback equipment, instruments, parapsychological aids for its students; and maintains a laboratory where tests and research are undertaken in the field of psychophysics.

**THE ROUNDTABLE OF THE LIGHT CENTERS** (psychic) /Miami, FL **(see 785)**

**MARTIN BUBER INSTITUTE** (holistic workshops) / Columbia, MD **(see 127)**

**INTERFACE** (multidisciplinary center) /Newton, MA **(see 131)**

**SIDDHARTHA FOUNDATION** (aura work) /Waltham, MA **(see 790)**

**(595) DREAM COUNSELLORS, INC.**
135 Madison Avenue
Albuquerque, NM 87123

(505) 265-0221

*C.C. Bateman, President*

Conducts lectures on dream interpretation, paranormal phenomena and altered states of consciousness. Drawing from the Tibetan science of "dream yoga," provides counseling to physicians, dentists, and psychologists on the application of dream interpretation as a diagnostic aid.

**CHRISTOS SCHOOL OF NATURAL HEALING** (natural healing) /Taos, NM **(see 135)**

**(596) DREAM DYNAMICS**
25 Sullivan Avenue
Farmingdale, NY 11735

(516) 249-3555

*Michael A. Daddio, Director*

Offers a series of weekly workshops at night in Dream Dynamics, the art of tapping dream energy for balanced expanded awareness and a deepening of the richness of living. The course series includes relaxation techniques, creative visualization, meditation, dream analysis, dreams in other cultures, and parapsychological aspects of dreams. Founded 1975.

**(597) CREATIVITY LABORATORIES**
A-1106
463 West Street
New York, NY 10014

(212) 989-1826

*Edward Eichel, Founder*

Developer of a group process aimed at building compatibility within the male-female relationship. The method works at releasing physical armoring; effecting an abreaction of emotional experiences that cause emotional defensiveness; integration of the physical, emotional, and mental aspects of being; and creating a compatible sexual orientation. The work, which is developed in part from the principles of Wilhelm Reich, is explained in detail in a book, *Psychosexual Integration*, available from the above address. Founded 1970.

**FRIENDS HOSPITAL** (horticultural therapy)/Philadelphia, PA **(see 1125)**

**ESOTERIC PHILOSOPHY CENTER** (educational center) /Houston, TX **(see 151)**

**(598) VIVAXIS ENERGIES INTERNATIONAL RESEARCH SOCIETY**
P.O. Box 718
Chemainus, British Columbia
Canada, VOR 1KO

*Francis Nixon, Director*

The research of the Vivaxis Energies International Research

Society is focused on basic environmental energies, forces that stimulate vital life, giving wave motions, which are recorded emanating from every normal, healthy person. The Society's motto summarizes its objectives: "Remove energy obstructions that hinder healing. Reinstate a strong wave field in your bone structure and you will find health is there all the time. The knowledge of the wavelengths of your Vivaxis forces is one important key that makes this objective possible."

*Vivaxis* is a coined word: *viva* (life), *axis* (center)—"Center of Life." The energies of Vivaxis are of prenatal origin; the atomic arrangement in the baby's bone structure reflects the geophysical magnetism of the place and time in which the baby's Vivaxis was created, shortly prior to birth. The Society publishes a newsletter as well as making available two books written by Francis Nixon, *Born to Be Magnetic*, Volumes 1 and 2, describing the development of this theory. A course is also available explaining this theory in greater depth as well as containing research information substantiating it. Membership is available by writing to the Society.

**SERENITY HEALTH EDUCATION CENTRE** (educational) /Vancouver, B.C., Canada **(see 159)**

**(599) SERENA**
55 Parkdale Avenue
Ottawa, Ontario
Canada, K1Y 1E5

(613) 728-6536

6646 rue St. Denis
Montreal, Quebec
Canada, H2S 2R9

(514) 273-7531

A family-planning information and counseling service with many existing centers and trained couples (write for list). Natural birth control with emphasis on the symptothermal test for ovulation.

**(600) AJAPA-BREATH FOUNDATION**
239 Mount Royal West
Montreal, 152 P.Q.,
Quebec, Canada

(514) 844-6023

Teaches a form of breathing designed to steadily increase the aspirant's energy and eventually effect a union with the Absolute. The Foundation maintains contact with the individual after training to provide any necessary guidance or assistance.

**INTERNATIONAL INSTITUTE OF INTEGRAL HUMAN SCIENCES** (educational) /Montreal, Quebec, Canada **(see 68)**

**(601) HYGEIA STUDIOS**
Brook House
Avening, Tetbury
Gloucestershire, England

*Theo Gimbel, Founder*

Residential weekend courses in color, sound, and prayer healing. Members have done research with mentally handicapped children and work closely with physicians and social workers in this and related fields. Manufacturers and distributors of products relating to color and sound.

**WESTBANK HEALING AND TEACHING CENTRE** (multidisciplinary treatment center) /Fife, Scotland **(see 163)**

**FREIDRICH HUSEMANN-KLINIK** (anthroposophical clinic) /West Germany **(see 817)**

**LUCAS KLINIK** (anthroposophical clinic) /West Germany **(see 814)**

## Journals and Publications

**BRAIN/MIND BULLETIN**/Los Angeles, CA **(see 184)**

**COMMON GROUND** (multidisciplinary source listings Bay area) /San Francisco, CA **(see 187)**

**NEW REALITIES** (psychic magazine)/San Francisco, CA **(see 802)**

**CO-EVOLUTION QUARTERLY** (new age) /Sausalito, CA **(see 190)**

**JOURNAL OF BORDERLAND RESEARCH**/Vista, CA **(see 804)**

**ALTERNATIVES JOURNAL** (multidisciplinary new age articles)/Miami, FL **(see 193)**

**EAST WEST JOURNAL** (multidisciplinary new age articles) /Brookline, MA **(see 195)**

**NEW AGE JOURNAL** (multidisciplinary )/Brookline, MA **(see 196)**

**(602) SCIENCE DIGEST**
224 West 57th Street
New York, NY 10019

(212) 262-4286

*Dick Teresi, Editor*

Articles and reports on many new developments in healing technology, life energies, and related fields. Recent articles have reported on Kirlian photography, ginseng, and futurism.

**SEEKER** (multidisciplinary newsletter directory NY area) /New York, NY **(see 202)**

**HUMAN DIMENSIONS** (journal of unusual parapsychology research) /Williamsville, NY **(see 203)**

**JOURNAL OF THE RESEARCH SOCIETY FOR NATURAL THERAPEUTICS** (multidisciplinary) / Dorset, England **(see 70)**

## Products and Services

**(603) PYRAMID PRODUCTS**
701 West Ivy Street
Glendale, CA 91204

(213) 240-0421

Distributor of pyramids, many pyramid accessories, and books on pyramids. Established 1970.

**(604) JOE DUNN SLOAN**
6315 Middleton
Huntington Park, CA 90255

(213) 589-1987

Distributor of the "D" and "S" cells, activated by light sensitive pigments. May be used in drinking water to clear bacteria as well as worn close to various parts of the body for a variety of purposes. Further information may be obtained by writing to Joe Sloan at the above address.

**(605) SUNIER PRODUCTIONS**
21 Stetson Avenue
Kentfield, CA 94904

(415) 457-2741

Distributors of "Sense Tapes," three-hour taped programs combining music and natural sounds to create a flowing, transporting aural environment.

**HEALTH RESEARCH** (books) /Mokelumne Hill, CA **(see 209)**

**BUTTERFLY MEDIA DIMENSIONS** (cassette tapes) /N. Hollywood, CA **(see 210)**

**(606) ANAND ELECTRONICS**
Box 2868
Oakland, CA 94618

Developer and distributor of the silent meditation timer.

**NEW DIMENSIONS FOUNDATION** (cassette tapes) / San Francisco, CA 94111 **(see 212)**

**COGNETICS** (cassette tapes) /Saratoga, CA **(see 214)**

**BIG SUR RECORDINGS** (audiovisual and cassette tapes) /Sausalito, CA **(see 1135)**

**QUINTESSENCE UNLIMITED** (multidisciplinary products) /Boulder, CO **(see 215)**

**HARTLEY FILM PRODUCTIONS** (audiovisual) /Cos Cob, CT **(see 219)**

**(607) THOTH LTD.**
102 Charles Street
Suite 20
Boston, MA 02114

Distributes pyramids, Reichian energy blankets, and the Samadhi Isolation Tank. The latter, developed by Dr. John Lilly, can be used as an adjunct to meditation, deep rest, and exploring unusual states of consciousness. Publishes the *Thoth Research Journal,* reporting on research findings in various heuristic fields, e.g., Kirlian, auras, pyramidology, and meditation.

**(608) THE PYRAMID CENTRE**
Box 26
34 Copley Street
Newton, MA 02158

(617) 969-6962

*Marion Greene, Distributor*

Distributes books on pyramids, and pyramid kits. The

pyramids can be used for meditation aids, preserving foods, and improving plant growth. The Centre also coordinates research findings on pyramid science.

**W.G. BAZAN** (books) /O'Fallon, MO **(see 224)**

**(609) QUEST FOR HEALTH**
P.O. Box 623
Radio City Station, NY 10019

(212) 989-6237

Distributor of circular minitrampoline exerciser; orgone energy blankets and collars, hats, knee pads, and mittens. Product information available on request.

**HERITAGE STORE** (Cayce) /Virginia Beach, VA **(see 230)**

**(610) TUESDAY ISLAND FARM**
RR #2 North Wallace
Nova Scotia, Canada

*Nancy and Daniel McNeil, Directors*

A $6 donation provides calculations for one year of your astrologically safe and fertile times, plus a booklet on the biological fertility cycle.

# Biomagnetics

*The following is a list of researchers in the field of biomagnetics. "Biomagnetics" is the study and application of magnets and magnetic energies on living systems. An important technique to be considered in the balancing and restoration of health to the human system.*

**(611) ALBERT ROY DAVIS RESEARCH LABORATORY**
520 Magnolia Avenue
Green Cove Springs, FL 32043

Research in biomagnetics.

**(612) BIOMAGNETICS INTERNATIONAL, INC.**
537 Florida Bank Building
Jacksonville, FL 32202

Researchers in biomagnetics.

**(613) DR. FREDERICK DOUGHTY BECK**
943 Jackson Avenue
New Orleans, LA 70130

Researcher in biomagnetics.

**(614) DR. AND MRS. ROBERT J. MORGAN**
County Bank Building
Delaware, OH 43015

Researchers in biomagnetics.

**(615) DR. HAROLD H.E. BROWNLEE**
86 Park Road South
Oshawa, Ontario, Canada

Researcher in biomagnetics.

**(616) BIOMAGNETICS AUSTRALIA, LTD.**
P.O. Box 292
Maroubra 2035
Sydney, Australia

*Kevin J. Dalton*

Researcher in biomagnetics.

**(617) DR. STEFAN N. NAYDENOV**
Aleksander Stamboliiski,
154-A, Sofia, Bulgaria

Researcher in biomagnetics.

**(618) DR. LEONARD J. ALLAN**
16 Lonsdale Avenue
Margate, Kent CT9 3BT
England

Researcher in biomagnetics.

**(619) DR. LESLIE O. KORTH**
"WENVOE"
159 St. Johns Road
Tunbridge Wells
Kent TN4 9UP, England

Researcher in biomagnetics.

**(620) DR. D.N. KHUSHALANI**
Rehmatbi Vadnagarwala Hospital
Calcutta, India

Researcher in biomagnetics.

**(621) DR. A.K. BHATTACHARYA**
Shastii Villa,
Naihati, India

Researcher in biomagnetics.

**(622) MAGNA INTERNATIONAL PRODUCTS, INC.**
Sakai 3-9-11
Musashino-Shi,
Tokyo, Japan

*Dr. Yoshio Seki*

Researcher in biomagnetics.

**(623) DR. IN SU KIM**
54-1, 2-ka, Myung-dong
Seoul, Korea

Researcher in biomagnetics.

**(624) PUERTO RICO SCIENTIFIC RESEARCH LABORATORY**
1707 Arkansas Street
San Gerardo, Rio Piedras,
Puerto Rico 00926

*Dr. Ralph U. Sierra, Director*

Researcher in biomagnetics.

**(625) VICTOR BEASLEY, PhD**
P.O. Box 420
Bridgetown, Barbados
West Indies

Researcher in biomagnetics.

# Toward A Medicine Of Subtle Energies

*William A. Tiller, PhD*

*Exploration of subtle energies functioning in Nature will lay the foundations for "subjective science" on an equal footing with our present "objective science." This subjective science will require a knowledge and stabilization of the mental and emotional fields of the participants as part of the overall experimental protocol.*

We may compare conventional scientific understanding of the universe to the visible tip of an iceberg. Although we have come to know that exposed tip very well, most of Nature is still hidden from us. History contains references to and speculation on many aspects of the hidden iceberg, and very recent research suggests some fascinating possibilities.

I have developed a new model of the universe on which a new medicine may be founded, based on certain major conclusions. We are elements of spirit, indestructible and eternal (multiplexed in the Divine), and contain a mechanism of perception—the mind, consisting of three levels: instinctive, intellectual, and spiritual. The mind, which is postulated to function in a six-dimensional space lattice, creates a vehicle for experience, and we, the spiritual being plus mechanism, invest ourselves in that vehicle, which runs a continuously programmed course. The "stuff" used for the construction of the vehicle (or stimulator) is of two conjugate natures: (1) that which is electrical, traveling at velocities less than electromagnetic light, and which has positive mass and energy, forms the physical part; and (2) that which is magnetic, traveling at velocities greater than electromagnetic light, and thus has negative mass and energy, forms the etheric part. The total sum of these two energies is zero, as is the sum of their entrophies; the total simulator (or vehicle) is created out of empty space through a fluctuation process and is just the world of appearances that we shape with our minds.

The conclusions are that we live in a multidimensional universe and are ourselves multidimensional beings comprised of a nontemporal part and a temporal part, as illustrated in Figure 1. The temporal portion, which is the simulator, is constructed from physical substance, which functions in the positive space-time frame (+ve S−T), and etheric substance, which functions in the negative space-time frame (− ve S–T). The being is interfaced with the simulator through the emotional circuitry of the system, which I think is fabricated from astral substance functioning in a transitional frame.

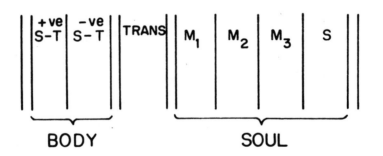

Fig. 1. Representation of being (soul) attached to the simulator (body) through the transitional frame as an interfacing network.

To illustrate the multidimensional aspect with a simple molecule like benzene, one would state that the *numina* of benzene has been probed with all the physical sensors of modern technology, and they have revealed the *phenomena* of benzene, i.e., the physical facet of the total "iceberg" that is benzene. In the future, as science learns to develop new categories of sensors, other facets of benzene will be revealed.

To illustrate the multidimensional aspects of the human species, it is perhaps beneficial to use a reaction type of equation (Eq. 1) to indicate the dynamic interplay among the different levels of the universe.

$$\text{Function} \rightleftarrows \text{Structure} \rightleftarrows \text{Chemistry} \rightleftarrows \begin{array}{c}\text{Positive}\\\text{Space-Time}\\\text{Energies}\end{array} \rightleftarrows \begin{array}{c}\text{Negative}\\\text{Space-Time}\\\text{Energies}\end{array} \rightleftarrows$$

$$\rightleftarrows \text{Mind} \rightleftarrows \text{Spirit} \rightleftarrows \text{Divine}$$

$$\text{(Eq. 1)}$$

In Equation 1, all the conventional energies (e.g., electromagentic and gravitational) function in the positive space-time frame, and the unconventional energies (e.g., magnetoelectric, levitational) function in the negative space-time frame. Generally, if there is an error in the function of a living organism, we trace it to a defect in its physical structure and trace that back to an imbalance in the chemistry of the substratum; we are only just beginning to recognize that perhaps the homeostasis at the chemical level depends on specific supportive energy field patterns at the positive space-time energy level. Homeostasis at this level depends on the energy field patterns of its substrate, i.e., the negative space-time frame. These patterns, in turn, are generated from the level of mind, which is imbedded in the frame of spirit, which is imbedded in the Divine. The system is totally interconnected, and a perturbation of any level sends waves of effect propagating both to the left and to the right on the reaction chain. In the past, we have attempted to rectify errors of function by inputs at the chemical level, becoming more and more sophisticated with our chemical inputs as both the system and the invader organism adapted itself to diminish the effectiveness of these inputs.

At this point, it is useful to recall Wolf's law for bone structure, stating that if a nonuniform stress is applied to the bone by the body for an extended period, the bone will grow new trabeculae (a type of bone girder) in the exact locations to best support this nonuniform stress distribution. The process probably occurs by the physical strain field interacting with electrostatic fields of the system, through piezoelectric effects, which produce changes there, and these changes cause ions and molecules to be transported to specific locations to such a degree that gelation and agglomeration occur into specific tissues and structures that comprise the trabeculae.

Carrying this idea further, mental stresses or aberrations can alter the curvature (or the detailed matrix) of negative space-time, causing alterations in both the curvature of positive space-time and in the magnetoelectric field patterns of etheric substance in the body. These, in turn, produce pattern correlations at the electromagnetic and other conventional energy levels in the physical body, which then alter the chemical flows, and so forth, leading to a concretization (or calcification) of the original mental stress at some physical locations of the body.

We must note that the removal of the body stress that created a certain pattern of trabeculae in a bone does not lead to the instantaneous dissolution of these trabeculae. Rather, they may disintegrate or dissolve very slowly (under the proper exercise) because of the molecular kinetics involved, and they may maintain the body in a distorted shape for a very long time, even if the initial physical cause is removed (rationale for Rolfing). The same situation is expected to occur for physical structures generated by emotional or mental stress patterns. Further, since these disharmonious patterns scatter energy from the main flow stream at the various levels already discussed, the removal of the anchoring patterns at the two ends of the chain will release the intervening pattern links, and more energy will be available for the organism's functioning.

The foregoing leads quite naturally to a perspective on healing: i.e., the perception that pathology can develop at a number of levels and that healing is needed at all of them to restore the system to a state of harmony. The initial pathology begins at the level of mind and propagates effects to both the negative space-time and the positive space-time levels. We then perceive what we call disease or malfunction at these levels and try to remove the effects by a variety of healing techniques.

The best healing mode is to help the person remove the pathology at the *cause* level and bring about the correction by a return to "right thinking." The next best healing mode is to effect repair of the structure at the negative space-time level. The next best level of healing is that which medicine practices today, wherein the structure is repaired at the positive space-time level. Since the energy structures at these different levels are coupled, repair at a lower level will still produce some feedback modification of energy structure at a higher level.

If harmony is not restored at the higher level, however, then a force will continue to exist for pathological development in the energy structure at a lower level. Of course, this force is basically like a thermodynamic potential to produce change so that the effects may be manifested or materialized in very different forms, depending on what alterations have already been made to the energy structures of the positive and negative space-time frames. The closest analogy to this occurs in the field of "phase equilibria" of materials. If you heat a complex alloy containing a number of chemical constituents to a high temperature so that it melts, then by cooling it again you produce a thermodynamic driving force for a phase change to one of several possible solid forms. By making very slight but specific modifications to the chemistry or cooling rate or other variables in the process, it is possible to change the type of solid phase that initially develops and the crystalline form that results.

The healer makes use of this extended energy structure of self to channel the needed frequency components of the needed energy at the particular dimensional level into the person being healed. Since the particular pathology is represented by a particular energy pattern and all patterns are formed by the superposition of waves, a pattern can be altered or completely eradicated by the input of the appropriate wave components at the appropriate intensity level. To do this effectively, a number of conditions need to be satisfied: (1) one must be able to generate or tap the needed wave components of the requisite type; (2) one must be able to tap these wave components from one's extended energy structure at the specifically needed ratios or relative intensities; (3) one must tap the requisite correction energy pattern at a high overall intensity, so that the healing needed is of short duration; (4) one must be sharply attuned to the person being healed, so that these energy components can be brought into that person's extended energy structure without scattering losses; and (5) the person being healed must have confidence in the healer, so that the healer's efforts are not mentally distorted or negated because of fears or doubts.

Equation 1 indicates that we can expect to see the introduction of new medical therapeutic devices designed to generate, restore, and sustain harmonious energy patterns at electromagnetic and other conventional energy levels. This will eventually be followed by families of devices for controlling the spectral flow of energy between the negative space-time frame and the positive, and eventually by devices for amplifying energy transfer from the mind frame into these two simulator frames. Of course, no matter how sophisticated these devices will eventually be, we must recognize that patients have free will and thus can impede the process with their own mental input if they so desire. Eventually, this psychophysiological factor will fully be taken into account as medicine realizes that when one enters the domain of *subtle energy therapies*, one moves into the domain of subjective science, where the mental and emotional states of the patient influence the process in lawful ways and thus are a necessary part of the protocol for achieving a given effect.

The body appears to contain a multidimensional antenna array for inside-outside connectivity which, at the physical level, takes the form of the autonomic nervous system. The loci of antenna elements on the surface of the skin appear to be the acupuncture point network. These are the points through which the energy pattern is radiated so that there is a greater skin conductance at these points (like a photoconduction effect in semiconductors and insulators). Researchers believe that one of the important power systems for this antenna array is the endocrine system, with its seven spatially distributed glands, serving not only to control the main chemical factories of the body but also as receptors and transmitters of subtle energies. Studies have shown that the seats of sensitivity for certain dowsing signals are the adrenal and pituitary glands. The endocrines also seem to serve as a bridge to other dimensions through connectivity with the chakras described in Eastern mystical literature. We can think of the endocrine-chakra pairs as transducers of energy between the physical and other dimensions of the universe.

A technique has been developed for monitoring the difference in the electrical characteristics, between the left and right sides of the body, of the acupuncture points at the ends of the meridians. If the standard deviation is greater than 1.21, an instability of the autonomic nervous system leading to the onset of disease for that meridian and that organ domain of the body is indicated. If the standard deviation is less than 0.5, a chronic disease is indicated. However, the strict correlation between these electrical indicators and Western medicine concepts of disease has not yet been accomplished—it is in progress. All the present modalities of acupuncture therapy show that they moderate the electrochemical potential of the tissue fluids at the acupuncture points and thus moderate the electrical characteristics of the antenna system in such a way as to restore functional balance. A mechanism for linking positive space-time and negative space-time disharmonious patterns has also been indicated.

In terms of therapy, we can readily see the connectivity between this model and polarity therapy, kinesiology, and vivaxis therapy, because they also deal with energy flows into and out of the body and use acupuncture points as the loci for strategic energy changes to the body. Devices designed for the restoration of this subtle energy balance have been in use for some time. Three of these are the Eeman's relaxation circuit, the Cayce radioactive appliance, and the Cayce wet cell appliance, which also appear to work in concordance with the proposed model. Since the negative space-time frame is in a type of mirror-image relationship to the positive space-time frame, homeopathic medicine fits quite naturally as the medicine needed for the etheric level of substance to restore proper function directly at that level and thus influence proper function at the physical level. Stepping further afield, radionic medicine deals with the interface between the mind dimensions and the negative space-time dimension. In the proper hands, radionic medicine appears to be an effective therapy at that level. We must learn much more about the negative space-time frame and its connective linkages, with both the frame of physical substance, on the one hand, and the frame of mental substance, on the other, before truly effective use of such techniques is possible. Since the techniques appear to violate the conventional view of reality, it is not surprising that they are considered quackery by the AMA and the FDA. It will require many years of effort and serious experimentation before the conventional view of medicine is replaced by such a new "world picture" that radionics techniques will be considered commonplace.

There is a truly great need for reliable experimental devices for monitoring body energies on successively more and more subtle levels. Measurements with these devices will help to forge the bridge between our present chemical modalities and our future modalities. The next step is to work with primarily physical-level monitoring devices (for example, Kirlian photography, acupuncture point and other skin monitors, electrostatic field monitors) and to provide a sound base from which to test our models. This step needs to be followed with biochemical and bioelectrical transducers (such as dowsing wands), deltron and magnetoelectric devices that reach into the negative space-time domain and lay a foundation for valid experimentation at that level. Finally, a family of devices that use and manipulate mental energies need to be studied in depth so that we can build a firm bridge from the point at which our consciousness is presently located to the fundamental level of our being—the spirit.

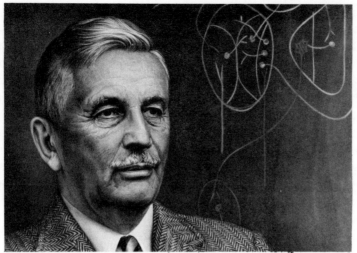

Harold Saxton Burr, PhD, E.K. Hunt Professor Emeritus, Anatomy, Yale University School of Medicine. Portrait by Artzybasheff; courtesy Yale University Art Gallery.

# The Fields Of Life

## Edward W. Russell, MA

*"It is even possible that science itself may be a symbol—a projection. In its aspiration to conquer the Universe and its desire to explode the cosmos, science may again be expressing those old desires mankind has had to achieve totality or wholeness."*

*Miguel Serrano*

In 1935, Dr. Harold Saxton Burr and Dr. F. S. C. Northrop, both of Yale University, first published their "electrodynamic theory of life." Since that time, the theory has been confirmed by thousands of experiments. Briefly, Burr (who died in 1973) and his colleagues discovered that all living forms—whether humans, animals, trees, plants, or lower forms of life—possess and are controlled by electromagnetic fields. These are the organizing "mechanisms" that keep all living forms in shape and build, maintain, and repair them through constant changes of materials. These organizing "fields of life"—or "L-fields"—can be measured and mapped with great precision by modern instruments.

A rough analogy may help the reader to visualize the function of these fields—the familiar school experiment with a magnet and iron filings. When a card held over a magnet is sprinkled with filings, the filings arrange themselves in a pattern that represents the lines of force of the magnet's field. However often the filings are changed, each set of filings will always assume the same pattern. Similarly, the L-fields—though infinitely more complicated—keep the ever-changing atoms, molecules, and cells of the living form in the same pattern.

The overall field of any given living form embraces many local "subfields" of the atoms, molecules, cells, and organs; the subfields interact to some extent with the overall field. Despite this "feedback" from the subfields, however, there is plenty of evidence that the overall field of the living form is primary and controls its component fields.

These L-fields can be measured with any good vacuum-tube or transistorized voltmeter of such high resistance that it draws virtually no current and therefore does not affect the voltage patterns in the field. These are DC potentials and have nothing to do with the brainwaves or with the currents measured by an electrocardiograph. Special electrodes of silver coated with silver chloride must be used. For precise readings of the field of the human body the electrodes are applied to the forehead and chest or palms—although it is possile to measure field voltage even with the electrodes very close to but not touching the skin. For special purposes they may be applied directly to some organ, but to get a less precise reading it is sometimes sufficient to dip a finger of each hand into two little dishes of saline solution connected to the voltmeter.

Through many years of painstaking and meticulous experimentation Burr and his colleagues made many important discoveries related to L-fields which demonstrate that the field *anticipates* physical events.

1. Measured over a period of a few weeks, L-fields of healthy men and women show regular cyclical rises and falls of voltage, which can be plotted in steady curves. These "peaks and valleys" of the voltage curves indicate the times when the individual is at his or her best and, conversely, times when vitality and efficiency are low. These curves can be projected and used to predict "highs" and "lows" weeks in advance. This knowledge could be of great value to those engaged in hazardous occupations; intelligently used, this discovery could save lives.

2. By measuring the voltage gradients in the L-field of a woman, it is possible to determine the moment of ovulation with great accuracy, for ovulation is preceded by a substantial rise in voltage, which falls rapidly to normal after ovulation. L-field measurements have revealed that some women ovulate over the entire menstrual cycle, and that ovulation may occur without menstruation, or menses without ovulation. The potential importance of this discovery for gynecology, family planning, and birth control is obvious.

3. Malignancies have been recorded electrically by L-field measurements before any clinical sign could be observed. This could prove a new tool with which to detect cancer early, when there is a better chance of treating it successfully.

4. Changes in the L-field of the body have been noted when wounds are healing. This offers the possibility of a reliable, simple way to measure the rate of healing, especially of internal wounds from operations.

5. Measurement of changes in the human L-field reveal the different effects of sleep, drugs, or hypnosis—another tool for medicine. A pupil of Dr. Burr, Dr. Leonard J. Ravitz, Jr., has actually measured the depth of hypnosis electrically.

6. Mentally unstable people display erratic voltage patterns in their L-fields before there are any obvious symptoms. This may make possible preventive mental health care.

7. Measurements of the L-fields of trees have revealed a relationship with both lunar cycles and with sunspots. If—as seems probable—such relationships can also be established with the human L-field, this will be important in the study not only of health and behavior, but also of physical problems that may arise in space exploration.

8. By measuring the L-fields of seeds, it is possible to predict how strong and healthy future plants will be.

9. Measurements of the L-fields of plants show that the change of a single gene in the parent stock produces profound changes in the voltage pattern. This discovery could be of great importance to the study of genetics in plants and animals.

10. Measurement of the voltages in different parts of the L-field of a frog's egg can show the *future* location of the frog's nervous system, indicating that the L-field of an egg serves as a "blueprint" or matrix for the organization of the form that will develop from the egg.

It should be obvious from this list—which is by no means complete—that the discovery of L-fields opens up vast possibilities for creative medical and biological research. Apart from further work on the discoveries summarized in the list, there are other opportunities for research. For example, there is some evidence that electrical treatment of the controlling L-field can reduce various physical ills. Alternating magnetic fields of certain specific frequencies applied to the L-field of the human body seem to reduce blood pressure and cholesterol levels. Wounds exposed to an electrical field reportedly heal faster. Clearly, the study of L-fields has much to contribute toward the evolution of new modes of healing.

## Research Information

(626) **EDWARD W. RUSSELL, MA**
"Tall Pines"
Hearthstone Ridge
Route, #1

Landrum, SC 29356

Will act as a central contact point to help researchers and physicians interested in the application and study of "L-Fields" (as it relates to the field of medicine) get in touch with one another. Serious inquirers please send self-addressed stamped envelope.

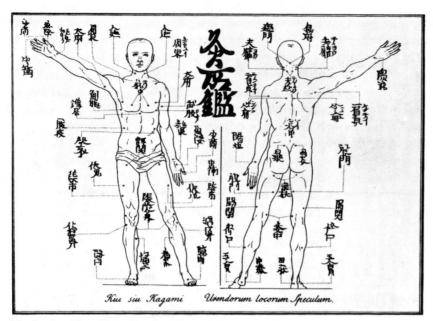

Moxibustion Chart. From: Engelbert Kaempfer's: *Histoire naturelle, civile, et écclesiastique de l'empire du Japon*, La Haye, 1929; courtesy, Univ. of California Press, from *The Yellow Emperor's Classic of Internal Medicine*. By Veith, Berkeley: 1970.

# Acupuncture In America

*David E. Bresler, PhD*
*Richard J. Kroening, MD*
*Michael P. Volen, MD*

For many years, occasional visitors from the West have returned from China with anecdotal reports of the successful use of acupuncture in the treatment of various medical problems. These reports remained largely curiosities in the United States until improvement of relations in the early 1970s brought new information which stimulated great interest in acupuncture.

Acupuncture has been practiced in China for over 3,000 years; its origins are lost in antiquity. Its endurance has been remarkable, considering the many cultural and political changes that have swept China. It is quite possible that more people have been treated by acupuncture in the course of human history than by any other formalized system of medicine. It is a complete and complex system of medicine, based upon the philosophy and world view of the culture from which it arose.

The classical Chinese conceptions of health and disease are intrinsically linked to the philosophical constructs of traditional Chinese thought. The ancient Chinese believed that the universe is permeated with a vital life force or energy (called *ch'i*), which circulates continuously through all living organisms. This energy was thought to follow specific pathways through the body—referred to as "meridians"—upon which the acupuncture "points" lie. Stimulation of specific acupuncture points was believed to affect the flow of ch'i in specific organ systems of the body.

Originally, twelve bilaterally symmetrical meridians were described, with each meridian named for one of the twelve major internal organs conceptualized by traditional Chinese medicine. In addition to these twelve paired meridians, two non-paired "control" meridians were described: the "Governing Vessel," which follows the spine and runs along the midline on the dorsal surface of the body, and the "Conception Vessel," which runs along the midline on the ventral surface of the body.

If the circulation of ch'i is impeded or blocked in a given meridian as a result of external events (such as trauma, cold, dampness) or internal factors (such as fear, anger, sorrow), an abnormal surplus or deficit of ch'i may result. This imbalance affects the entire organism and is ultimately manifested by the presence of pain or disease. Utilizing a variety of diagnostic techniques, the traditional acupuncture practitioner first attempts to identify the nature of the imbalance of energy and then selects the appropriate acupuncture points on the basis of this evaluation. Depending on the problem, the points selected may be stimulated by acupuncture (the insertion of fine, solid needles), moxibustion (heating with mugwort, a traditional Chinese herb), or acupressure (massage). Modern technology also made available a variety of new techniques, including electrical stimulation of the needles, ultrasound stimulation, and even laser beam stimulation.

A considerable amount of research has now been conducted to explore the possible mechanisms of action of acupuncture. In particular, neurophysiological research on the nature of pain has produced several theories that attempt to explain the analgesic effects of acupuncture. Most theories of acupuncture have focused on the nervous system, and abundant scientific evidence indicates that acupuncture points represent neural receptors. In addition, recent investigations have also raised the intriguing possibility that the pain-relieving effects of acupuncture may be produced by stimulating the release of naturally occurring morphine-like substances in the central nervous system.

At present, no single explanation of the phenomenon of acupuncture has been generally accepted, and it is quite possible that a number of different factors may be involved, including a complex mobilization of the immune/inflammatory system, peripheral neural stimulation, and subtle psychological factors.

At present, the widest application of acupuncture in America has been for treatment of patients with chronic pain. When performed by well-trained, experienced therapists, acupuncture is a safe and effective treatment modality that often provides significant and long-lasting pain relief to patients with headaches, osteoarthritis, neuralgia and neuritis, low back and other musculoskeletal pain problems. Other types of medical problems may also respond to acupuncture, but very little research has been conducted in this country concerning acupuncture therapy for problems other than chronic pain.

Acupuncture is employed widely in China and elsewhere in the world for treatment of a great variety of medical problems. It is also considered to be a sophisticated form of preventive medicine; it may be used to maintain health as well as to treat disease. An ancient Chinese aphorism states, "The superior acupuncturist treats before illness is manifested; the inferior acupuncturist treats illness he was unable to prevent." In light of its strong emphasis on nutritional, environmental, and psychological factors, as well as physical symptoms, acupuncture may also be considered one of the earliest systems of wholistic* or integral medicine.

In Chinese medicine, all bodily processes are described in terms of the interaction of opposing *yin* and *yang* forces. The goal of medical care is to maintain or restore energy balance between yin and yang, thus ensuring proper health. This concept of yin-yang balance is analogous to the modern Western concept of homeostasis.

The conceptual similarities are most clear when one considers the sympathetic and parasympathetic divisions of the autonomic nervous system. Overactivity of the sympathetic nervous system produces what the Chinese might call "excess yang" ailments, whereas overactivity of the parasympathetic nervous system produces "excess yin" ailments. Yin and yang may also be reflected by opposing flexor and extensor muscles, the manner in which blood sugar is regulated by insulin and glucogen, and by the way in which central nervous system activation and sleep are regulated by norepinephrine and serotonin. It is intriguing to consider the possibility that many "incurable" ailments related to lack of homeostatic balance may someday be routinely treated by acupuncture therapy.

Traditional Chinese medicine approaches the concepts of health and disease from a totally different perspective than Western medicine, thus its ideas and terminology often seem strange or unfamiliar to most Western physicians. In addition, Western medicine has become increasingly specialized, and it has not been clear where acupuncture, which approaches the treatment of the patient as a whole, should fit into this system of specialization. Thus, many physicians, while interested in the potential applications of acupuncture, are not sure how it could be included in their own medical practice and few have access to formal training programs.

---

*Spelled holistic in original text.

The legal status of acupuncture continues to be quite confused, with different states enacting widely differing laws regulating its practice. Despite its long history and overwhelming scientific evidence of its efficacy, the American Medical Association and the Food and Drug Administration continue to insist that acupuncture be considered an "experimental" form of treatment. Because of this position, the Medicare and Medicaid agencies, as well as most health insurance carriers, will not provide reimbursement for acupuncture therapy, thus limiting its availability to those people fortunate enough to be able to pay for it.

It is hoped that this situation will change as acupuncture is more thoroughly investigated in this country. Acupuncture research is now being conducted at a number of medical schools in the United States, and although there is still disagreement as to its mechanism of action, most physicians who have seriously investigated acupuncture agree that it is a safe and effective form of therapy.

It seems strange that acupuncture has been less readily available in the United States, with its sophisticated health care system, than in most other countries of the world. However, as new state laws are enacted to set standards for practice, and more and more people are helped, acupuncture may soon find a home in America as well.

## Groups and Associations

### (627) ACUPUNCTURE RESEARCH INSTITUTE
Alumni Association
P.O. Box 7534
Long Beach, CA 90807

(213) 860-3666

Provides information for physicians about acupuncture training programs and research projects. Maintains list of active members. Publishes newsletter, *Meridian*.

### (628) NATIONAL ACUPUNCTURE ASSOCIATION
P.O. Box 24509
Los Angeles, CA 90024

(213) 477-4343

Conducts basic training program for physicians and lay professionals. Disseminates information about acupuncture to physicians and the general public. Maintains list of active members, available on request.

### CENTER FOR INTEGRAL MEDICINE/Pacific
Palisades, CA (see 57)

### (629) UNITED ACUPUNCTURISTS OF CALIFORNIA
125 Quincy
St. Mary's Square
San Francisco, CA 94108

(415) 434-2545

Represents interests of traditional acupuncturists; concerned with promoting legislation and policy changes to make acupuncture legal.

### (630) NEVADA BOARD OF CHINESE MEDICINE
201 South Fall Street
Carson City, NV 89701

(702) 885-4800

State certifying agency; provides information about licensing requirements for acupuncturists in the State of Nevada.

### (631) NATIONAL ACUPUNCTURE RESEARCH SOCIETY
1841 Broadway
New York, NY 10023

(212) 582-0331

Conducts training program in acupuncture for physicians and other health care professionals.

### (632) ACUPUNCTURE ASSOCIATION
34 Alderney Street
London, SW1V 4EU
England

Tel: 01-834-3353

Maintains list of acupuncturists practicing in Great Britain.

## Schools, Centers, and Clinics

### PSYCHOSOMATIC MEDICINE CLINIC/Berkeley, CA (see 78)

### (633) ACUPUNCTURE PROJECT
Franz Hall A-181
University of California
School of Medicine
Los Angeles, CA 90024

(213) 825-4833

*David E. Bresler, PhD, Director*

A team of doctors offers professional training to medical, dental, and psychology students as well as resident physicians and dentists. An Acupuncture Clinic, a division of the Project, provides treatment for a wide variety of pain-related disorders and is conducting clinical research focusing on acute and chronic pain disorders including heacaches, facial and dental pain syndromes, arthritis, and nerve injuries. The Project is supported by patients and by donations from interested groups and organizations.

**(634) CENTER FOR CHINESE MEDICINE**
P.O. Box 32072
Los Angeles, CA 90032

(213) 282-2141

*John F. Chow, PharmD, MD, Medical Director*

Established for the purpose of facilitating information exchange between East and West relating to Chinese medicine. Provides basic educational training in acupuncture and related fields of Chinese medicine; both professional and lay workshops are offered. Acupuncture referrals are made on request. The Center maintains a speakers' bureau and publishes a newsletter, *Acupuncture News.* Founded 1974.

**KHALSA MEDICAL AND COUNSELING ASSOCIATES**/Los Angeles, CA **(see 92)**

**McCORNACK CENTER FOR THE HEALING ARTS**/Mendocino, CA **(see 95)**

**(635) ACUPUNCTURE WHOLISTIC CENTER**
822 South Atlantic Boulevard
Monterey Park, CA 91754

(213) 289-3621

*Pedro Chan, Director*

Practice of acupuncture and herbal medicine.

**GEORGE OHSAWA MACROBIOTIC FOUNDATION**/Oroville, CA **(see 535)**

**(636) ACUPUNCTURE AND HERBS RESEARCH**
4465 Rolfe Road
San Diego, CA 92117

(714) 270-4971

*Tomson Liang, CA*

Acupuncture clinic providing treatment for pain from arthritis, injury, surgical recovery, headaches including migraine, eyestrain and cancer. Uses herbs for reducing blood fats, relieving prostate congestion and easing hot flashes without estrogen. Also acts as a distributor for electrical acupuncture equipment without needles, ginseng and other Chinese herbs, books and pamphlets on current health related methods and herbs. Consults with MD's on problems treatable with acupuncture and herbs, and offers private tutoring in acupuncture and electrical acupuncture.

**AGE OF ENLIGHTENMENT CENTER FOR HOLISTIC HEALTH**/San Diego, CA **(see 104)**

**SAN DIEGO NATURAL HEALTH CLINIC**/San Diego, CA **(see 108)**

**(637) ACUPUNCTURE RESEARCH INSTITUTE**
9375 San Fernando Road
Sun Valley, CA 91352

(213) 768-3000

*Willem H. Khoe, MD, President*

Teaches ancient and modern acupuncture to professionals. Public education is offered on a monthly basis. Founded 1972.

**SCHOOL OF ACTUALISM**/Valley Center, CA (also Escondido, La Jolla, Los Angeles, San Francisco, and Santa Ana, CA) **(see 783)**

**(638) INSTITUTE OF PNEUMOLOGY**
5524 MacArthur Boulevard, N.W.
Washington, DC 20016

(202) 363-2455

*James H. Johnson, MD, Director*

Holistic family medical clinic emphasizing acupuncture and nutrition.

**(639) EMORY UNIVERSITY**
School of Dentistry
1462 Clifton Road, N.E.
Atlanta, GA 30322

*Atten: Lindsey M. Hunt, PhD, Acupuncture Research Project*

Research in the physiological evaluation of dental anesthesia.

**EXPANSION**/Bedford, MA **(see 1090)**

**(640) MASSACHUSETTS GENERAL HOSPITAL**
32 Fruit
Boston, MA 02114

*Atten: Gene Smith, PhD, Acupuncture Research Project*

Research studies of acupuncture in dental pain.

**ACUPUNCTURE CENTER OF MASSACHUSETTS**/Newton, MA **(see 130)**

**(641) NEW ENGLAND SCHOOL OF ACUPUNCTURE**
5 Bridge Street
Watertown, MA 02172

(617) 924-7900

*James Tin Yau So, ND, Principal*

A faculty of Eastern and Western practitioners offers the serious student of Oriental medicine a firm foundation in acupuncture. The program presently offered is a ten-month intensive in classical and modern European acupuncture. The school is legally licensed to teach Oriental medicine. Founded 1975.

**(642) RYODORAKU RESEARCH INSTITUTE OF NORTH AMERICA, INC.**
8133 Wornall Road
Kansas City, MO 64114

(816) 361-4077

Offers a PhD program in medical acupuncture for qualified MDs, DOs, DDSs, DMDs, DVMs, and PhDs. Requirements include 100 hours of clinical acupuncture practice and completion of a dissertation.

**CENTRAL BERGEN COMMUNITY MENTAL HEALTH CENTER**/Paramus, NJ **(see 1112)**

**INSTITUTE FOR SELF DEVELOPMENT**/Manhasset, NY **(see 137)**

**(643) ACUPUNCTURE CENTER OF NEW YORK**
426 East 89th Street
New York, NY 10028

(212) 534-6800

*Ralph Sepson, MD, Medical Director*

Comprehensive medical examination, and if indicated, treatment in acupuncture and moxa is given.

**NEW YORK STAR CENTER** (Actualism) /New York, NY **(see 783)**

**(644) EAST-WEST ACADEMY OF HEALTH PRACTICES**
2710 Northeast Broadway
Portland, OR 97232

(503) 282-6035

*Beth Gilbert, Coordinator*

Provides training in acupuncture theory; Swedish, acupressure, reflexology, and polarity massage, nutrition, and yoga.

**DALLAS STAR CENTER** (Actualism) /Dallas, TX **(see 783)**

**SUNSHINE MEDICAL SHOW**/Seattle, WA **(see 156.1)**

**(645) UNIVERSITY OF WASHINGTON**
School of Medicine
Seattle, WA 98195

*Atten: C. Richard Chapman, PhD, Acupuncture Research Project*

Research in acupuncture and perception of dental pain.

**PAIN AND HEALTH REHABILITATION CENTER**/La Crosse, WI **(see 157)**

**COLD MOUNTAIN INSTITUTE**/Vancouver, B.C., Canada **(see 1130)**

**(646) INTERNATIONAL INSTITUTE OF ORIENTAL MEDICINE**
Thorne House
Gerrards Cross
Berks, England

*J.D. Van Buren, DO, ND*

Professional course on acupuncture; curriculum study covers a period of 3 years.

**(647) THE COLLEGE OF TRADITIONAL CHINESE ACUPUNCTURE**
St. Albans House
Royal Leamington Spa
Warwickshire, England

Tel: Leamington 39347

*J.R. Worsley, President*

Provides theoretical, practical and clinical training in acupuncture to the levels of Licentiate, 2½ years, Bachelor, 4½ years, and Doctorate, 7½ years. Founded 1968.

*AFFILIATE CENTER*

**THE CENTER FOR TRADITIONAL ACUPUNCTURE, INC.**
The American City Building
Columbia, MD 21044

(301) 997-3770

**SWEDISH HERBAL INSTITUTE** (research) /
Gothenburg, Sweden **(see 554)**

## Journals and Publications

**(648) THE AMERICAN JOURNAL OF ACUPUNCTURE**
1400 Lost Acre Drive
Felton, CA 95018

Professional publication on acupuncture and related topics.

**MERIDIAN** (acupuncture newsletter) /Long Beach, CA **(see 627)**

**BRAIN/MIND BULLETIN**/Los Angeles, CA **(see 184)**

**(649) JOURNAL OF ACUPUNCTURE AND ELECTROTHERAPEUTICS RESEARCH**
Pergamon Press
Maxwell House, Fairview Park
Elmsford, NY 10523

*Yoshiaki Omura, MD, ScD, Editor-in-Chief*

Headington Hill Hall
Oxford, OX3 OBW, England

International journal with articles on the medical, physiological, legal, and historical aspects of acupuncture.

**(650) AMERICAN JOURNAL OF CHINESE MEDICINE**
Box 555
Garden City, NY 11530

(516) 248-0930

Concerned with comparative study of medicine, health care, and policy. Interest is focused on technical and scientific aspects of indigenous medical practices, including drug plants, acupuncture, and other modalities.

## Products and Services

**(651) CHAN'S CORPORATION**
2930 West Valley Boulevard
Alhambra, CA 91803

(213) 281-1610

Carries a complete supply of acupuncture books, charts, needles, instruments, moxa, and models.

**(652) BIO-INSTRUMENTATION, INC.**
7260 Evanston Place
Goleta, CA 93107

(805) 968-8778

Distributor of electroacupuncture equipment with and without needles.

**(653) B.X. & L. INDUSTRIES, INC.**
17905 Sky Park Boulevard, Suite K
Irvine, CA 92707

(714) 979-4755

Distributes frequency modulated acupuncture stimulators, needles, charts, manikens, books, and staple guns.

**(654) O-MATIC, INC.**
902 East Holt Avenue
Pomona, CA 91767

(714) 629-3910

Distributors of automated meridian readout machines and electroacupuncture (no needle) equipment.

**ACUPUNCTURE AND HERBS RESEARCH**/San Diego, CA **(see 636)**

**(655) CADRE**
124 28th Avenue
San Mateo, CA 94403

(415) 341-4204

Distributes a complete line of books, charts, needles, and electronic acupuncture equipment.

**(656) GENERAL MEDICAL INDUSTRIES, INC.**
969 Barcelona Drive
Santa Barbara, CA 93105

(805) 687-0483

Distributes instruments for transcutaneous nerve stimulation (TNS), electrosleep, and acupuncture.

**COGNETICS** (cassette tapes) /Saratoga, CA **(see 214)**

**(657) IONLAB, INC.**
13617 Sherman Way
Van Nuys, CA 91405

(213) 765-2327

Distributor of "acu-aids," 6 x 6 mm adhesive squares each containing a tiny steel ball for continuous acupressure stimulation at specific acupuncture points.

**(658) ACCU-TUBE CORPORATION**
2960 South Umatilla Street
Englewood, CO 80110

(303) 761-2258

Distributes and manufactures electronic acupuncture equipment and needles.

**(659) TRUELINE INSTRUMENTS, INC.**
P.O. Box 1357
Englewood, CO 80110

(303) 781-6621

Distributes acupuncture needles, charts, and electronic instruments.

**(660) INTERNATIONAL ACUPUNCTURE PRODUCTS, LTD.**
P.O. Box 3212
Darien, CT 06820

(203) 655-0800

Distributes acupuncture charts, electric stimulators, needles, and books.

**(661) PEKING BOOK HOUSE**
1520 Sherman Avenue
Evanston, IL 60201

(312) 491-0477

Distributor of acupuncture books and equipment direct from the Peoples' Republic of China.

**(662) LITERATURE SEARCH PROGRAMS**
MEDLARS Management Section
National Library of Medicine
8600 Rockville Pike
Bethesda, MD 20014

(301) 496-6193

A series of four bibliographical searches available in the field of acupuncture.

**(663) NATIONAL INSTITUTE OF GENERAL MEDICAL SCIENCES**
National Institutes of Health
Bethesda, MD 20014

(301) 496-7373

*Atten: Emilie Black, MD, Director, Clinical and Physiological Sciences*

Supplies grants to researchers wishing to engage in research in acupuncture for the relief of pain. Further information may be obtained by writing to Dr. Black at the above address.

**(664) FRIENDSHIP INTERNATIONAL DIVISION, SOBIN INTERNATIONAL**
Sobin Park
Boston, MA 02210

(617) 268-5100

Distributors of acupuncture demonstration models from the People's Republic of China.

**(665) DOCTORS SUPPLY COMPANY**
24028 Union
Dearborn, MI 48124

(313) 278-2840

Distributes full line of acupuncture books and supplies.

**(666) PROFESSIONAL MEDICAL DISTRIBUTORS, INC.**
Jaesic Industrial Co., Inc.
29830 Beck Road
Wixom, MI 48096

(313) 624-6413

Manufacturer of apparatus for acupuncture point detection and treatment.

**(667) LYCEE TRADING CORPORATION**
P.O. Box 206
East Northport, NY 11731

(516) 249-4929

Publisher of acupuncture books and charts and distributor of needles, moxa, and electrostimulators.

ASI (publishing co.) /New York, NY (see 227)

**(668) HSINHUA TRADING LIMITED**
2216 24th Avenue N.W.
Calgary, Alberta, Canada T2M 1Z7

(403) 289-4913

Distributors of electro-acupuncture equipment, needles, and moxa direct from the Peoples' Republic of China.

**(669) NIKKA OVERSEAS AGENCY, LTD.**
378 Powell Street
Vancouver 4, British Columbia
Canada

(604) 684-4155

Distributes electronic acupuncture equipment for Ryodoraku treatment (see 642) as well as other acupuncture materials and supplies.

**(670) INTERTRONIC SYSTEMS LIMITED**
980 Alness Street #15
Downsview, Ontario
Canada M3J 2S2

(416) 661-3902

Distributes full line of electronic biomedical acupuncture equipment.

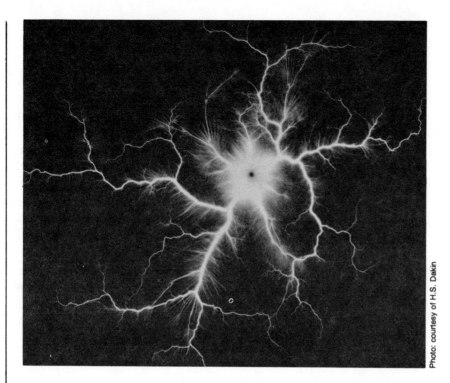

# Aeroiontherapy

*Felix G. Sulman, MD, DMD*

Air ion formation begins when high atmospheric energies released by thunderstorms or hot dry winds act on gaseous molecules to eject an electron. The displaced electron attaches itself to an adjacent molecule, transforming it into a negative ion, whereas the original molecule, deprived of its balanced "dipole moment," now turns into a positive ion. [The word *ion* was coined by the English physicist Michael Faraday (1795–1867), who by identifying ions with the ancient Greek Ionians intended to stress their ability to migrate.] The atmosphere contains a large number of electrically charged oxygen or water particles, "air ions," which are classified into three groups: small, intermediate, and large. Only small ions, composed of electrically charged clusters of molecules of atmospheric gases (0.001 to 0.003 $\mu$m in diameter) with great mobility (1 cm/sec) and an electric charge per ion of $(15.9)10^{-20}$ coulomb, are used for ion therapy.

Ions are attracted to naturally occurring molecular groups; thus, the body's ability to incorporate them is not surprising. When oxygen is resorbed via the lung alveoles, the ionized molecules are taken up like the normal oxygen molecules and pass into the blood corpuscles. The red blood corpuscles, whose hemoglobin is oxygenated by the air during inspiration, also receive the ionized oxygen. The negative charge is carried throughout the body, whereas the positive charge may attack the blood platelets (thrombocytes) which in sensitive patients release an irritating hormone, serotonin. All investigators agree that, in general, negative ions are beneficial and positive ions harmful to the recipient. Moreover, people can be exposed to negative ionization, in reasonable quantities, day and night without doing any harm, provided that no significant quantities of ozone are produced (no more than 0.1 part per million).

Exposure to atmospheres containing high densities of positive air ions releases serotonin, which produces dryness, burning and itching of the nose, nasal obstruction, headache, dry, scratchy throat, difficulty in swallowing, dry lips, dizziness, difficulty in breathing, and itching of the eyes. The pioneer research of A. P. Krueger in Berkeley has thus opened the way to our understanding of ionization mechanisms. He has shown that negative air ions do not produce this unpleasant serotonin syndrome; rather, they act directly on the respiratory enzyme, cytochrome oxidase, and promote cell respiration.

Positive air ions release serotonin, which may produce a number of complaints, such as difficulty in breathing and asthma attacks. Rheumatic people feel their joints, as well as insomnia, irritability, and tension. Migraine patients suffer from severe attacks of headache with nausea and vomiting, and optical disturbances. Heart cases complain of palpitations, heart pain, and edematous swellings. Women before the age of menopause complain of hot flushes with sweat or chills. Hay fever patients get bad attacks of rhinitis with conjunctivitis, even when it is not hay fever season. Giddiness, tremor, and balance disturbances may appear, as well as diarrhea and a constant desire to urinate. The hostile positive ions can be neutralized by modern apparatuses which emit a surplus of negative ions and neutralize the positive ions.

Negative ionization for therapeutic purposes is derived from ionizing sources: e.g., an electric tension of 5 to 10 kV with a needle at its end which emits up to 50 times more negative than positive ions. "Corona discharge" produces a strong ozone current which disappears at a distance of 1 meter.

Negative ions abolish the adverse effects of the positive ions. However, not everyone enjoys negative ionization. Only 30 percent of the population need negative ionization; another 30 percent feel well if the amount of negative ionization in the air is increased. There still remain 40 percent who do not notice negative ionization. However, a patient who does not need ionization will not be harmed by it. The patient who does need it will feel the benefit within a few minutes and report an easing of the various complaints mentioned above.

A number of conditions indicate ionotherapy.

1. *Suffering from Weather Changes*. Weather fronts produce positive ions and release serotonin, leading to the numerous ailments mentioned earlier.
2. *Vegetative Effects*. Vegetative distony, a disturbance of the autonomic system, can be brought about by daily stress which culminates in the same symptoms as those previously described. In 50 percent of cases it may be provoked by the release of serotonin. There exists, therefore, the possibility of prophylactic treatment by negative ionization, which lowers the serotonin content of the blood. Another effect of lack of negative ionization is claustrophobia. Negative ionization can abolish the feeling of oppression patients experience in work rooms, bedrooms, or badly ventilated dwellings.
3. *Burns*. Burns have become an important chapter in plastic surgery. Treatment aims at reducing serotonin release and bacterial infection of the skin graft to a minimum. Negative ionization can fulfill both these demands, since it suppresses the release of serotonin and the Brownian molecular movement of bacteria. The result is a 70 percent reduction of the bacterial flora in the patient's room. (This anti-bacterial effect is now being put to use in cold storage plants and refrigerators.)
4. *Miscellaneous*. Ionizing apparatuses have also been recommended for combating other diseases where serotonin may be the cause, such as thromboembolism, heart ailments with breathlessness, migraine, habitual serotonin abortion in women, asthma, hay fever, and allergic skin conditions.

We have recently investigated the psychic effects of the ionizing apparatuses in our laboratories. The EEG, after negative ionization, shows an advance of the normal alpha rhythm from the occipital brain to the forebrain, which promotes the conception of ideas; a stabilization of the frequency at 10 hertz, which indicates relaxation; and an increase of amplitudes, which improves work capacity. Last but not least, there occurs a synchronization of the right and left brain hemispheres, which means a balancing of the personality.

## Groups and Researchers

(671) **ALBERT P. KRUEGER, PhD**
University of California (Berkeley)
Earl Warren Hall
School of Public Health
Berkeley, CA 94720

Involved in air ion research.

(672) **THE AMERICAN INSTITUTE OF MEDICAL CLIMATOLOGY**
1023 Welsh Road
Philadelphia, PA 19115

(215) 673-8368

*George King, Executive Director*

Promotes the sciences of bioclimatology and biometeorology by organizing, conducting, and correlating pertinent studies on the relationship between weather and climate and life in all its phases. The scope of the investigations includes all measurable, observable, or otherwise determinable meteorotropic, psychotropic and physiological effects of the atmosphere. Specialized application of the Institute's program are in the fields of medicine, rheumatology, psychology, air pollution, medical hydrology, and institutional and industrial planning. The AIMC sponsors meetings, seminars, and lectures and provides library assistance and disseminates papers of pertinent interest. Membership is open to individuals who possess a BS degree or its equivalent and maintain some competence in fields related to medical climatology.

### (673) FELIX G. SULMAN, MD, DMD
Bioclimatology Unit
Department of Applied Pharmacology
Hebrew University
Hadassah Medical Center
Jerusalem, Israel

Involved in air ion research.

### (674) INTERNATIONAL SOCIETY OF BIO-METEOROLOGY
Hofbrouckerlaan 54
Oegstgeest (Leiden)
The Netherlands

*Dr. S.W. Tromp, Secretariat*

The general purpose of the Society is the development of biometeorology. This is accomplished within ten permanent study groups. These are (1) effects of heat and cold on man and animals; (2) effects of altitude on man and animals; (3) effects of climate on human health and disease; (4) effects of weather on animal disease and reproduction; (5) effects of weather and climate on plants; (6) architectural, urban, and engineering biometeorology; (7) biological effects of natural electric, magnetic, and electromagnetic fields; (8) physical, physiological, and therapeutic effects of ionized air and electroaerosols; (9) biological rhythms with special reference to environmental influences; and (10) physicochemical and biological fluctuating phenomena. The Society publishes a quarterly journal, *The International Journal of Biometeorology,* and organizes an international congress every three years. Founded 1956.

SWEDISH HERBAL INSTITUTE (research) / Gothenburg, Sweden (see 554)

## Journals and Publications

### (675) G.W.K. KING ASSOCIATES
Newton, PA 18940

(215) 968-4483

Publisher of bibliographies and research papers on ion research in collaboration with the American Institute of Medical Climatology (see 572).

### INTERNATIONAL JOURNAL OF BIOMETEOR-OLOGY/The Netherlands (see 674)

## Products and Services

QUINTESSENCE UNLIMITED (consciousness tools) /Boulder, CO (see 215)

### (676) HEALTHION CO.
910 East Evans Avenue
Denver, CO 80210

(303) 733-2915

Disseminates information on negative ion technology, and manufactures negative ion instruments and measuring devices for home, car, and office.

### (677) M-TRON INDUSTRIES, INC.
100 Douglas
Yankton, SD 57078

Manufacturer of air ionizing apparatus (under the name of building outfits and kits).

### (678) BATTELLE MEMORIAL INSTITUTE
Pacific Northwest Laboratories
Battelle Boulevard
Richland, WA 99352

(509) 946-2121

*Dr. A.P. Wehner*

Developer of air ion aerosol units.

### (679) ELCAR
5620 Bois Franc
Montreal, Quebec
Canada H4S 1A9

Manufacturer of air ionization generators and electronic air purifiers.

### (680) MEDION
Oxted P.O.B. 1
Surrey, England

Markets the MEDICOR line and an ionizer which emits ions in six different directions, helpful where several people are sitting around a table.

### (681) MEDICOR
P.O.B. 150,
Budapest, 1389
Hungary

Manufactures desk model, car model, and fan ionizers.

### (682) AMCOR
Herzlia,
P.O.B. 337,
Israel

Manufactures air ionization units for use in motor cars, and combination air conditioning/air ionization units, some specific for asthmatics.

### (683) KROPF
Anker Str. 4
Bern, Switzerland

Manufacturer of the Ion Detector Vitar-14 for the measurement of ion flux by transistorized neon lamps with a short aerial. Also manufactures an aesthetic, effective air ionizer which can be combined with an air filter and a deodorant air refresher.

### (684) MULTORGAN
Magliaso,
Switzerland

Manufactures small air ionizers for home or car.

### (685) TRAFOTEX
Van den Berg,
8116 Wuerenlos,
Switzerland

Manufactures a car model ionizer which can sustain a negative or neutral charge in a car with open windows.

### (686) BENTAX
C.J. Habicht
Bentax A.G. 8000-Zürich,
Switzerland

Manufacturer of room ionizing apparatuses for large offices and factory rooms, as well as for tunnels and refrigeration store houses.

### (687) KATHREIN
82-Rosenheim
West Germany

Manufactures ionometers for the measurement of high ion concentrations.

### (688) GTB (Gesellschaft für Technische Beratung)
Gutenberg Str. 134,
Stuttgart, West Germany

Manufacturer of room ionizing devices for large rooms, factories, and refrigeration store houses, as well as a smaller unit (the Jonotron).

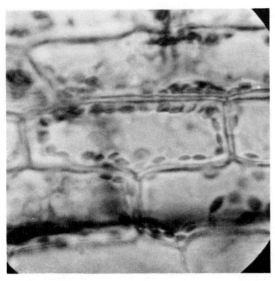

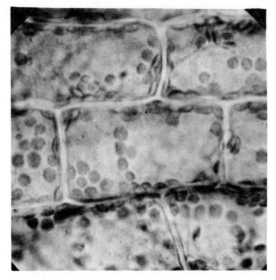

FIGURE 1: Under normal sunlight chloroplasts move around the inside of a plant cell in an orderly fashion.

FIGURE 2: Under red light chloroplasts cluster in corners or cut across the middle of the cell.

# The Effects Of Light On Health

*John N. Ott, ScD (Hon.)*

One of the most interesting developments in medicine during the past few years has been the introduction of light therapy (or phototherapy) for a number of therapeutic uses. Phototherapy is now being used in place of a complete blood transfusion for the treatment of neonatal hyperbilirubinemia, or jaundice, in premature babies. The use of light for the treatment of jaundice may have been practiced originally in India by midwives, who placed unclothed jaundiced infants in the sunlight to cure them. The use of artificial light to treat jaundice traces back to the work done in 1958 by Dr. Richard J. Cremer, of Harefield Hospital in Middlesex, England. Dr. Cremer showed that the serum bilirubin levels that cause jaundice could be lowered in infants by exposing them either to sunlight or to artificial blue light. The accepted alternative treatment for severe cases, blood transfusion, carries considerable risk.

Photochemotherapy has also been introduced as a treatment for psoriasis. Both Thomas Fitzpatrick at Massachusetts General Hospital in Boston and Professor Klaus Wolff at the University Dermatology Clinic in Vienna have pioneered the use of an orally administered drug (methoxsalen) which is specifically activated by long-wavelength ultraviolet or black light. The afflicted areas are then exposed to the light in what looks something like a telephone booth.

Dr. Troy D. Feller of Baylor College of Medicine reported to the 120th annual meeting of the American Medical Association on a new light therapy for treating herpes virus. A certain kind of dye that absorbs light is applied to the skin lesion, which is then exposed to daylight-type fluorescent light. This process is referred to as "photodynamic inactivation." Logically, if a particular ailment can be treated with certain wavelengths of light, living under an artificial light source lacking these wavelengths might contribute to causing the ailment in the first place. Conversely, long-term exposure to low-level or trace amounts of any radiation in excess of normal could produce abnormal responses or side effects over an extended period of time.

What all this means is that it now appears that there are biological responses to trace levels of radiation comparable to the equivalent trace levels in chemistry. Not long ago, one part per million was considered fairly insignificant and very difficult to measure accurately. But then it was discovered that one part per ten million, one part per billion, and one part per trillion can produce significant biological responses. Methods have been developed to measure these trace levels in chemistry, but as yet there are no methods to measure such low levels of radiation in light sources. We can only observe the reactions on various biological reactors such as bean plants, laboratory animals, and school children.

The effects of sunlight, both beneficial and harmful, on the human skin have long been recognized. However, more recently, neurochemical channels leading from the retina to the pituitary and pineal glands have been reported. These master glands control the endocrine system, which produces and releases the hormones that control body chemistry. Thus, the basic principles of photosynthesis in plants, sometimes referred to as the conversion of light energy into chemical energy, appear to carry over into animal life—a fact that has not previously been recognized.

Since the beginning, life on this earth has evolved under the full spectrum of natural sunlight. Recent experimental studies have indicated, through sensitive photoreceptor mechanisms, specific endocrine responses in both the skin and the retina to narrow bands of wavelengths within the entire electromagnetic spectrum and not just to the difference between light and dark. Various skin and suntan lotions block certain light rays from penetrating the skin, and ordinary glass in windows, windshields, and eyeglasses filter most of the ultraviolet from entering the eyes. Artificial light sources also grossly distort the natural spectrum of light entering the eyes. Certain areas of the spectrum are very weak or even totally lacking, whereas other areas of the spectrum contain very strong peaks of energy. Thus, a condition can develop which is now referred to as "malillumination," a form of optical malnutrition. Moreoever, manmade radiation from TV sets, fluorescent tubes, radar and radar ovens, telephone microwave relay towers, computers and office machines using cathode-ray tubes, and other similar electronic devices are creating levels of artificial radiation many times greater than the natural general background radiation.

A serious question now exists as to what this relatively recent drastic change in our light and radiation environment may have on human health and behavior. In the field of time-lapse photography it has been observed that plants produce only staminate blossoms under ordinary cool-white light; with daylight white, they produce only pistillate blossoms. A controlled study by the Department of Biology at Loyola University in Chicago has shown that different kinds of lights influence the sex of tropical fish. Today the chinchilla industry is obtaining approximately 95 percent of a given sex, depending on the lights used in the breeding rooms.

In 1964 an article in *Time* linking listlessness among children with excessive TV viewing led the Environmental Health and Light Research Institute to conduct an experiment to determine whether there might be any basic physiological responses in plants or laboratory animals to some sort of radiation being emitted from TV sets. We set up a large-screen color TV; one half of the picture tube was covered with 1/16 inch of solid lead (a common xray shield), and the other half was covered with ordinary heavy black photographic paper that would stop all visible light but allow other radiation to penetrate. We placed pots containing bean seeds directly in front of the TV and others outdoors at a distance of 50 feet from the greenhouse where the TV set was located. At the end of 3 weeks the young bean plants outdoors and those in front of the lead shield showed approximately 6 inches of apparently normal growth. The plants in the pots shielded only by the black photographic paper showed an excessive vinelike growth ranging up to 31.5 inches. Furthermore, the leaves of these plants were all approximately three times as large.

These results prompted us to set up a similar experiment using white laboratory rats. The thickness of the lead shield was increased to 1/8 inch. Two cages, each containing two rats approximately 3 months old, were placed directly in front of the color TV tube, one on the paper-covered side, the other by the lead shield. The picture was turned on for 6 hours each weekday and 10 hours on Saturday and Sunday (the sound was turned off). The rats protected only by the paper showed abnormally stimulated activities for 3 to 10 days and then became progressively more lethargic. After 30 days they were extremely lethargic; it was necessary to push them to make them move. This experiment was repeated three times, giving the same results.

This color television happened to be set up 15 feet from our animal breeding room, with two ordinary building partitions in between. We soon observed that our animal breeding program, which had been going on very successfully for 2 years, was completely disrupted. Whereas rat litters had previously averaged eight or more young, this figure immediately dropped off to one or two, and many of these did not survive. After the TV set was removed, it took approximately 6 months before the breeding program was back to normal. This information, presented to the House Subcommittee on Public Health and Environment, led the way to the 1968 Radiation Control Act.

In another experiment we observed rats and mice kept under different types of fluorescent lights. The most significant abnormal conditions were found in the animals under pink fluorescent (rats and mice are nocturnal and do not see into the far red end of the spectrum); the abnormal responses consisted of excessive calcium deposits in the heart tissue, smaller number of young in the litters and lower survival rate, significantly greater tumor development or cancer, plus a strong tendency toward becoming irritable, aggressive, and cannibalistic. All evidence points to the fact that having laboratory light sources under scientific control is absolutely crucial; indeed, all past, present, and future research, on humans as well as animals, may be invalid if it does not take into consideration the intensity and wavelength distribution, as well as the periodicity of light, as an important variable.

In 1964, the European Society for the Study of Drug Toxicity reported that the amount of light that mice were subjected to proved to be an important factor in the toxicity level of the drugs tested. It seems logical that light could similarly influence the effectiveness of other nutritional elements, including vitamins or drugs like tranquilizers. If the specific wavelengths to which a certain vitamin reacts are of very low energy or totally lacking in an artificial light source, then a megadose would be required to bring about a normal reaction. If the wavelength-absorption characteristics of a food or drug happen to coincide with a peak of energy in an artificial light source, then the result could be an overreaction or an allergic type of response.

During the 1972–1973 school year the EHLRI undertook a study of the effects of lighting on behavioral problems of first grade students. In a pilot project conducted in four windowless elementary classrooms, children showed dramatic reactions to an improved lighting environment. Under their normal classroom lighting, some first graders in the study demonstrated nervous fatigue, irritability, lapses of attention, and hyperactive behavior. After full-spectrum lighting was installed with lead foil shields over the cathode ends of the fluorescent tubes to stop suspected soft radiation and an aluminum screen grid over the entire fixture to stop known RF radiation (characteristic of all fluorescent tubes), a marked improvement appeared in the youngsters.

That the improvement occurred when that part of the visible spectrum which is lacking in standard artificial light sources was supplied and excessive radiation was eliminated seems to indicate that hyperactivity may be a radiation stress condition. Thus far hyperkinesis has primarily been attributed to minimal brain damage or chemical imbalances and controlled by means of psychoactive drugs (as many as one million children in the United States are now relying on such drugs). Recent evidence also suggests that food additives may be a factor. Just as certain drugs increase susceptibility to sunburn, artificial flavorings and especially coloring materials, because of their greater absorptive and reflective characteristics, could cause a similar abnormal reaction to excessive peaks of light energy.

Evidence is accumulating that the harmful biological effects of artificial light sources and low levels of manmade radiation may be more far-reaching than anyone has suspected. If these factors lead to hyperactivity and learning disability in young children, what might be their contribution to the more serious problems of alcoholism, drug addiction, crime, and violence confronting modern civilization? Phototherapy researchers intend to find out.

## Groups

**(689) CENTER FOR LIGHT RESEARCH**
Roswell Park Memorial Institute
666 Elm Street
Buffalo, N.Y. 14263

(716) 845-2300

Engaged in the study of the effects of light and radiation on health and behavior. Main areas of concern include the effects of light and radiation in tumor development and cancer, as well as behavioral problems and learning disabilities in children.

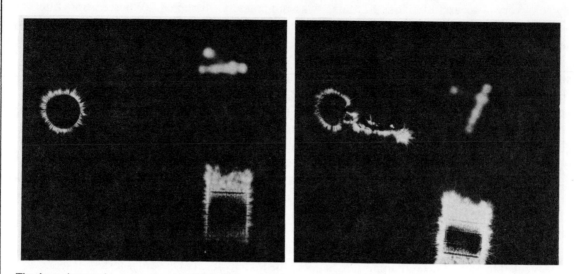

The above photographs were produced by Uri Geller in a preliminary experiment with high voltage photography conducted by J.L. Hickman. The picture on the left was the control photograph. In the picture on the right, the watch (the square glowing object) and Geller's fingertip were placed as before but this time Geller was concentrating on "shooting energy toward the watch" (subject's words) . . . the evidence from these experiments should be considered as preliminary and tentative . . . rather than as a basis for definitive answers, regarding the nature of biophysical energy. Courtesy H.S. Dakin Co., from *High Voltage Photography*. San Francisco: H.S. Dakin Co., 1974

# Kirlian Photography: An Update
*William W. Eidson, PhD and David L. Faust*

Information about Kirlian photography (KP) first became available in 1963 when the Foreign Technology Division of the Air Force translated "Photography and Visual Observations by Means of High-Frequency Currents," by Semyon D. Kirlian and his wife, Valentina. Originally, the paper was published in the *Russian Journal of Scientific and Applied Photography and Cinemaphotography* in 1961 (now available from National Technical Information Services as AD-299 666). There was no interest in this paper in the United States until May 1970 when Sheila Ostrander and Lynn Schroeder published *Psychic Discoveries Behind the Iron Curtain*. Their best-selling book, now in its 17th printing, is the single most important factor in the development of the controversy surrounding Kirlian photography.

The controversy centers on Russian claims and speculation that KP is a technique amplifying the presence of a "living plasma" or "bioplasma" which is similar to the solid state plasma known in conventional physics. Ostrander and Schroeder interpreted "bioplasma" as a "life force," and after interviewing Russian researchers, they reported that KP displays human beings as "a spectacular panorama of colors, whole galaxies of lights . . . all shining and twinkling . . . multicolored flares . . . and that those flares are indicators of the health or mental state of the person photographed.

The characteristics of the photographs agree quite closely with those attributed to a "life force" reported for thousands of years by many cultures and observed by the psychically gifted. However, generally accepted medical and scientific schools of thought do not support a "life force" hypothesis.

Size, structure, brightness, and color of the "life force" envelope, or "aura," differ from person to person. That difference reveals physical, emotional, and psychic details of body and mind functions. Faith healers, for example, show a dimming of their "aura" after the "laying on of hands," suggesting that the "life force" has been transferred to the patient whose "aura" brightens and changes in pattern.

In the United States and many parts of the world the experimental techniques called Kirlian photography display size, structure, brightness, and color variations, both in living and nonliving specimens. However, research shows that these variations are related to more than 25 other conditions, including details of equipment construction and adjustment, as well as the atmospheric environment. Thus, when a living system is studied, the analysis required to investigate a "life force" influence is extremely complex since it must be filtered out from a myriad of photographic effects produced by known physiological changes (e.g., perspiration).

The basic process that interacts with the object being photographed is a high-voltage electrical discharge. A large-scale phenomenon exist in the form of natural atmospheric lightning. On a personal scale, we often experience the phenomenon in the form of the discharge of static electricity when we touch an uncharged or oppositely charged object after walking across a synthetic carpet on a dry day. The area on your finger from which the spark jumps to the object, is the area that initially interested the Kirlians, in 1939.

We might think of the spark discharge as a simple phenomenon and the information available from its interaction as trivial, but close examination allows no such conclusion. Sophisticated analysis replaces the simplified view of spark discharges with a variety of additional discharge processes known as "corona."

Though much has been written since 1970 about work attempting to replicate the Kirlians' experiments in the United States, the literature generally can be characterized as limited in scope, technically shallow, often motivated by psychic claims and thus unaccepted by mainstream scientific publications with two exceptions. In July 1973, Boyers and Tiller published an article in the *Journal of Applied Physics* about physical parameters that can influence Kirlian photography. On October 15, 1976, Pehek, Kyler, and Faust published an article in *Science* about the modulation of corona discharge images by water vapor on and within the surface of specimens that they had studied. It is most important to understand that both of these articles only lay groundwork for closer consideration of Kirlian photography rather than closing all issues as some popular press accounts have indicated. It is also important to recognize that the standard physics, electrical engineering, and biomedical literature has literally thousands of articles and books which provide useful information bearing on Kirlian photography.

Work to date suggests that water dynamics of a living system may be sensed over 10,000 times faster than that of previously known systems. This should add valuable baseline information to well-accepted electrophysiological measurements such as skin resistance or EEG. We already know that the skin, which is actually the body's largest organ, reflects internal conditions. Therefore, psychological and disease specific claims may be supported by this aspect of KP alone.

Beyond the moisture-sensing properties of KP, as seen in the West, the Kirlians' 1961 statement still stands: "Having studied specimens with varying geometrical configurations, together with their [optical] spectrums and their dynamics of development, it is apparently possible to make judgments about the biological and pathological states of an organism and its organs." The spectral changes [color] observed in Western photographs are virtually all associated with photographic film curling or moisture, or both. The Kirlians are describing essentially a fluorescence and phosphorescence, in the visible and ultraviolet, of cell components of the living specimen. This information is usually obscured by Western KP techniques. The diagnostic value of this information is still to be realized, but it appears that clinical evaluation of advanced instrumentation systems will soon take place.

We should note that instruments inspired by the Kirlians' work involve a number of dominant effects that depend on subtle changes in the experimental design (e.g., electrode geometry, high-voltage waveform); this is the reason for much of the confusion the field of KP has experienced. In fact, ironically, specialized experimental designs using Kirlian photography techniques may be useful in exploring, with true scientific rigor, the very "psychic phenomenon" that was responsible for the earlier difficulties with the scientific community which KP researchers encountered. Moisture-sensing properties may be valuable in investigating the rapid and quite significant water loss (order of pounds) by the human body, which reports indicate occurs during psychic feats (e.g., psychokinesis). Likewise, the extreme sensitivity of the process to changes in dielectric properties may allow examination of phenomena which appear to influence the electromagnetic permittivity of space (e.g., "out-of-body projection" using an assumption of space polarization bias).

Dr. Ioan Dumitrescu, a Romanian researcher, has noted five basic effects under the general heading of "electronography" (a KP inspired technique) and has announced cancer detection capability.

They have already examined 6000 people by this technique. Russians, Inyushin and Chekorov, in their book *Biostimulation through Laser Radiation and Bioplasma* (translation by Hill and Ghosal, Denmark) make some important comments: "In conclusion, we consider it essential to briefly dwell on some interpretations of the Kirlian effect which appeared recently in foreign publications [referring to USA media ] gas discharge luminescence [corona ] taking place around the human finger and its light effects was called 'bioplasma' . . . this is in principle incorrect." In our work we have not once shown that the Kirlian effect is an oblique method of uncovering some of the properties of bioplasma. "Only on the basis of quantitative evaluation of the luminescence . . . is it possible to obtain reliable information about the processes taking place in plants and man. The diagnostic value of the Kirlian effect does not arouse doubt."

Kirlian photography holds promise as an important new medical diagnostic tool, but more basic research is needed before the potential of this new tool is fully realizable. If foreign claims are proved to be accurate, Kirlian photography may well expand our knowledge of living systems with an impact comparable to the xray.

## Groups and Researchers

(690) **DAVID E. LORD, PhD**
Lawrence Livermore Laboratory
University of California
P.O. Box 808
Livermore, CA 94550

(415) 447-7011

Researcher in Kirlian photography and material science studies.

(691) **THELMA MOSS, PhD**
Neuropsychiatric Institute
Center for Health Sciences
University of California
Los Angeles, CA 90024

(213) 825-0080

Researcher in Kirlian photography.

(692) **GARY K. POOCK, PhD**
U.S. Naval Postgraduate School
Monterey, CA 93940

(408) 484-1892

Research in Kirlian photography; real time studies in 16-mm black and white and color with image intensification. Several publications available.

(693) **WILLIAM A. TILLER, PhD, Professor and Chairman**
Department of Material Science and Engineering
Stanford University
Palo Alto, CA 94305

(415) 497-3901

Active in all areas of Kirlian photography research; list of publications available on request.

(694) **HENRY S. DAKIN**
3101 Washington Street
San Francisco, CA 94115

(415) 931-2593

Researcher in all facets of Kirlian photography and energy field studies.

**BORDERLAND SCIENCES RESEARCH FOUNDATION** /Vista, CA **(see 586)**

(695) **HENRI MONTANDON, PhD**
5620 Greenspring Avenue
Baltimore, MD 21209

(301) 664-4818

Researcher in experimental psychology and Kirlian photography.

(696) **HARRY S. KYLER, PhD**
837 Lafayette Drive
Mount Laurel, NJ 08054

Researcher in Kirlian photography and experimental psychology.

(697) **BENJAMIN SHAFFIROFF, MD**
2202 Quentin Road
Brooklyn, NY 11223

(212) 339-3888

Researcher in Kirlian photography.

(698) **INTERNATIONAL KIRLIAN RESEARCH ASSOCIATION**
411 East Seventh Street
Brooklyn, NY 11218

(212) 854-5196

*Edward Graff, Executive Director*

An international group of research scientists and physicians involved in correlating, standardizing, and promoting all phases of research into Kirlian photography. Research members receive a mailing list of all other members. There are annual scientific conferences, and in progress are a controlled laboratory and the development of audiovisual teaching materials. The Association also publishes a monthly newsletter. Founded 1974.

(699) **CECILE RUCHIN**
26 Gramercy Park
New York, NY 10003

(212) 475-6763

Researcher in holography and Kirlian photography.

**(700) RICHARD DOBRIN, PhD**
Energy Research Group
137 Bowery
New York, NY 10002

(212) 966-6425

Researcher in Kirlian photography, atomic, solid state, radiologic physics, and energy fields.

**(701) YOSHIAKI OMURA, MD, ScD**
800 Riverside Drive
New York, NY 10032

(212) 928-0658

Researcher in Kirlian photography and acupuncture.

**(702) DAVID SHEINKIN, MD**
Mt. View Medical Building
Mount View Road
Nyack, NY 10960

(914) 358-6800

Clinical studies in the potential of Kirlian photography for medical diagnosis in preventive medicine.

**(703) AL HULSTRUNK, PhD**
RD 2, Box 101
Rexford, NY 12148

(518) 371-2659

Researcher in Kirlian photography.

**(704) MARGARET ARMSTRONG, RN, PhD**
University of Rochester
School of Medicine and Dentistry
School of Nursing
Rochester, NY 14642

(716) 275-5305

Research in Kirlian photography combined with clinical studies in experimental physiology.

**(705) PAUL SAUVIN**
16 Merritt Avenue
White Plains, NY 10606

(914) 949-9557

Researcher in Kirlian photography.

**HUMAN DIMENSIONS** (unusual parapsychology research) /Williamsville, NY **(see 588)**

**(706) WILLIAM JOINES, PhD**
Department of Electrical Engineering
Duke University
Durham, NC 27706

(919) 684-3123

Researcher in Kirlian photography and biomedical engineering studies; graduate research encouraged.

**(707) DAVID L. FAUST**
3900 Chestnut Street, Apt. 812
Philadelphia, PA 19104

(215) 382-8118

Researcher in Kirlian photography and instrument development.

**(708) WILLIAM EIDSON, PhD, Chairman,**
Department of Physics,

Drexel University
32nd and Chestnut
Philadelphia, PA 19104

(215) 895-2707

Head of multidisciplinary research team conducting activities in all areas of Kirlian photography from clinical studies to material science as well as instrument development. List of publications available on request with self-addressed stamped envelope.

**(709) DAVID B. CAMMACK AND WAYNE RICHARD**
P.O. Box 6153
Princess Ann Station
Virginia Beach, VA 23456

(804) 425-9371

Conducts research in Kirlian photography in the areas of psychology, childbirth, and parapsychology.

**(710) SCOTT HILL, MEE**
Physics Laboratory I
University of Copenhagen
H.C. Orsted Institute
Universitetsparken 5
DK-2100 Copenhagen O, Denmark

Researcher in Kirlian photography, biophysics and psychotronics.

**(711) DENNIS MILNER, PhD**
Department of Industrial Metallurgy
Birmingham University
Birmingham, England

Researcher in Kirlian photography and subtle energies.

**(712) IOAN F.L. DUMITRESCU, MD**
Ministry of Chemical Industry
Center for Work Protection and Hygiene
Bucharest 31,
Str. Pop de Basesti 59
Romania

Clinical studies in Kirlian photography and electrography.

## Journals and Publications

**BRAIN/MIND BULLETIN**/Los Angeles, CA **(see 184)**

**JOURNAL OF BORDERLAND RESEARCH**/Vista, CA **(see 804)**

**OSTEOPATHIC PHYSICIAN** (multidisciplinary journal) /New York, NY **(see 376)**

**HUMAN DIMENSIONS JOURNAL**/Williamsville, NY **(see 203)**

## Products and Services

**COGNETICS** (cassette tapes) /Saratoga, CA **(see 214)**

**QUINTESSENCE UNLIMITED** (consciousness tools) /Boulder, CO **(see 215)**

**HARTLEY FILM PRODUCTIONS** (audiovisual) /Cos Cob, CT **(see 219)**

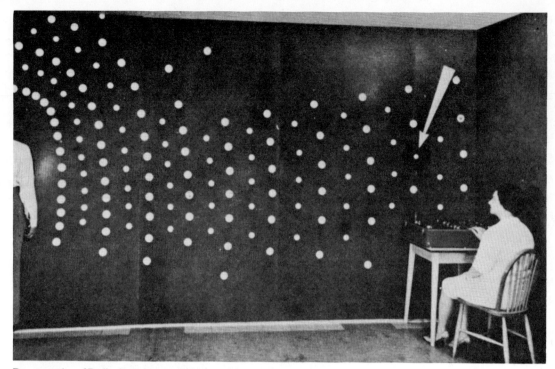

Demonstration of Radionic equipment relative to picking up the human force field; courtesy Delawarr Laboratories, Oxford England.

# Radionics: A Modern Instrumentalized Therapy

*Marjorie de la Warr*

Radionics is the modern name for special methods of medical and veterinary diagnosis and treatment that have been known since early in this century. (These methods can also be applied to the stimulation of agricultural crops and to the elimination of pests; when used for this purpose, the methods are sometimes also known as Radiurgics.)

Radionics has for part of its pedigree the background of radiesthesia, which is older than the pyramids of Egypt and, for that matter, the science of modern medicine based on pharmaceutical remedies. Perhaps the best-known and least disputed of all the radiesthesia methods is water divining, using the hazel twig, where it is irrefutable that the twig reacts to the emanations of the subterranean water.

In the nineteenth century, the German Baron von Reichenbach discovered a peculiar kind of force—which he termed "odic force" which could be conducted along wires, focused by a lens or distorted by a candle flame. But the basic phenomena of modern Radionics were discovered early this century by Dr. Albert Abrams of San Francisco, whom Sir James Barr, a past president of the British Medical Association, has described as "by far the greatest medical genius the profession has produced for half a century."

As Abrams had qualified in California before he was old enough to receive a medical diploma, he learned German and graduated in medicine with the highest possible honors from Heidelberg University. He then did postgraduate work in Heidelberg, Berlin, Paris, and London. In 1897 Sir J. J. Thompson discovered the electron, and a few years later Sir Ernest Rutherford showed that all atoms consist of a central nucleus surrounded by a "cloud" of electrons in constant motion. Abrams was profoundly impressed by these discoveries and was eager to try to correlate the laws of biology with the laws of physics.

By nature and through training Abrams was an exceptionally perceptive and persistent observer. In

1910, while examining a patient with a cancerous ulcer on the lip, he detected a small area of the abdomen which gave a dull note when percussed with his fingers. After further tests he made the remarkable discovery that the dull note could only be detected when the patient was facing west. He deduced that he was dealing with a phenomenon of an electronic nature which was influenced by the earth's magentic field.

The idea came to him to use a wire to connect his patient to the forehead of a healthy young man. When he did so, he found that the "radiations" from the patient induced a dull note in the same area of the young man's abdomen. Further tests revealed that the patient need not be connected to the young man or even present. A sample of the patient's blood at the far end of the wire was enough to induce a reflex action in the abdominal muscles of the young man and evince a dull note.

Convinced that he was dealing with some kind of electronic radiation, he tried interrupting the wire with rheostats and found that these could be used to "tune out" or measure the "radiations" from diseased blood. He named his discovery the Electronic Reactions of Abrams, or E.R.A.

He then tried samples of blood from patients suffering from a variety of diseases and found that all of these induced dull notes in specific areas of a healthy abdomen. Furthermore, he found that if he placed a specific for a given disease—say, quinine for malaria—in proximity to the blood sample, the dull note disappeared. This discovery led him to apply E.R.A. to the *treatment* of disease. With the aid of one of the foremost electronic experts of the time, he produced an instrument called the "Oscilloclast" in which radiations from the circuit, which included rheostats, were superimposed on pulses of negative potentials and of radio frequencies. He found that, by applying these radiations to patients, he could cure certain diseases.

Of course, the radiations from diseased blood are not electronic in the accepted sense of the word; they are radiations in a different—and more subtle—"energy spectrum." And they can only be detected by their effect on the human mind and nervous system.

In the modern detection method, the human abdomen had been replaced by a rubbing-plate or by a pendulum of the kind used by dowsers. In both cases the mind and nervous system of the operator are involved. With the rubbing-plate—usually rubber on one plate of a condenser—the mind of the operator induces an effect at the fingertips, which causes them to stick. The operator's mind also actuates the pendulum. Radionic instruments merely serve to focus the operator's mind, which serves as a kind of radar, receiving return "signals" from the patient's subconscious.

Ruth Drown, Guyon Richards and others followed the guidelines set by Abrams and made valuable contributions. Then, in World War II, George de la Warr and his wife founded the Delawarr Laboratories at Oxford, England and for many years vigorously developed the new science of Radionics.

With improved instruments, based on the Abrams principles, they felt the need for more accurate "rates" to represent the emanations of diseases. A series of bacteria cultures were placed, in turn, in the instrument. Mrs. de la Warr would then focus her mind on whatever particular bacteria was being "rated" and would turn the first dial till she got a reaction on the rubber diaphragm. She would then turn the other dials in sequence, noting the figure on each at which she got a reaction.

In this way she was able to determine "rates," sometimes with an accuracy of nine digits, and eventually established 4,000 "rates."

de la Warr felt that the instrument needed a stabilizer and found that a bar magnet would serve this purpose. In 1943, therefore, he modified the diagnostic instrument by inserting a bar magnet upright between the two wells of the instrument which by a knob could be made to rotate until it took up the position where it had a stabilizing effect. This very simple addition to the instrument proved the most important additional development and is incorporated into all the subsequent apparatus invented.

At the same time the tuning-dials were standardized on all instruments so that the same rates could be used on any instrument.

This brief account of the historical background of Radionics is, of course, incomplete and cannot do justice to all the developments which have taken place at the Delawarr Laboratories in the years since they were founded.

Radionic diagnosis and treatment are based on the fact that all substances radiate an energy which can be detected by the human mind with the aid of Radionic instruments. In the case of the hydrogen atom, the wave of energy is sinusoidal in form. But the more complex the substance the more complex the wave-form.

Any variation in the substance, caused by impurities or composition, will show as variations in the wave-form. Such variations can be detected and measured by the diagnostic instrument, by calibrating them against the standard "rates" of pure substances.

de la Warr postulated that the diagnostic instrument is analogous to the "read off" stage of a computer, which is activated when resonance is obtained between the radiations from the specimen and the dial settings of the diagnostic instrument. He thought that the reaction on the rubber diaphragm, signalling this resonance, took place through the operation of the pacinian corpuscles—the mecanoreceptors—which are located in the fingertips.

Further studies have suggested that the sensory receptors of the skin act as transducers which convert one form of energy into another; and that the pacinian corpuscle can both receive and transmit sensory data.

Radionic diagnosis and treatment are hard for some to understand because they usually employ specimens from the patient who need not be physically present. This is possible because radionic emanations are "non-spatial" they are at the patient and at the specimen. No time, therefore, is taken for these radiations to pass from the patient to the specimen or from the patient to the treatment instrument or *vice versa*.

It should be emphasized that a radionic diagnosis is not the same as a medical diagnosis, though the two may coincide. The difference is that a radionic diagnosis detects abnormalities in the energy field of the patient, which may or may not be reflected in physical symptoms. A radionic diagnosis is concerned with basic causes and can often detect trouble *before* physical symptoms are evident.

Some criticise Radionics because not all individuals can operate the rubber detector that is the most important part of the diagnostic instrument because without it information cannot be produced. Observations carried out over the past 30 years at the laboratories at Oxford seem to indicate that approximately 70 percent of individuals who try out the diagnostic instrument can be taught to use the rubber detector, whereas the remaining 30 percent cannot, whatever their own desires and feelings may be. This, of course, applies to other forms of indicating devices of a like nature such as the pendulum and the divining rod and therefore the radionic diagnostic instrument is not alone in this form of criticism.

As far as is known, no other center similar to the Laboratories at Oxford exists for the purpose of carrying out research on the general principles and applications, the design, development, and manufacture of instruments intended to display radionic principles and on the desirability of maintaining a large radionic practice in order to implement the work mentioned previously.

## Groups and Associations

**HUNA INTERNATIONAL** (unusual energies) /Santa Monica, CA **(see 591)**

(713) **CLARK ENTERPRISES**
P.O. Drawer I
Marble Falls, TX 78654

(513) 593-5454

*Lt. Col. I.B. Clark, USMS, Ret'd, Director of Research*

Consultants in radiesthesia and radionics as well as radionic locating service; wholesale distributors of radionic equipment and supplies.

(714) **DELAWARR LABORATORIES, LTD.**
Raleigh Park Road
Oxford, OX2 9BB
England

Tel: 0865-48572

*Leonard P. Corte, Director*

The laboratories operate on three levels. A clinical radionics practice supplemented with color therapy, vibration therapy (for musculo-skeletal conditions), and magnetic therapy for altering blood chemistry and relieving vasomotor conditions such as hay fever and asthma has been in existence since 1943. The Laboratories also conduct both original and corroborative research. Finally, they serve as manufacturers of radionics instruments for both research and clinical practice.

The Laboratories' Information Service publishes a newsletter, and distributes books and reprints on radionics. Write for details on membership and their information service. Founded 1943.

## (715) THE RADIONIC ASSOCIATION

Field House
Peaslake
Guildford, Surrey GU5 9SS
England

Tel: Dorking 730080

*John Wilcox, Secretary*

Dedicated to protecting and promoting the practice of Radionics as an honorable and skilled profession, to promote research, and to encourage communication with individuals in related fields. The Association is a professional society of qualified radionic practitioners, while simultaneously, a society of laymen interested in Radionics wishing to keep in touch with the development of the subject. The activities of the Association include the publication of a journal, *Radionics Quarterly,* and the annual conference, at which scientific papers are read. The Radionic Trust also maintains a training program for individuals wishing to become qualified practioners, and distributes radionic instruments to members of the school and to qualified practioners. An extensive list of books and publications on Radionics is available to the public through mail order. Founded 1943.

### REPRESENTATIVE PRACTITIONERS OF THE RADIONICS ASSOCIATION

Mrs. C.N. Gulson and Mrs. S.E. Janssen
P.O. Box 59
St. Ives, New South Wales 2075
Australia

Mrs. M.R. Morrison
P.O. Box 121
Christie's Beach
South Australia 5165

Mr. D.C. Willis
5661 Westhaven Road
West Vancouver
British Columbia V7W 1T7
Canada

Mr. A.J. Burson
12A Adelaide Road
Newton, Wellington
New Zealand

Joyce Conradie, HD
82 Briley Court
Jager Street
Hillbrow, Johannesburg 2001
South Africa

Mrs. E. Johnson
8 Rue du Theatre
1820 Montreux
Switzerland

Dr. A.W.K. Scheller
213 Rotenburg
Mauerseeweg 14
West Germany

## Journals and Publications

**NEW AGE JOURNAL** (multidisciplinary) /Brookline, MA **(see 196)**

**HUMAN DIMENSIONS** (multidisciplinary journal) / Williamsville, NY **(see 203)**

**RADIONICS QUARTERLY**/Surrey, England **(see 715)**

**DELAWARR LABORATORIES NEWSLETTER**/ Oxford, England **(see 714)**

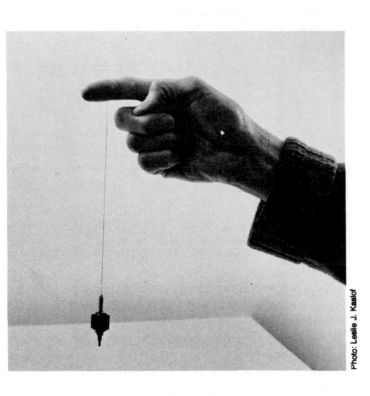

Photo: Leslie J. Kaslof

# Radiesthesia – Psionic Medicine

*Aubrey Westlake, MB, BChir*

*Rhabdomacy*—the old term for water divining—may be defined as "the use of the divining rod (traditionally a forked hazel twig) for discovering subterranean water or mineral ores." The first mention of its use for these purposes in England was in 1683, but it was certainly in practical use in much earlier times—e.g., in ancient Egypt.

In 1867, Prof. William Barrett started to make a careful and comprehensive investigation of the phenomenon of dowsing; in 1926, he published his findings in *The Divining Rod*. Dowsing thus became a legitimate subject for scientific study, and in 1933 Colonel Bell founded the British Society of Dowsers to inquire further into the whole subject, both in theory and practice, and, if possible, to find an explanation in terms of modern physics.

It soon became evident, however, that the subject lay outside ordinary scientific explanation and, moreover, had a scope that extended beyond locating water, mineral ores, or oil. Certain French priests who were dowsers found that they could use dowsing for medical purposes—to divine disordered states of the physical body. This was the beginning of medical dowsing, or radiesthesia.

In 1939, Dr. Guyon Richards formed the Society for the Study of Radiesthesia and gathered around him a remarkable group of doctors to explore the rich potentialities of the new concepts. They made considerable progress in refining techniques for diagnosis and treatment, and they collected and assessed research data. Medical dowsing was further advanced in America through the work of Dr. Albert Abrams, the founder of radionics—instrumental radiesthesia.

Since then the main advance has been twofold: (1) a greater understanding has been gained of what dowsing is. It has become clear that we are dealing with a hitherto unrecognized sense, supersensible in its nature, which operates on the physical-etheric level. This special sense is known as the "radiesthetic faculty," and there is growing evidence that it can be used successfully in the investigation of many other problems of the contemporary world. (2) measurement has been introduced and refined, so that it is now possible to compare and assess data, thus establishing a scientific basis for clinical work.

Although radiesthesia has become the most advanced aspect of dowsing, it is still only in the early stages of development. In the future it may open up an entirely new aspect of the art and science of fundamental healing.

Psionic medicine is essentially an attempt to restore to modern medicine its indispensable and necessary counterpart, that aspect mainly lost sight of in the materialistic—one might also say mechanistic—trends of contemporary scientific medicine, limited as it is to knowledge of the physical body provided by physical sense perception alone, augmented though it may be by all sorts of instrumentation of the greatest possible ingenuity and complicity, operated and controlled by brilliant intellects.

Thus psionic medicine, as its name implies, seeks to restore to materialistic medicine, through the use of a new supersensory sense (the radiesthetic or dowsing faculty), a dimension it has largely lost—a dimension not only vital to the recovery of the art of medicine, but which alone can give real meaning and understanding to its science. If this dimension can be restored, then it will be possible once again to have a true comprehensive science and art of healing in a fundamental sense.

As a new dimension, psionic medicine is thus not just an alternative form of healing, but the starting point of the supersensible and spiritual complement that will make sense of the whole, on all planes of consciousness.

The main progenitor of psionic medicine and its practical application has been Dr. L. George Laurence, who after a lifetime of practice and experience in orthodox medicine, came to a realization: "I did not know *why* people were ill, and was reduced to treating signs and symptoms without a real clue to fundamental causation." It was not until late in Laurence's medical career that he joined the Medical Society for the Study of Radiesthesia, and here he found the missing concepts in medicine he had been seeking. He then set out to develop them. His work has resulted in the integration of his findings into a unified whole, which he named psionic medicine.

The first step was devising a technique using a special diagnostic pattern and the radiesthetic faculty by which deviation from the point of dynamic balance can be determined in degrees, plus and minus; the therapeutic remedy (usually homeopathic) is what rectifies this departure from the norm. The whole pattern then becomes an indication of the restoration to health by a true balance of the three factors involved—the patient, the cause, and the right remedy. Diagnosis and treatment are thus ascertained by the same procedure.

Laurence adapted McDonagh's Unitary Theory of Disease, which postulates that all diseases are merely aspects, in various ways and forms, of unbalance, or—to use his term—aberration of the protein of the body, and that no disease can be cured unless and until the balance is restored, that is, the aberration is corrected. The main aberration, according to McDonagh, is either overcontraction or overexpansion of the protein as a whole or any of its parts. Laurence showed that the factors responsible for the aberration include the toxic factors of our polluted environment, as well as earlier factors first postulated by Hahnemann, the founder of homeopathy.

Laurence also incorporated Hahnemann's miasmic theory of chronic disease. In the last eleven years of his life Hahnemann devoted himself to the problem of the causation of chronic disease to discover "why homeopathic remedies then known failed to cure, thoroughly and forever, certain chronic diseases," and he sought "a complete and correct idea of the true nature of those thousands of chronic ailments which remain uncured in spite of the incontrovertible truth of the homeopathic doctrine." He came to the conclusion that "The first condition of finding out was to discover all the ailments and symptoms inherent in the unknown primitive malady." But what was this primitive malady? According to Hahnemann, "It owed its existence to some chronic miasm." He was in fact speaking much more truly than even he knew, as it was impossible for him to be more precise with the limited medical and scientific knowledge of those times. But radiesthetic research has shown that these miasms undoubtedly exist and underlie most chronic disease, and can be passed on from one generation to another by etheric heredity.

Laurence found in the course of his psionic research that, in addition to these inherited miasms, there are also acquired miasms, or, as Laurence prefers to call them, "retained toxins of acquired infections"—especially that of measles. These "toxins" or "hangovers" can themselves be responsible for quite serious ailments but when acquired in addition to any hereditary miasm may cause serious departures from normal health. It is just as important to eliminate these acquired toxins as it is to get rid of any hereditary miasms, if one is to deal adequately with the symptoms and manifestations of any disorder, subacute or chronic.

It was also left to Laurence, 120 years later, to find the solution to the problem that had defeated Hahnemann—how to get rid of the miasms. This Laurence did furst by utlizing McDonagh's theory in a practical way. He argued that if miasms have the power to produce aberrations in the protein of the body, it followed, according to homeopathic principles, that if we could potentize protein we might have a powerful and far-reaching means of adjusting these fundamental imbalances of the protein. This proved to be the case, but it still left problems, and something that would go even deeper was evidently needed. DNA and RNA, recent discoveries of the organic chemists, turned out to be what were required, and the homeopathic potentization of these substances proved to be the fundamental remedies Hahnemann had been seeking.

All these discoveries gave a new dimension to homeopathy, which Dr. Laurence found, generally speaking, was the treatment of choice, when determined radiesthetically; for the potentized remedies of homeopathy are found to be the vehicles for conveying the supersensible healing force necessary for the correction of the protein imbalances, and he found in practice that the dynamic balance can in fact be restored by such remedies and a real cure obtained. This is because the homeopathic medicines work by virtue of the specific "vital essence"—the *vis medicatrix*—of each remedy, which has been "liberated" to some extent by the act of potentization (i.e., by dilution and succussion) from its ordinary materialized form and has thus become supersensible in nature and able to work therapeutically on that level.

And finally Laurence found in the "spiritual science" of Rudolf Steiner the knowledge necessary for an understanding of the fourfold makeup of man (physical body, etheric body, astral body, and ego) and the true nature of the healing force (*vis medicatrix natura*) as being an aspect of the etheric formative forces.

Some of the special features of this integration are:
1. It is essentially simple, both in theory and practice, and requires the minimum of equipment and apparatus.
2. Accurate assessment can very rapidly be made of fundamental causal factors—environmental, hereditary, internal.
3. The very earliest departures from health can be detected, thus providing a true preventative medicine, and this is especially so in the detection and elimination of hereditary miasms in children, thus breaking this hereditary chain for the first time in history.
4. There is hope for chronics, as the cause of the chronicity can be diagnosed and eliminated, so that further degeneration is arrested and restoration made possible. Experience in very many cases has proved conclusively how important it is to eliminate causation before treating symptoms.
5. Treatment is entirely individual and consists essentially in stimulating and cooperating with the healing forces of the body.
6. The course and results of therapy can be monitored radiesthetically during the whole period of treatment and necessary adjustments made with confidence.

## Groups and Associations

(716) **AMERICAN SOCIETY OF DOWSERS**
Danville, VT 05828

(802) 684-3417

An open membership, nonprofit, educational, scientific society dedicated to advancing the practice and science of dowsing (radiesthesia) in the United States. The Society publishes a quarterly, *The American Dowser*, for its membership, and holds annual conventions in mid-September at Danville, Vermont. A large selection of books on dowsing and related subjects, as well as pendulums and divining rods, may be ordered through the Society at the above address (Atten: Paul J. Sevigny, Supply Division). Founded 1961.

(717) **THE PSIONIC MEDICAL SOCIETY**
34 Beacon Hill Court
Hindhead, Surrey
England

*George Laurence, President*

Established as a registered charity for the purpose of pursuing research into the causes of chronic and 'incurable' disease and the advancement of, and training in, methods of diagnosis and treatment. The Institute holds examinations and maintains a register of qualified members. Membership is confined to qualified medical and dental practitioners who have undergone the necessary training and have satisfied the examiners of their competence in the techniques of psionic medicine. (In psionic medicine diagnosis is made with the aid of medical dowsing and treatment is with homeopathic preparations.) Publishes journal.

## Schools, Centers, and Clinics

(718) **UNIVERSITY OF THE TREES**
P.O. Box 644
Boulder Creek, CA 95006

(408) 338-3855

*Christopher Hills, Founder*

Courses and instruction in all aspects of radiesthesia and related fields. Publishers of the book *Supersensonics* as well as many other titles. Has available a complete line of radiesthesia equipment and pendulums.

**HUMAN DIMENSIONS INSTITUTE-WEST**/Ojai, CA **(see 588)**

**SAN DIEGO NATURAL HEALTH CLINIC**/San Diego, CA **(see 108)**

**SCHOOL OF SCIENTIFIC NUTRITION**/Albuquerque, NM **(see 501)**

**ALTERNATIVE HEALTH EDUCATION CENTER/**
Rochester, NY **(see 143)**

**RAMANA HEALTH CENTRE**/Hants, England **(see 161)**

**THE COMPANY OF SOMATOGRAPHERS** (psychophysical treatment and radiesthesia)/London, England; New York, NY **(see 845)**

**WESTBANK HEALING AND TEACHING CENTRE/**
Fife, Scotland **(see 163)**

## Journals and Publications

**JOURNAL OF BORDERLAND RESEARCH**/Vista, CA **(see 804)**

**NEW AGE JOURNAL** (multidisciplinary)/Brookline, MA **(see 196)**

**HUMAN DIMENSIONS** (multidisciplinary journal)/ Williamsville, NY **(see 203)**

**THE AMERICAN DOWSER** (journal)/Danville, VT **(see 716)**

**JOURNAL OF THE PSIONIC MEDICINE SOCIETY**/Surrey, England **(see 717)**

## Products and Services

**UNIVERSITY OF THE TREES** (pendulums)/Boulder Creek, CA **(see 718)**

**BORDERLAND SCIENCES RESEARCH FOUNDATION** (books)/Vista, CA **(see 804)**

**CLARK ENTERPRISES** (radiesthesia and radionics)/ Marble Falls, TX **(see 713)**

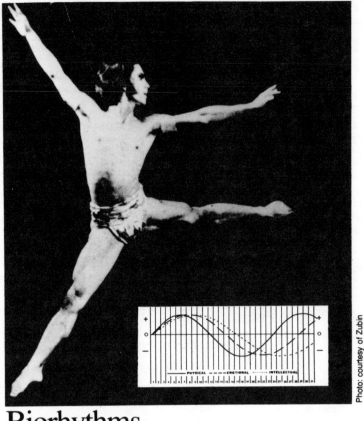

Photo: courtesy of Zubin

# Biorhythms

*Bernard Gittleson*

*"One does not need to have lived a long span of life before one comes to realize that life is subject to consistent changes. Even if someone could live a life completely devoid of outside influences, a life during which nothing whatever disturbs the mental or physical aspect, life would nevertheless not be the same day after day."*

Dr. Herman Swoboda

The theory of biorhythm holds that when a person is born, the trauma of leaving the safe and warm confines of the mother's womb sets in motion a series of three cycles which will continue to reoccur at regular intervals until death. These are the physical cycle (23 days long), the emotional cycle (28 days long), and the intellectual cycle (33 days long). One half of each cycle places the individual in a negative or low position. It is while crossing the middle of each cycle, either from high to low or from low to high, that the individual experiences an unstable or "critical" period. During this period accidents occur or, conversely, the individual may excel beyond his or her expectations. With the conjunction of the cycles, critical days occur during 20 percent of the total time.

The biorhythm theory evolved through the work of a series of researchers. The "father" of biorhythm theory was Dr. Herman Swoboda, who, as a professor of psychology at the University of Vienna, kept detailed records between 1897 and 1902 on the onset and development of inflammations, fevers, heart attacks, asthma, and other illnesses. As the data accumulated, a pattern began to emerge, which led Swoboda to propose that man experiences internal cycles of 23 and 28 days. His findings were published in his first book, *Die Perioden des Menschlichen Lebens* [*The Periodicity in Man's Life*], and later in his most important work, *Das Siebenjahr* [*The Year of Seven*]. In the latter book, Dr. Swoboda applied mathematical analysis to the basic concept of repetitive cycles and drew upon the experiences of hundreds of families to conclude that most major events in life fall on a given sequence of days.

Although Swoboda is clearly considered the initial proponent of biorhythm (or bionomy, as he called it), he was by no means the only major contributor. In 1900, Dr. Wilhelm Freeze at the University of

Berlin found and documented cases of children developing illnesses at periodic intervals. Bolstering his medical knowledge with the psychoanalytical expertise of his colleague and friend Dr. Sigmund Freud, Freeze theorized that there exists a 23-day physical cycle and a 28-day sensitivity cycle. In 1928, Dr. Alfred Teltscher, a faculty member of the engineering department of the University of Innsbruck, carried out experiments using 5,000 students. After observing and recording the behavioral patterns of so large and diverse a group, Teltscher was able not only to confirm the existence of a physical and emotional cycle but also to speculate that yet another cycle, an intellectual cycle of 33 days, exists. Noting that each student experienced clearly defined peaks and valleys in his or her intellectual capacity, he postulated that a third cycle must be at work.

Perhaps the most complex early founder of biorhythm was a German physician named Wilhelm Fleiss. Fleiss, as a nose and throat specialist, found that many of his young patients would show symptoms of an illness a given number of days after being exposed to a contagious disease. The uncanny repetitiveness of these patterns led Fleiss to delve into the past histories of many of his patients, tracing their periods of illness from the day of birth. After six years of evaluating thousands of case histories, Fleiss published his first book, *Der Ablauf das Lebens* [*The Course of Life*], in which he asserts that a 23-day and a 28-day rhythm are fundamental to the understanding of life processes.

As a contemporary and close friend of Freud, Fleiss speculated on the causes of certain human characteristics. He believed very strongly that each individual inherits both male and female traits and is therefore internally bisexual. Transferring this concept to his study of periodic rhythms, Dr. Fleiss concluded that the 23-day rhythm is actually masculine in origin, while the 28-day rhythm is essentially a feminine trait. Because of their inherent bisexuality, both males and females experience both rhythms.

Like Swoboda, Fleiss was defeated by his own affinity for accumulating data. His pages and pages of numerical tables, charts, calculations, and conclusions proved too cumbersome for the medical hierarchy of his day. The concept of internal rhythms was difficult enough for people to accept without having to endure the mathematical configurations that supposedly served as proof.

Though the means of understanding biorhythms has been made less complicated over the past fifty years, some skepticism remains. Alfred Judt, a German mathematician, and, later, Hans R. Freuh, a Swiss engineer, simplified the long and laborious mathematical tables that proved to be Fleiss's undoing. Hand-operated slide rules gave way to electronic calculators and computerized readouts. Now that researchers possess all the necessary tools to investigate the existence of biorhythms properly, they may be able to convince the public in general and the scientific community in particular.

The difficulties that arise in trying to prove the biorhythm theory are attributable to the fact that biorhythm, like psychology, sociology, and political science, is an empirical science; that is, assumptions are made based on observation, not on experimentation. Thus, even at this stage there is still no definitive proof that biorhythm exists; yet it is clearly beyond the hypothetical stage, for thousands of well-documented cases already support the theory.

The medical and scientific communities are not unfamiliar with bodily cycles: body temperature varies about 2 degrees every day, starting below the normal 98.6 in the morning and rising above it in the evening; the liver converts glycogen to glucose at different rates during a given day, with a maximum at about 5:00 P.M. and a minimum at about 4:00 A.M.; heartbeat, blood pressure, kidney function, and hormone output show marked differences at different periods of the day. However, the 23-, 28-, and 33-day concurrent cycles described by the biorhythm theory have yet to be acknowledged, despite impressive evidence.

Dr. F. Wehrli of Locarno, Switzerland, writes in the preface of the book *Biorhythm* by Hans J. Wernli that he used biorhythms in his hospital for over 15 years in an effort to ascertain the best days for performing elective surgery. He performed over 10,000 operations without a single failure or complication (normally, he points out, complications arise in 30–60 percent of surgical cases). He attributes his success to his use of biorhythms.

Dr. Robert A. Reismann of the Hahnemann Medical College and Hospital writes in the *Annals of Clinical and Laboratory Science:* "Regardless of skepticism and considering all theories, conjectures and facts about biorhythms offered by so many for so long, there is something to it.'' This conclusion follows a rather lengthy discussion of biological rhythms, in which Reismann proposes a relationship between biorhythms and periodic diseases. Sufferers of periodic fever, peritonitis, hereditary angioedema, and psychoses have been found to experience seizures and symptoms every 14 days, or concurrently with the critical period in the emotional biorhythmic cycle. Furthermore, Dr. Reismann points to the 8- to 10-day cycles for estrone excretion, 7-day cycles of ketosteroids, and 20-to-22-day cycles for changes in plasma testosterone and indications that, indeed, ''these facts implicate the omnipresence of biorhythms.''

Harold R. Willis, Assistant Professor of Psychology at Southern State College, has done extensive research into the relationship between biorhythms and medically related deaths. A study was conducted in 1973 in which 200 hospital deaths were recorded and analyzed (for the purpose of reliability, subjects who died when 70 years of age or older were excluded from the study). Willis found that of the 200 cases studied, 112 patients (or 56 percent) died on critical days. A second study conducted on an additional 120 cases in 1974 resulted in similar findings: 62 patients (or 52 percent) died on critical days.

Small-scale but no less significant research has been done involving almost every area of physiological and mental health. Dr. Lucien Sansouci, a consultant to a state mental hospital in Rhode Island, found that several of his most schizophrenic patients shifted into violent behavior when their emotional cycles were in a critical period. Dr. Philip A. Costin, former medical director of the Canadian Air Force, conducted a number of studies and was able to correlate feats of heroism, acts of cowardice, and suicides with the cyclic ups and downs of military personnel.

An even greater interest in biorhythms has been shown in the area of safety management. This interest is not surprising, in view of the fact that increased safety leads to greater productivity and hence, in industry, greater profit. Mr. Robert Schwarz, president of the Bureau of Indian Affairs in Portland, Oregon, conducted a study of the workers in his charge and found that between 41 and 73 percent of all self-inflicted accidents occurred when the victim was ''critical'' in at least one of his or her biorhythms. Pfizer, Inc., a leading pharmaceutical company, initiated a safety program based largely on biorhythm, and according to Safety Manager Aldo Osti, ''Accidents dropped almost 60 percent.'' Russell K. Anderson, former president of Russell K. Anderson Associates, Safety Engineers, investigated over 300 accidents in four different areas of industry: a metalworking plant, a chemical plant, a textile mill, and a knitting mill. Anderson found that almost 70 percent of the accidents caused by human factors occurred on a critical day in the victim's cycle (the figure for mechanical accidents was even higher).

Not only is further scientific and medical research needed, it presents intriguing possibilities. If we are indeed emotionally unstable during our critical periods, then the neurohumors secreted by our nerve endings should increase. If this hypothesis is found to be true, one cycle might find universal acceptance. Similar experiments could be conducted into the ATP levels in the mitochondria of muscle cells at different periods and the changes in secretions by the thyroid and the adrenal medulla. Such research could indicate that internal changes do occur during periods that coincide with changes in our biorhythm cycles. The concept seems feasible, and the possibilities for exploration are infinite.

## Researchers, United States and Canada

(719) **RUSSELL ANDERSON**
1228 Yosemite Drive
Colorado Springs, CO 80910

Researcher in biorhythm.

(720) **GEORGE THOMMEN**
2433 Brazilia Drive
Clearwater, FL 33515

Researcher in biorhythm.

(721) **DAVID SMITH**
Kosmos International Horizon
3930 First National Bank Tower
Atlanta, GA 30319

(404) 658-1475

Researcher in biorhythm.

(722) **BERNARD GITTLESON**
119 West 57th Street
New York, NY 10019

Researcher in biorhythm.

(723) **ROBERT SCHWARTZ**
Bureau of Indian Affairs
Box 3785
Portland, OR 97403

Researcher in biorhythm.


(724) **LUCIEN SANSOUCI, PhD**
41 Thomas Street
Woonsocket, RI 02895

Researcher in biorhythm.


(725) **DAVID HUMPHREY**
1203 East 33rd Street
Texarkana, TX 75501

Researcher in biorhythm.


(726) **KEITH HENSCHEN, MD**
College of Health
University of Utah
1400 East Second, South
Salt Lake City, UT 84112

Researcher in biorhythm.


(727) **PHILIP COSTIN, MD**
10 Driveway North
Ottawa, Canada

Researcher in biorhythm.


# Journals and Publications

**BIORHYTHM NEWSLETTER**/New York, NY **(see 729)**

# Products and Services

(728) **AIRLIGHT**
602 East Micheltorena
Santa Barbara, CA 93103

(805) 966-6000

Commercial biorhythm computation service. One year's chart, $5. Also send birthdate.


**QUINTESSENCE UNLIMITED** (consciousness tools)/ Boulder, CO **(see 215)**


**JAPAN PUBLICATIONS** (book publisher)/Elmsford, NY **(see 872)**


(729) **BIORHYTHM COMPUTERS, INC.**
298 Fifth Avenue
New York, NY 10003

(212) 977-9566

Has available a one year computerized biorhythm chart with interpretations. Publishes a monthly newsletter featuring the latest news and developments in the field of biorhythms. Distributes various biorhythm devices and graphs.


(730) **VILLAGE PLANETAIRE, INC.**
322 Est Villeneuve
Montreal, Quebec H2T 1L8
Canada

Commercial biorhythm computation service. Also conducts research to verify the existence of a 4th cycle, 38 days long, related to intuition, telepathy and ESP energies.


**COMPANY OF SOMOTAGRAPHERS**/England; New York, NY **(see 845)**


**INTERNATIONAL SOCIETY OF BIOMETEOR-OLOGY**/The Netherlands **(see 674)**

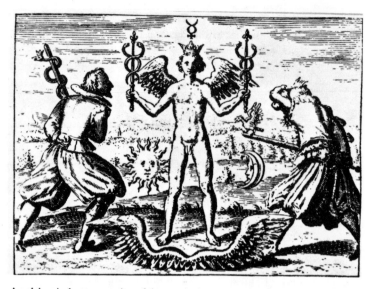

An alchemical representation of the ventricular system. According to F. Basilius Valentinus. The lateral and fourth ventricles are represented as two contesting swordsmen, with Mercury as the third ventricle in equilibrium between them. From, *Man Grand Symbol of the Mysteries, Gems of Thought In Occult Anatomy*. By Manly P. Hall, Los Angeles: Philosophical Research Society, 1972.

# Astrology And Medicine
*Mario Jones, MD*

*"We all live under the haunting fear that something may corrupt the environment to the point where man joins the dinosaur as an obsolete form of life. And what makes these thoughts all the more disturbing is the knowledge that our fate could perhaps be sealed twenty or more years before the development of symptoms."*

*Dr. David Price, of the United States Public Health Service*

In the classical world astrology and medicine were nearly one. Both disciplines, based on scientific observations and hypotheses but very humanistic in their goals, tried to understand man as an entity and in relation to the rest of the universe. Until recently, traditional medicine was a highly personal relationship between healer and patient; subjective psychological and spiritual understanding was used to direct and reinforce scientific techniques. Caught in the wave of technology and superspecialization of our time, medicine lost track of the whole person. A new discipline, psychosomatics, emerged to remind us that disease and total personal needs are inseparable—as is shown in astrological analysis, in which body and soul are symbolized by the same factors.

The aim of medical astrology is, in the words of an early theorist, H. G. Muller-Freywardt, MD, to help to "find the way out of a crisis," using the anamnesis, or personal history of the patient. An isolated chart can foster great theoretical discussions but can also lead to perfectly sensible, logical, and wrong conclusions unless it is related to the client's problem. Medical astrology is not a game to surprise and astound with the revelation of circumstances of which the patient is well aware, but a serious discipline that correlates the problem with the astrological chart and then finds the possible solutions and long-range prognosis. The practitioner's role is not to astound the patient with brilliant technical conclusions, but to look at the problems with compassion and do his or her utmost to restore the patient's confidence and peace of mind.

The modern study of medical astrology is in its infancy. The available literature is very limited, because valuable research can be done only by those who have a working knowledge of astrology, biology, pathology, and psychology. Another obstacle is the great number of different astrological schools that have tried astromedical research. Most of the work of the ancient physician-astrologers has been lost, destroyed, or perhaps even suppressed, and what little we have is of little value: isolated clues, no standardization of problems, incomplete data, obsolete interpretations of good and bad (benign and malefic influence of planets and aspects), and reliance on such slippery concepts as hyleg and anareta make these works true historical curiosities.

A modern attempt to organize medical astrology into a body of knowledge susceptible of methodic, practical, team-oriented research has been made by the Cosmobiological School of Aalen. Relying heavily on the midpoint structures, this school investigated correlations with biological functions and general pathology, and in 1950 Muller-Freywardt wrote an article on the "cosmobiological correspondences of the human body," which became the cornerstone of modern medical astrology.

Muller-Freywardt defines the following points:

1. The scope of astrology in medicine (he stresses the importance of the anamnesis and the goal of helping a patient out of a crisis);
2. The astrological chart as the basis for an individual therapeutic prescription;
3. Three planetary pairs as *general* combinations of disease: Mars/Neptune, Saturn/Neptune, and Sun/Neptune (active structures of these pairs do not mean disease, but when disease is present, one, two, or all three are active);
4. The importance of the personal points (Midheaven, Ascendant, Sun, Moon); also, the Node as a personal point; and
5. The biological and medical interpretation of the planets and personal points.

Further research in cosmobiology revealed many other significant combinations, some quite certain, others still being methodically researched.

To the premises of cosmobiology we can add Uranian astrological factors to enrich the interpretation with planetary pictures and Uranian house theory. These methods provide basic, specific parameters that can be examined objectively by a number of independent observers and probably analyzed statistically.

This research has already given us many practical applications, but there is much to be done. Astrology has been concerned for a long time with disease, but not with normal physiological functions; these remain to be studied. The only modern work in astrological anatomy is that published by Reinhold Ebertin (*The Combination of Stellar Influences*), and although is it quite accurate, it will have to be revised before it can be universally acceptable.

A new dimension in astrology that is very important in astromedical research has been opened by the theory of harmonics, pioneered by John Addey. Harmonic charts can define a problem with extraordinary accuracy and clarity, and can be very helpful in the study of many biological functions for which the astrological parameters are still obscure.

Though often overlooked, psychology is very important in medicine, and in medical astrology it is indispensable. Astrology shows how psychological and somatic considerations in disease go hand in hand. A psychological definition is necessary to know how the disease is going to affect the total life of the patient and to find appropriate therapeutic means. Unfortunately, the difficulties redouble; if to the many different astrological approaches we add the diverse psychological systems, we end up with a distinct approach for every astrologer, a state of confusion that can lead to a number of valid approaches to the patient's problem, but not to a systematic study of psychosomatic disease (and maybe this is an inherent problem of astrology as a symbolic discipline). Some astrologers base all medical interpretations on psychological factors, but this is wrong, for though we can certainly identify psychological trends of disease, we don't know what biological system is going to respond unless we make a physiological analysis. Psychic and somatic must be studied simultaneously.

Finally, the concept of "environment" plays an outstanding role. This is not only the individual psychosomatic condition of the patient but also the general milieu in which his or her life unfolds—social, professional and material values, needs, problems, friends, associates, etc. Environment must be correlated to the given problem and to the astrological chart, because a reading, besides being astrologically valid, has to make sense in view of the client's problems. This takes us back to our basic need; a sound anamnesis. We must know as much as possible about our client before validating an interpretation and making future projections.

Medical astrology can help in the following areas:

1. *General Evaluation:* Astrology can give a fast overall view of the patient's strong and weak points, past, present, and future range of problems, and the possible areas of affliction. In conventional medicine this would take an almost lifelong acquaintance of physician and patient.

2. *Diagnosis:* The precise pathological diagnosis of an illness belongs now to technical medicine. Astrology can be of great help in differential diagnosis directing the clinician to a particular area when the case is obscure.

3. *Treatment:* Astrology can be very helpful in the selection of therapy—be it allopathic, homeopathic, herbal, or mechanical—and in the selection of an appropriate time for radical therapeutic measures such as surgery.

4. *Prognosis and Timing:* Here astrology reigns supreme. It can give a very clear projection of the present problem (a "prognosis," rather than a "prediction"). It can define with amazing accuracy crisis during an illness and long-term possibility of a recurrence.

5. *A Health Plan for Life:* A good general evaluation (astrological and environmental) can outline a definite plan of living for a particular person; activities, diet, special precautions, etc. Since astrology and environment have to be evaluated together, and environment can change from time to time, it is not advisable to make projections way into the future. They should be restricted to relatively short periods of time—a year at most, or even six months.

Medicine, over and above the study of disease, should be one of the most important branches in the general study of man. Curing disease and healing wounds is only a part of it; even more important is understanding patients and helping them, even if they can't be cured. Here astrology can be extremely useful, both in theory and practice.

The use of astrology by serious practitioners with a solid medical background cannot but help the art and practice of medicine.

## Groups and Associations

(731) **NATIONAL COUNCIL FOR GEOCOSMIC RESEARCH, INC.**
436 West 22nd Street
New York, NY 10011

(212) 989-5088

*Charles Emerson, Director*

Maintains information on cooperative research in medical astrology. Also publishes the *Journal of the National Council for Geocosmic Research,* of which the 1975-1976 issues had articles on medical astrology.

## Centers and Clinics

**CHURCH OF GENTLE BROTHERS AND SISTERS** (educational center)/San Francisco, CA **(see 109)**

**NURSE CONSULTANTS AND HEALTH COUNSELORS**/San Francisco, CA **(see 112)**

**DESERT LIGHT FOUNDATION** (holistic clinic and school)/Albuquerque, NM **(see 134)**

**EUGENE CENTER FOR THE HEALING ARTS/** Eugene, OR **(see 148)**

**ASSOCIATION FOR DOCUMENTATION AND ENLIGHTENMENT, INC.** (psychic research and healing center)/Virginia Beach, VA **(see 796)**

**HOME CENTER** (wholistic treatment center)/Virginia Beach, VA **(see 155)**

## Journals and Publications

**JOURNAL OF THE NATIONAL COUNCIL OF GEOCOSMIC RESEARCH**/New York, NY **(see 731)**

**SEEKER** (multidisciplinary newsletter directory NY area)/New York, NY **(see 202)**

## Products and Services

**TUESDAY ISLAND FARM** (astrological birth control chart)/Nova Scotia, Canada **(see 610)**

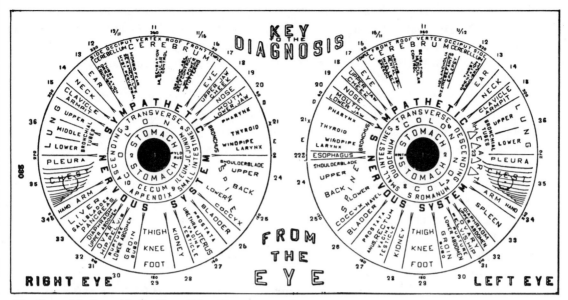

The Chart originally used by Dr. Henry Edward Lane; courtesy Bernard Jensen, from *The Science and Practice of Iridology*. By Bernard Jensen. Escondido, CA: Bernard Jensen Publishing Co., 1952.

# Iridology: Its Origin, Development, And Meaning
*Bernard Jensen, DC, ND*

Iridology, also known as irisdiagnosis, irisology, iroscopy, iris science, and diagnosis from the eye, is based on the findings of Ignatz von Peczely of Hungary, a physician and surgeon, and N. Liljequist of Sweden, a minister.

Both worked independently, unaware of each other's efforts. Von Peczely wrote a treatise on the subject in 1868, and his first and only book was published in 1880; a book by Liljequist appeared in 1871. Both are credited as being discoverers of diagnosis from the iris. Von Peczely investigated how signs in the iris reveal changes in bodily conditions; Liljequist was more interested in how the lines of colored areas in the iris indicate administration and retention of various drugs and chemicals in the body.

The basic premise of iridology is that each organ of the body is represented by an area of the iris. Charts made to show such areas present the organs with the pupil area corresponding to the navel; the organs occupy areas in the iris in relation to the position they occupy with regard to the naval and the medial and lateral aspects of the body. Blue, brown, and intermediate (a mixture of blue and brown), with many variations of shades depending on the intermingling of races and peoples, are considered to be normally colored irises. Variously colored spots found in the iris, such as red, white, yellow, green, rust colored, and variations of these colors, are indicative of mineral or drug deposits in parts of the body corresponding with the area of the iris in which the spots are found.

Iridology presents four classifications of pathology:

1. High white in the blue eye or high yellow in the brown eye is indicative of acute inflammation.
2. Grayish white in the blue eye or slightly dull yellow in the brown eye is indicative of subacute inflammation.
3. Dark gray in the blue eye or very dull yellow in the brown eye is indicative of chronic conditions.
4. Black in either blue or brown eye is indicative of extreme degeneration and destruction of tissues. It does not offer information as to specific diseases but is considered to present information relating to disturbed organic (structural) and/or functional (working) behavior.

In surveying the iris, attention is given to the purity or brightness of the coloring. In a state of good health, the colors are bright and clear; in ill health or a toxic condition, the colors are defiled and dull. In the blue iris, acid or toxic irritation is manifested by a white sheen superimposed over the basic blue (the iris has been described as looking as if a beaten egg white had been splattered over it); in the brown iris there is murkiness and the appearance of yellow or light brown tinting.

The texture of the iris provides most interesting information, thought to be unobtainable from any other source. The texture may show the fineness of woven silk or the coarseness of burlap. If the fibers composing the iris are closely woven (like silk) and extend into the pupillary area, this indicates inherent strength, a strong constitution, and good recuperative ability; thus we can be sure that the individual's resistance is good and that he or she will respond to proper treatment. Loosely woven fibers indicate a general lack of inherent strength (referred to as inherent weakness), a poor constitution, and slow recuperative or regenerative ability. Moreover, the absence of closely knit fibers in a particular area of the iris indicates an inherent weakness of the particular part of the body that the area represents.

Distortions or irregularities in the ring or "autonomic wreath" (which appears about one-third of the distance from the pupil to the edge of the iris), gives information as to the condition of the autonomic nervous system. Regularity of the ring or wreath indicates normal nerve tension. Distortion indicates atonic (lacking power or tone) or spastic (cramped or tensed) conditions in the part of the body corresponding to the iris area where the distortion occurs.

The appearance of what are known as nerve or cramp rings (referred to in ophthalmology as contraction furrows) is of great interest, as it indicates the state of tension existing in the tissues of the body. Of course, the contraction furrows that appear in the skin of a healthy young child upon motion of the underlying tissues are not permanent. However, the contraction furrows that appear permanently in the skin of the aged or debilitated depict waning life and lost flexibility of body tissues. So it is with the contraction furrows of the iris: when manifested permanently, they become nerve or cramp rings and indicate that the organs involved are aging.

Iridological diagnosis can also indicate an approaching general or nervous prostration long before there are very definite physical manifestations. In this condition there appear radiating lines throughout the iris which converge at the autonomic wreath and appear superimposed on the fibers of the iris. Moreover, iridology can determine channels of toxic absorption from the intestinal tract into the tissues of the body, by observing the presence of deep grooves which look as if the tissues had been sliced like a pie; these are known as *radii solaris* ("rays of the sun"), or "spokes."

The practitioner may also determine a patient's progress, and even predict and evaluate a "retracing" or healing crisis that is in store. Rather than having to rely on numerous time-consuming tests and on the patient's statements as to reactions and feelings, iridologists are able—by observing a change from dark gray to grayish white, or from grayish white to clear bright white—to foresee the retracing process or healing crisis that it is on its way before it is actually physically demonstrated.

Of course, it is not possible to discuss detail here. A good course in iridology comprises no less than a hundred hours of lecturing and demonstration, and for the practitioner to attain high proficiency, such a course must be supplemented by years of clinical experience. While much information has been developed since the inception of the procedure in 1868–71, there is still much more to be determined. Iridologists hope that interest in this work will continue unabated and will ultimately elevate iridology to the level of importance it should occupy in every practitioner's procedure, and that public demand will be aroused to compel its advantageous use.

## Groups and Associations

(732) **WORLD IRIDOLOGY FELLOWSHIP**
3673 Glenfeliz
Los Angeles, CA 90039

*Dr. John Arnold*

Association of practitioners engaged in the practice of iridology. Memberships available. Also publishes journals.

## Schools, Centers, and Clinics

**BERKELEY HOLISTIC HEALTH CENTER**/Berkeley, CA (see 76)

**HIDDEN VALLEY HEALTH RANCH** (resort and fasting)/Escondido, CA **(see 166)**

**ISLA VISTA OPEN DOOR MEDICAL CLINIC**/Isla Vista, CA **(see 85)**

**OPEN EDUCATION EXCHANGE**/Oakland, CA **(see 100)**

**EAST-WEST ACADEMY OF HEALING ARTS**/San Francisco, CA **(see 110)**

**HOLISTIC LIFE UNIVERSITY** (multidisciplinary workshops)/San Francisco, CA **(see 111)**

**DESERT LIGHT FOUNDATION** (holistic clinic and school)/Albuquerque, NM **(see 134)**

**PREVENTIVE MEDICINE CLINIC**/Bellevue, WA **(see 156)**

## Journals and Publications

**WELL-BEING MAGAZINE** (natural healing)/San Diego, CA **(see 186)**

**COMMON GROUND** (multidisciplinary directory of San Francisco Bay Area)/San Francisco, CA **(see 187)**

**ALTERNATIVES JOURNAL** (multidisciplinary new age articles)/Miami, FL **(see 193)**

## Products and Services

(733) **BERNARD JENSEN, DC, ND**
Route 1, Box 52
Escondido, CA 92025

(714) 749-2727

Source of books, charts, and supplies for iridology.

Jensen, Bernard, *Science and Practice of Iridology*. Text for the study of iridology. $18.50. Available from above address.

Jensen, Bernard, *Jensen's Iridology Manual*. Explanation of lesions with 36 slides for study. $26.00. Available from above address.

**HEALTH RESEARCH** (books)/Mokelumne Hill, CA **(see 209)**

# V
# BIOFEEDBACK AND
# SELF-REGULATION

---

Biofeedback

Self-Health: From Pain To Health Maintenance

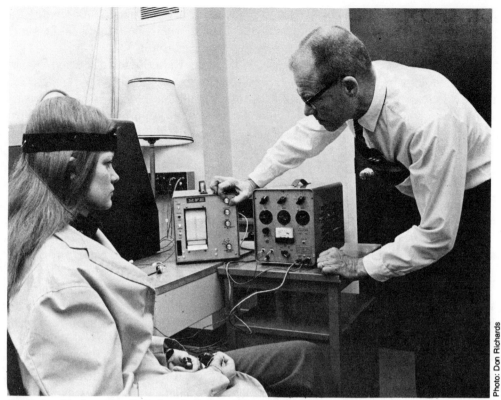

Research subject receiving EEG theta-feedback training by Elmer Green in a study of imagery associated with creative insights.

# Biofeedback

*Elmer Green, PhD*

*Biofeedback* is generally defined as the presentation to a person of ongoing biological information, such as heart rate, usually by means of meters, lights, or auditory signals, so that he or she can become aware of inside-the-skin behaviors. Biofeedback *training* means using the information in learning how to self-regulate the biological process being displayed. Although these kinds of definitions are most often used, there are some qualifications.

If one wants to make self-regulation truly voluntary and not dependent on a machine, it is necessary to be conscious of what the feedback represents. Biofeedback of autonomic processes presents to the cerebral cortex (the main area of consciousness in humans) information that usually is fed back almost entirely to subcortical brain centers. Blood flow in the various parts of the body and in various organs, for instance, is continuously and sensitively monitored by an internal feedback system that sends signals to an unconscious subcortical control center, the hypothalamus, and not until large temperature changes occur (due to blood flow changes) does the cortex become aware. For example, the average person without training cannot tell within 5.0°F what the hand temperature is, and cannot control hand temperature, but when a great deal of hand-temperature information is fed to the cortex, by the use of a temperature indicator that provides a just noticeable difference of 0.01°F, then the average person can learn to increase hand temperature at will within a couple of days.

Our primitive ancestors, with a life expectancy of perhaps twenty years, did not have much use or need for conscious inside-the-skin information in order to survive in a struggle with outside-the-skin nature, but our present-day problems are almost the reverse of theirs. Our stress is not from the physical world as much as from the psychological world, and feedback of inside-the-skin information is useful for control of inside-the-skin stress responses. In this regard, some of our problems with stress seem to be tied to the fact that we still have the caveman and cavewoman bodies of our ancestors. Many anthropologists point out that no significant changes have taken place in the gene pool for ten thousand years—some say fifty thousand—and that we still handle most stress with our "fight or flight" brain, the limbic system, sometimes called the visceral brain or the emotional brain.

The Biofeedback Society of America (founded in 1969 as the Biofeedback Research Society) invented the modern terminology in the field, but the earliest date for the use of biofeedback was at least as long ago as the development of yoga for control of certain autonomic processes of the body. In learning to control blood flow in the limbs, for instance, the color of the skin provided visual feedback as an indication of success. This is definitely biofeedback; information that was usually unconscious became detectable to the eye, and was fed to the cortex via the optic nerve. Such a feedback system was relatively inefficient because of low sensitivity, but nowadays sensitive electronic thermometers make learning easy.

The fact that it is quite easy to learn with biofeedback to control certain autonomic functions raises a question: How does biofeedback work? As a possible answer, consider figure 1. Sensory perception of outside-the-skin (OUTS) events, stressful or otherwise (upper left box), leads to a physiological response along arrows 1 to 4. If the physiological response is "picked up" and fed back (arrow 5) to a person who attempts to control inside-the-skin (INS) behavior, through imagining and visualizing a desired change, then arrows 6 and 7 come into being, resulting in a "new" limbic (emotional) response. This response in turn makes a change in "signals" transmitted along arrows 3 and 4, modifying the original physiological response. A cybernetic loop is thus completed, and the dynamic equilibrium (homeostasis) of the system can be brought under voluntary control. Biofeedback practice, acting in the opposite way to drugs, increases a person's *sensitivity* to INS events, and eventually arrow 8 develops, followed by the development of arrows 9 and 10. External feedback is then unnecessary, because direct perception of INS events becomes adequate for maintaining self-regulation skills. Physiological self-control through classical yoga develops along the route of arrows 7-3-4-9-10-7, but for control of specific physiological and psychosomatic problems biofeedback training seems more efficient.

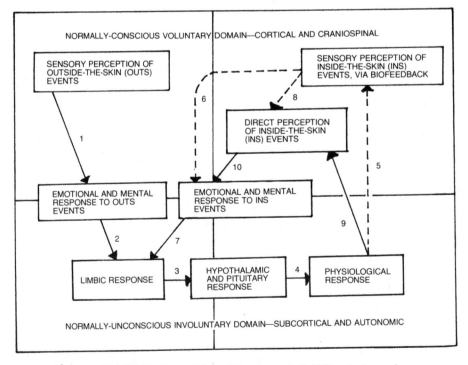

Fig. 1. Simplified Operational Diagram of Self-Regulation of Psychophysiological Events and Processes. SOURCE: Nils O. Jacobson, ed. *New Ways to Health* (Stockholm: Natur och Kulfur, 1975). Courtesy Elmer Green.

The main scientific question about biofeedback, and yoga too, seems to be, How does visualization, or imagination of a change in physiological processes, get converted into an actual physiological process? Along the same vein: How does an "organ-specific formula" (a phrase from J.H. Schultz's *Autogenic Training)* make a change in an organ? And again, how do John Basmajian's and Bernard Engel's biofeedback training methods, respectively, lead to control of firing in single motor nerve cells and in specific sections of the heart? The answer may be, of course, that mind and body are made of the same basic substance, and that if we can regulate mind, we can regulate body. Whatever the case, it is clear that much interesting research remains to be done.

## Groups and Associations

**(734) BIOFEEDBACK SOCIETY OF AMERICA**
Psychiatry C268
University of Colorado Medical Center
4200 East Ninth Avenue
Denver, CO 80220

(303) 394-7054

*Francine Butler, Executive Director*

An open forum for the exchange of ideas, methods and results of biofeedback and related studies. Emphasis is primarily on scientific and clinical investigations of human behavior and human potential, both in experimental and applied settings. The Society is involved in promoting biofeedback by maintaining high clinical standards, by developing and coordinating research, and by meetings, workshops, and publications. There are annual professional workshops (four days each fall) and scientific meetings. The Society publishes *Biofeedback and Self-Regulation*, the official journal, and a quarterly newsletter, *Biofeedback*. Membership is open to professionals interested in the scientific and clinical applications of biofeedback. Founded 1971.

*AFFILIATE AND STATE ASSOCIATIONS*

**ARIZONA BIOFEEDBACK SOCIETY**
P.O. Box 10741
Phoenix, AZ 85064

*Atten: Harry Edwin Smith*

Member of The Biofeedback Society of America.

**BIOFEEDBACK SOCIETY OF CALIFORNIA**
2043 Pine Street
San Francisco, CA 94115

(415) 921-5455

*Leslie Tauber, Executive Director*

An open forum for the exchange of ideas, methods, clinical experience and results of biofeedback and related disciplines. Members have demonstrated professional competence in biofeedback for one or more years, and are licensed or certified for their professions where required. Associate Memberships and Supporting Affiliate status are also available. Member of The Biofeedback Society of America.

**MIDWEST BIOFEEDBACK ASSOCIATION**
161 East Erie Street
Chicago, IL 60611

Member of The Biofeedback Society of America.

**ILLINOIS BIOFEEDBACK SOCIETY**
P.O. Box 8
Glenwood, IL 60425

*Atten: Alan Long, PhD*

Member of The Biofeedback Society of America.

**INDIANA BIOFEEDBACK SOCIETY**
Community Hospital of Indianapolis
1500 North Ritter Avenue
Indianapolis, IN 46219

(317) 353-1411

*Atten: Jerry E. Wesch, PhD*

Member of The Biofeedback Society of America.

**KANSAS BIOFEEDBACK SOCIETY**
Holtz Hall
Kansas State University
Manhattan, KS 66502

*Atten: Tim Lowenstein*

Member of The Biofeedback Society of America.

**LOUISIANA BIOFEEDBACK SOCIETY**
810 East 70th Street
Shreveport, LA 71106

*Atten: Tom Staats*

Member of The Biofeedback Society of America.

**MICHICAN BIOFEEDBACK SOCIETY**
University of Michigan, Mason Hall
Ann Arbor, MI 48104

(313) 764-1817

*Atten: James Papsdorf*

Member of The Biofeedback Society of America.

**NEW MEXICO BIOFEEDBACK SOCIETY**
Southwest Mental Health Center
555 North Main
Las Cruces, NM 88001

(505) 524-9601

*Atten: Barbara Gilmore*

Member of The Biofeedback Society of America.

**NEW YORK BIOFEEDBACK SOCIETY**
2152 Muliner Avenue
Bronx, NY 10462

(212) 822-7040

*Atten: Andrew Cannistraci, DDS*

Member of The Biofeedback Society of America.

**EASTERN BIOFEEDBACK SOCIETY**
83-91 Woodhaven Boulevard
Queens, NY 11421

(212) 846-2889

*Atten: Henry Meyers*

Member of The Biofeedback Society of America.

**TENNESSEE BIOFEEDBACK SOCIETY**
Union Square Building
2670 Union Avenue
Memphis, TN 38112

(901) 458-1181

*Atten: Eric Theiner*

Member of The Biofeedback Society of America.

**BIOFEEDBACK ASSOCIATION OF ALBERTA**
Department of Educational Psychology
University of Alberta
Edmonton, Alberta, Canada T6G 2G5

*Atten: George Fitzsimmons, PhD, President*

Member of The Biofeedback Society of America.

**LA SOCIETE DE REFROACTION DE QUEBEC**
(Biofeedback Society of Quebec)
822 Est Sherbrooke
Suite 400
Montreal 132, Quebec
Canada

*Atten: F. Poirier, MD*

Member of The Biofeedback Society of America.

**AUSTRALIAN BIOFEEDBACK SOCIETY**
c/o Bio-Cybernetic Systems
GPO, Box 7030
Sydney, 2001 Australia

*Atten: Ralph Henderson, National Secretary*

Member of The Biofeedback Society of America.

## Schools, Centers, and Clinics

**RIGGS AND ASSOCIATES** (psychotherapy)/
Anaheim—San Diego, CA **(see 1046)**

**PSYCHOSOMATIC MEDICINE CLINIC**/Berkeley,
CA **(see 76)**

**(735) AWARENESS DEVELOPMENT LABS INC.**
16055 Ventura Boulevard, Suite 930
Encino, CA 91436

(213) 986-9555

*Robert M. Tutone, PhD, Director*

Offers full spectrum biofeedback training (EMG, EEG, temperature), instruction in systematic relaxation and au-

togenic training, behavior modification, and ongoing therapeutic groups. Referrals for diagnosed psychosomatic disorders are accepted, and comprehensive programs for stress and weight control are available.

**MEDICINE HOLISTICS** (workshops)/Fresno, CA **(see 83)**

**WHOLISTIC MEDICINE AND PERSONAL GROWTH CENTER**/Hawthorne, CA **(see 84)**

**(736) A.H.C. BIOFEEDBACK TRAINING**
1516 Westwood Boulevard, Suite 207
Los Angeles, CA 90024

(213) 475-9213

*Janet Bright, Co-founder*

Holistically oriented pilot biofeedback clinic, established to augment medical treatments, develop health maintenance programs for industry and other groups, qualify biofeedback trainers, and to collect research data on biofeedback. The staff have diverse backgrounds, and are interested in the applications of biofeedback to psychotherapy, medical problems, and encounter groups.

**BIOFEEDBACK RESEARCH INSTITUTE**/Los Angeles, CA **(see 747)**

**HOLISTIC HEALTH CENTER** (treatment and education)/Los Angeles, CA **(see 90)**

**INSTITUTE FOR CREATIVE AGING** (geriatric)/ Malibu, CA **(see 94)**

**HEART HAUS CENTER** (holistic center)/Mill Valley, CA **(see 1056)**

**WELLNESS RESOURCE CENTER** (preventive)/Mill Valley, CA **(see 96)**

**NOVATO INSTITUTE FOR SOMATIC RE-SEARCH**/Novato, CA **(see 836)**

**AUTOGENIC HEALTH CENTER**/Oakland, CA **(see 98)**

**OPEN EDUCATION EXCHANGE** (holistic)/Oakland, CA **(see 100)**

**SAN ANDREAS HEALTH CENTER** (educational and therapy)/Palo Alto, CA **(see 101)**

**SACRAMENTO MEDICAL PREVENTICS CLINIC**/ Sacramento, CA **(see 103)**

**AGE OF ENLIGHTENMENT CENTER FOR HOLIS-TIC HEALTH** (Transcendental Meditation and treatment)/ San Diego, CA **(see 104)**

**CHILD PSYCHOLOGY INSTITUTE OF SAN DIEGO**/San Diego, CA **(see 1058)**

**SAN DIEGO NATURAL HEALTH CLINIC**/San Diego, CA **(see 108)**

**BIOFEEDBACK INSTITUTE OF SAN FRANCISCO**/ San Francisco, CA **(see 1059)**

**HOLISTIC LIFE UNIVERSITY** (multidisciplinary workshops)/San Francisco, CA **(see 111)**

**NURSE CONSULTANTS AND HEALTH COUNSELORS** (educational)/San Francisco, CA **(see 112)**

**(737) PHYSIOBEHAVIORAL TRAINING LABORATORY**
649 Irving Street
San Francisco, CA 94122

(415) 664-1464

*Jimmy Scott, PhD, Director*

Utilizes brain wave, skin temperature, muscle, and GSR biofeedback training modes to deal with a large variety of physiobehavioral complaints. Special programs are run for weight control, assertiveness behavior, and general stress reduction. The biofeedback training is supplanted with dietary surveys, blood chemistry tests, and hair analysis to establish the nutritional status of the patient. Founded 1973.

**PSYCHOTHERAPY AND GROWTH CENTER**/San Jose, CA **(see 1066)**

**ASSOCIATED PSYCHOLOGISTS OF SANTA CLARA**/Santa Clara, CA **(see 114)**

**FAMILY PRACTICE CENTER**/Santa Rosa, CA **(see 116)**

**STAMFORD CENTER FOR THE HEALING ARTS** (wholistic church clinic)/Stamford, CT **(see 121)**

**MANKIND RESEARCH FOUNDATION** (heuristic research)/Washington, DC **(see 122)**

**PSYCHOPHYSICS FOUNDATION** (heuristic research)/Miami, FL **(see 594)**

**(738) BIOFEEDBACK MEDITATIONAL TRAINING CENTER**
1505 Greenwood Road
Glenview, IL 60025

(312) 724-2273

*Rudolph M. Ballentine, MD, Director*

Founded by Swami Rama, the Center integrates biofeedback training with expert instruction in yogic breathing and relaxation practices. Biofeedback training is offered for specific problems such as headaches, circulatory problems, and muscle tension. Emphasis is placed on going beyond the clinical use of biofeedback to its development as an adjunct to meditation and a tool for exploring altered states of consciousness. Founded 1972.

**HIMALAYAN INSTITUTE COMBINED THERAPY CENTER** (wholistic clinic)/Glenview, IL **(see 125)**

**CENTERS FOR HEALTH AND LIFE** (educational and treatment)/Des Moines, IA **(see 126)**

**(739) BIOFEEDBACK INSTITUTE**
126 Harvard Street
Brookline, MA 02146

(617) 738-4502

*Buryl Payne, PhD, Director*

Integrates biofeedback training with gestalt, bioenergetics, behavior modification, assertiveness training and hypnosis. Problems dealt with include hypertension, insomnia, anxiety, and phobias.

**INSTITUTE FOR PSYCHOENERGETICS** (mind body program)/Brookline, MA **(see 128)**

**NEW ENGLAND CENTER** (multidisciplinary center)/Leverett, MA **(see 843)**

**MEDITATION CENTER**/Minneapolis, MN **(see 1108)**

**CENTRAL BERGEN COMMUNITY MENTAL HEALTH CENTER**/Paramus, NJ **(see 1112)**

**INSTITUTE FOR SELF DEVELOPMENT** (workshops and treatment)/Manhasset, NY **(see 137)**

**NEW AGE HEALTH FARM**/Neversink, NY **(see 172)**

**BEHAVIOR THERAPY CENTER OF NEW YORK** (psychotherapy)/New York, NY **(see 1115)**

**(740) BIOFEEDBACK STUDY CENTER OF NEW YORK**
55 East Ninth Street
New York, NY 10003

(212) 673-4710

*Lowell K. Cohn, Director*

Maintains a clinic for patients referred by doctors, dentists, and psychologists. Treatment, in consultation with the individual's physician, is offered for essential hypertension, migraine, Raynaud's disease, bruxism, and vascular disorders. The center also holds professional seminars and workshops, serves as consultant to groups interested in setting up their own biofeedback programs, and accepts individual clients interested in personal growth. Founded 1975.

**BIOMONITORING APPLIANCES** (equipment and treatment)/New York, NY **(see 757)**

**(741) INNER SPACE UNLIMITED, INC.**
Beach Road, Brayton Park
Ossining, NY 10562

(914) 762-4646

*Adam Crane, Founder*

Offers a training program designed to assist the client in taking responsibility for his/her health development. ISU serves the medical community by offering training for MDs, psychologists, and other professionals in biofeedback training as an aid to therapy for psychosomatic disorders. Also consults, designs, and installs biofeedback facilities for medical and research applications, and offers a full line of commercial biofeedback instruments.

**PSI CENTER** (clinic and treatment)/Cincinnati, OH **(see 145)**

**ALETHEIA PSYCHO-PHYSICAL FOUNDATIONS** (voluntary control of internal states)/Grants Pass, OR **(see 795)**

**PAIN AND HEALTH REHABILITATION CENTER/** La Crosse, WI **(see 157)**

**YORK UNIVERSITY** (parapsychology)/Downsville, Ontario, Canada **(see 68)**

**SWEDISH HERBAL INSTITUTE** (research)/ Gothenburg, Sweden **(see 554)**

## Journals and Publications

**BRAIN/MIND BULLETIN**/Los Angeles, CA **(see 184)**

**(742) BIOFEEDBACK NETWORK**
P.O. Box 816
Greenburg, KS 67054

(316) 723-2272

*E.W. Rakestraw*

Newsletter to help stimulate interest in new biofeedback products. Books and information available.

**(743) BIOFEEDBACK AND SELF REGULATION**
Plenum Publishing Corporation
227 West Seventeenth Street
New York, NY 10011

(212) 255-0713

*Johann Stoyva, PhD, Editor*

Interdisciplinary quarterly for the review and rapid dissemination of information in biofeedback and self-regulation.

## Products and Services

**(744) AQUARIUS ELECTRONICS**
P.O. Box 96
Albion, CA 95410

(707) 937-0064

Distributes a full line of biofeedback equipment.

**(745) AUTOGENIC SYSTEMS, INC.**
809 Allston Way
Berkeley, CA 94710

(415) 548-6056

One of the nation's largest biofeedback companies, provides quality professional instruments.

**(746) BIO-FEEDBACK TECHNOLOGY, INC.**
10612-A Trask Avenue
Garden Grove, CA 92643

(714) 537-3800

Manufacturers of research biofeedback instrumentation, feedback encephalographs, feedback myographs, differential thermometers, GSR's and electroenterographs.

**(747) BIOFEEDBACK RESEARCH INSTITUTE, INC.**
6325 Wilshire Boulevard
Los Angeles, CA 90048

(213) 933-9451

Professional biofeedback instrumentation (EEG, EMG, GSR, thermal, integrator) as developed at the Institute's clinical and research center. Founded 1969.

**(748) BIOFEEDBACK ELECTRONICS, INC.**
P.O. Box 1491
Monterey, CA 93940

(408) 373-2486

Manufactures portable biofeedback systems to monitor temperature, GSR, pulse, blood pressure, intestinal peristalsis, respiratory sounds, and plethysmography, together with cassette recordings to instruct patients in the details of biofeedback conditioning.

**BUTTERFLY MEDIA DIMENSIONS** (cassette tapes)/ N. Hollywood, CA **(see 210)**

**CENTER FOR HEALTH EDUCATION** (cassette tapes)/Palo Verdes, CA **(see 211)**

**(749) ELECTRO LABS**
P.O. Box 2386
Pomona, CA 91766

(714) 624-0393

Involved in biofeedback research; developer of programs for back pain and childbirth relaxation.

**(750) SELF CONTROL SYSTEMS**
Box 6462
San Diego, CA 92106 ·

(714) 224-5281

Specializes in clinical EMG instruments, home trainers, portable, dental, multi-channel and group biofeedback EMG's.

**COGNETICS** (cassette tapes)/Saratoga, CA **(see 214)**

**(751) BIOFEEDBACK SYSTEMS, INC.**
2736 47th Street
Boulder, CO 80301

(303) 444-1411

First company to offer commercially available biofeedback equipment (1968). Continues innovation in new system concepts and software.

**HARTLEY FILM PRODUCTION** (multidisciplinary audiovisuals)/Cos Cob, CT **(see 219)**

**(752) NEURONICS, INC.**
104 East Oak
Chicago, IL 60611

(312) 649-1400

Developer of the multi-physiomonitor, the sleep-dream monitor, and the plethysmomonitor. Inquire for further information.

**(753) MEDICAL DEVICE CORPORATION**
1555 North Bellefontaine Street
Indianapolis, IN 46202

(317) 637-5776

Manufactures physiological trend indicators for use in

thermal biofeedback and physiologic control training utilizing registration of topical skin temperature changes.

## (754) SYSTEC, INC.
500 Locust Street
Lawrence, KS 66044

(913) 843-8844

Supplies biofeedback equipment to the professional community.

## (755) CYBORG CORPORATION
342 Western Avenue
Boston, MA 02135

(617) 782-9820

Distributes research and clinical biofeedback equipment, sponsors seminars and workshops throughout the country, and distributes over 30 cassette tapes on the use of biofeedback.

## (756) THE BOSTON DESIGN COMPANY
Seven Harvard Square
Brookline, MA 02146

(617) 738-4500

Distributes the DESIGN 5, GSR (Galvanic Skin Response) biofeedback units.

## (757) BIOMONITORING APPLICATIONS, INC.
270 Madison Avenue
New York, NY 10016

(212) 258-2724

Distributors of audio cassette programs for biofeedback, yoga, and other relaxation techniques. Specific programs are geared to curb smoking behavior, insomnia, and overweight. There is also a complete line of books and publications on biofeedback and related areas. BMA also offers symposia and practical instructions by leading behavioral therapists and researchers on key topics of clinical interest associated with biofeedback and its applications.

## (758) BIOFEEDBACK COMPUTERS, INC.
420 Laurel Avenue
Cheltenham, PA 19012

(215) 379-8536

Devoted to research and development of clinical biofeedback instrumentation.

## (759) COULBOURN INSTRUMENTS, INC.
Box 2551
,Lehigh Valley, PA 18001

(215) 395-3771

Modular analog and digital logic system designed to permit an easy, non-technical understanding of its workability.

## (760) BIOSCAN CORPORATION
6842 Westover
Houston, TX 77017

(713) 645-2427

Manufactures portable EEG, EMG, and temperature biofeedback instruments, computer based biofeedback and data acquisition systems, and cassette tape instructional programs.

## (761) NARCO BIO-SYSTEMS, INC.
7651 Airport Boulevard
Houston, TX 77017

(713) 644-7521

Biofeedback systems for EEG, EMG, and temperature. The Projector Physiograph and Cassette Data Recorder provide a method of viewing and storing data.

## (762) LAWSON ELECTRONICS
P.O. Box 711
Poteet, TX 78065

(512) 742-3587

Distributes low-cost biofeedback equipment.

## (763) MOTION CONTROL, INC.
1005 South 300 West
Salt Lake City, UT 84101

(801) 364-1958

Involved in biomedical engineering, prosthetic limb research and associated product development.

## (764) J & J ENTERPRISES
Route 8
Box 8102
Bainbridge Island, WA 98110

(206) 842-2360

Manufacturer of low cost biofeedback equipment.

## (765) THOUGHT TECHNOLOGY
2193 Clifton Avenue
Montreal, Quebec
Canada H4A 2N5

(514) 484-0305

Distributes compact GSR equipment.

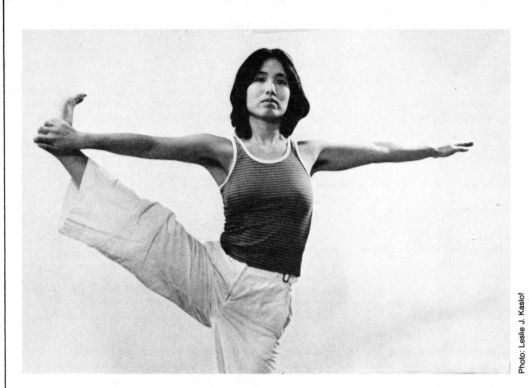

Photo: Leslie J. Kaslof

# Self-Health: From Pain To Health Maintenance

*C. Norman Shealy, MD*

Since 1972 the Pain and Health Rehabilitation Center has tried a wide variety of techniques aimed at teaching chronic pain patients how to gain control over their otherwise untreatable pain. The techniques thus developed are applicable to all persons and offer a comprehensive self-health program.

The essentials for self-health are:

1. Proper nutrition and habits (primarily this requires eating a wide variety of proteins and fresh fruits and vegetables and avoiding table sugar, caffeine, and nicotine).
2. Good sanitation.
3. Light (allowing an adequate amount of full-spectrum light to enter your eyes to help balance the hypothalamus).
4. Physical exercise:
   a. Full limbering of all the joints, muscles, and tendons daily (just think about and explore every body part).
   b. Strengthening of heart and lungs (the aerobics program of Dr. Kenneth Cooper offers the best physical exercise for heart and lungs).
5. Self-health training (biogenics):
   a. Components—The most important and specific aspect of the comprehensive self-health program represents a synthesis of many disciplines, including:
   *Emil Coué's autosuggestion*
      Over 60 years ago, Emil Coué, a French pharmacist, demonstrated that positive affirmations were capable of healing many individuals. His best-known phrase was: "Every day in every way I am getting better and better." But his contribution was much broader. Perhaps his most important philosophy is expressed in the statement "When there is a conflict between will and

imagination, imagination always wins.''

*Autogenic training*

Beginning in the early 1900s, J. H. Schultz developed on the basis of feelings reported by hypnotized patients a *focused*, alert concentration exercise which led to physiologic balance, or homeostatis. His phrases:

My arms and legs are heavy and warm;

My heartbeat is calm and regular;

It breathes me;

My abdomen is warm;

My forehead is cool;

My mind is quiet and still.

When individuals had trained with these phrases for six months, 80 percent reported marked improvement.

*Progressive relaxation*

During the same period of time, Edmond Jacobson elaborated his techniques for deep physical relaxation, which provides systematic voluntary muscle contraction followed by relaxation. Working in this way through every muscle group, general homeostatis is achieved, and 80 percent of patients with a wide variety of symptoms improve.

*Psychosynthesis*

Simultaneously, Roberto Assagioli, an Italian psychiatrist, was developing his elaborate humanistic psychotherapeutic program. He worked to strengthen the will and to turn patients to spiritual awareness.

*Insight Exercises*

Gestalt and Jungian techniques designed to help patients develop emotional or psychological insight are an integral part of the mental exercise training. Patients need to learn that emotional hang-ups need to be *examined*, dealt with, and resolved in a loving, joyful way. Patients must really *experience* the emotional balance.

*Biofeedback Training*

Most biofeedback is quite nonspecific and primarily proves to patients that they can mentally control body processes. This feedback gives them faith to continue using the mental exercises.

b. Process—How to do the program yourself:

*Relax*

How you relax is not important, but relaxation is. The most simple technique is to repeat to yourself ''I am'' as you breathe in, ''Relaxed'' as you breathe out. Within 5 minutes almost everyone is relaxed.

*Balance feelings in the body*

Whenever one area of the body is more involved in the stress response than others, it *feels* tense or absent (or has a ''block''). By tuning in to each part of the body and noting whether it is relaxed, you can consciously relax that area. This may be done by mentally feeling the heartbeat in that area; by tensing muscles in that area and then relaxing them; or by just imagining that you are *breathing through* that area.

*Balance emotions*

At this stage you consciously examine anger, fear, depression, guilt, etc., and make an intelligent, willful decision to resolve the problem and to create emotional joy, happiness, compassion, forgiveness, and love. And do it.

*Program yourself to accomplish a goal*

*Verbally:* Use a short positive phrase (healing mantra) which expresses the desired goal *as if accomplished:* i.e., ''My blood pressure is normal.''

*Visually:* Create a visual image of yourself as having accomplished your goal. This may be done either symbolically or literally but must be positive, definite, and experienced.

*Become spiritually attuned*

Be aware that *you* are something beyond body, mind, and emotions. Tune in to your ideal, super, inner essence or spirit. Be aware that your inner self is magnificent, wise, and loving.

It is best to *practice biogenics daily,* ten to fifteen minutes three times a day or twenty minutes twice a day. It is also good to pause frequently during the day and take just a minute or two to breathe deeply and relax.

For individuals with no real illness, the simple practice program can change a "tense, nervous" individual into a calm, relaxed, and effective one. Patients with chronic disease or pain will need much more intense training, a minimum of 40 to 90 hours, preferrably under professional guidance.

Using the system outlined, almost everyone can become more relaxed, less anxious and tense, happier, more balanced physiologically, and thus assured of the best chance of maintaining health.

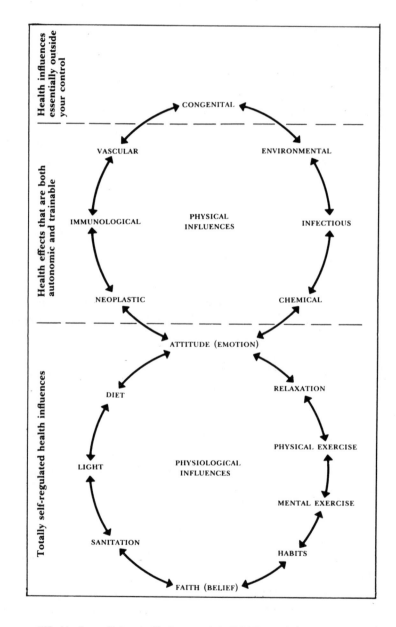

"Health, Stress Relaxation" chart; courtesy Dial Press, from *90 Days to Self-Health.* By C. Norman Shealy. New York: Dial Press, 1977.

# VI
# PSYCHIC AND SPIRITUAL HEALING

———

Unconventional Healing

The Potential Use Of Therapeutic Touch In Healing

Anthroposophical Medicine

Edgar Cayce And Wholistic Medicine

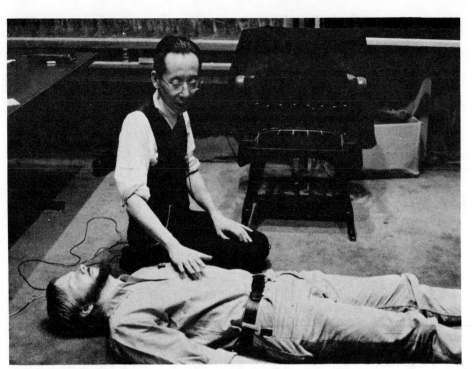

Demonstration of palm healing, by Michio Kushi, photo courtesy of East West Foundation.

# Unconventional Healing
*Olga N. Worrall, PhD, DHL*

*"The more I observe and study things the more convinced I become that sorrow over separation and death is perhaps the greatest delusion. To realize that it is a delusion is to become free. There is no death, no separation of the substance."*

*Mahatma Gandhi*

Unconventional healing is the art of restoring a person (or other living entity) to a condition of health through the use of powers usually attributed to the Supreme Being and various saints. This art has been given many names, such as faith healing, spiritual healing, psychic healing, magnetic healing, New Thought healing, laying on of hands, use of the sacraments—the list is potentially endless.

Unconventional healing operates in many ways, and in its broadest interpretation is at work in every case of recovery from disease. It would be difficult to prove that unconventional healing is not being applied at the same time as medical treatment, and who is to say that the hands of the Lord or saints do not work through and with doctors and nurses to contribute to the recovery of the patient?

Unconventional healing is usually interpreted as the restoration of health without the assistance of medical or other treatment. However, in practically every case of illness, medical or other treatment has already been administered before unconventional healing is requested. Thus, if a patient recovers when unconventional healing is added to the medical or other treatment, the recovery may be the result of the combination of the two methods; unconventional healing may only have been instrumental in tipping the scales in favor of recovery.

There is no reason to eliminate correct medical treatment while the patient is receiving unconventional healing; the two are complementary and compatible. Healers can work in harmony with the medical profession.

Everything in nature is according to law. It is impossible to break any of nature's laws. We live according to the laws of health or the laws of disease. We cannot break the laws of health; rather, we may choose to live according to the laws of disease. Unconventional healing is a natural phenomenon. It occurs strictly in accordance with natural laws. Someday, science will discover those basic laws and the mechanisms which make possible the seemingly impossible and presently unexplainable healing of disease by means other than those used by the conventional healing arts. We will then, no doubt, have a new name for an art that has been practiced successfully for thousands of years. In the meantime, the absence of specific knowledge pertaining to the laws governing unconventional healing gives rise to conjecture.

Over the years healers have developed a theory on how this power works, a working hypothesis founded on observation of results. There exists a field of energy akin to life itself around and about us, "paraelectricity." We draw our daily supply of energy from this inexhaustible storehouse. When we insulate ourselves by wrong thinking or wrong living from this source of supply, we become sick. Expended energy returns to the source. If we expend more energy than we take in, we become tired and listless; we are like batteries that need recharging. Rest and sleep are the usual methods used to recharge the human battery. In sickness, something has interfered with the recharging, and more than rest and sleep are required to restore the health potential.

Medical therapy may remove the interference completely or in part, and the human battery will be able to take more or less full charge again. If medical therapy is not successful, however, then supplementary treatment must be provided. Unconventional healing can be a supplementary treatment.

For complete healing to be manifested, a perfect balance of all systems must be brought about, on all levels of man's being—spiritual, mental, and physical. All forms of therapy that can beneficially be applied to restore the balance of health can simultaneously be used on a patient, where possible, for each complements the other, and all methods, including unconventional healing therapy, simply influence the mechanisms that must work harmoniously together to maintain the balance of health.

# The Potential Use Of Therapeutic Touch In Healing

*Dolores Krieger, RN, PhD*

Touch as a therapeutic adjunct reaches exceedingly far into the history of man's concern for man. Touching another person, with a strong intent to help or to heal that person, has been known by a variety of names in diverse cultures; for many centuries in the Western civilizations it has been known as the laying on of hands.

Touching those who are ill has always characterized nursing. Usually this touching occurs during an attempt to soothe or otherwise relieve the discomfort associated with illness. Although it has generally been acknowledged that this personalized interaction frequently is therapeutic, substantive study of its nature has been remarkably sparse.

Evidence of this singular expression of man for man reaches back into antiquity, as is seen in the ancient traditions handed on from teacher to pupil in India and Tibet, in the early rock carvings of Egypt and Chaldea, in the writings of both the old and new Judeo-Christian testaments, and in the accounts of certain historical figures, such as the Roman emperors Vespasian and Hadrian, or the Norwegian King Olaf. In fact, the laying on of hands was known as the "king's touch" in early France and England, as the touch of kings of that period was considered especially good for the curing of goiter, scrofula, and other throat ailments. There are actual instances recorded where more common folk who were also able to demonstrate this ability were suspected of coveting the throne. During the Middle Ages innumerable accounts of healing by laying on of hands appear in church histories in the West. It is, however, a commentary on these times to note that healing outside the church was looked upon with suspicion and thought to be witchcraft.

In more recent times, Mesmer taught what he called the "projection of animal magnetism" through the hands. The technique was so widely practiced and studied in Europe during the nineteenth century that several governments passed strong laws restricting the practice of magnetic healing to qualified medical practitioners. In the twentieth century, with the development of powerful medical technologies, and because the process underlying the laying on of hands has been resistant to accepted scientific methodologies, interest and practice in this manner of healing declined steadily.

One of the first in the West to revive scientific interest in healing by the laying on of hands was Bernard Grad, a biochemist at McGill University. In 1964 he conducted double-blind experiments using the services of a renowned healer, Oskar Estebany. Grad soaked barley seeds in a saline solution to simulate a "sick" condition, then divided them into experimental and control samples. The experimental group was irrigated by water from flasks that had previously been held by Estebany in a manner similar to the way in which he did the laying on of hands; the control sample was irrigated with untreated water. Grad found that the treated seeds in the experimental group had a faster rate of growth, their sprouts had a greater net weight, and they had significantly more chlorophyll content than the control group.

Working from Grad's data, I have tried to determine significant physiological indices that would reliably reflect the interaction between a healer's treatment by the laying on of hands and ill human subjects. Using a frame of reference derived from comparative studies of Eastern religions, I noted that the literature, particularly of India and Tibet, elucidated the personalized interaction involved in the act in a way that lent itself to the development of a paradigm that might be analyzed in the Western mode.

One aspect of the concept of "energy" in the East is *prana*, the organization that underlies the life process, and this feature of energy seems pertinent to the dynamics underlying the personalized interaction upon which the laying on of hands appears to be based. The word *prana* derives from *pra* ("forth") and *an* (which denotes "to breathe," "to move," or "to live"). In Eastern literature the term *prana* has two meanings. In its more subtle sense, prana refers to the life breath sent out from the spiritual plane of individuals to all the lower levels of their existence. The second reference applies specifically to physical inhalation and exhalation. Prana is said to be solar in origin and intimately connected with what we in the West call the oxygen molecule.

Healthy people are considered to have an overabundance of prana, whereas ill people have a deficit. Prana utilizes the breathing, the blood, or the nerves as conductors. Pranic flow is amenable to direction and manipulation by what is currently called ''mind control'' in the West. Thus, healers are individuals whose health gives them access to an overabundance of prana, and whose strong sense of commitment and intention to help the ill give them a certain control over the projection of this vital energy flow. Patients being thus helped would acquire the projected prana via a biological pathway sensitive to oxygen uptake.

A physiological index that serves as a dependent variable sensitive to treatment by the laying on of hands is the patient's hemoglobin. Hemoglobin, a component of the red blood cells, is one of the body's most sensitive indicators of oxygen uptake and very accessible for study. Furthermore, the biochemical configuration of the porphyrin structure in hemoglobin, which is important to the function of hemoglobin as a very efficient conveyor of oxygen to the tissues, resembles the chlorin of chlorophyll in that both the nature and arrangement of their side-chains are very similar, and they are derivative of the same biosynthetic pathway. The major difference is that the structure in chlorophyll is patterned around an atom of magnesium, while the porphyria in hemoglobin has an atom of iron at its center. One of the findings Grad reported in his study of the effects of laying on of hands on barley seeds was the increased chlorophyll content. Since hemoglobin contains the corresponding tetrapyrrole that is effective in man, it seems reasonable that it should be the appopriate test object for human subjects.

In 1971, I did a pilot study involving the laying on of hands in a homogeneous group to test three substantive hypotheses: whether (1) in the experimental group the post-test mean hemoglobin values would be greater than the pre-test mean hemoglobin values; (2) in the control group there would be no significant difference between the post-test mean and the pre-test mean hemoglobin values; and (3) the post-test mean hemoglobin value of the experimental group would be greater than the post-test means of the control group.

These results were replicated in a full-scale study done in 1972 and 1973. In all of these studies, Estebany acted the role of the healer. I proposed in a report to the American Nurses Association Council of Nurse Researchers that a further replication of the study be conducted in which nurses would be placed in the role of healer using this mode of therapeutic touch. A further study was designed to meet this commitment in 1974.

The statistical analysis supported the hypotheses put forward by this study. A significant change in the mean hemoglobin value occurred in the group of patients who were treated by nurses doing therapeutic touch (by chance the change could have happened only once in a thousand times); on the other hand, a comparable group of patients who were given routine nursing care showed no significant change in their hemoglobin value after routine nursing care. Since serious effort was made to rule out known major intervening variables, the data lends itself to positive suggestion that subtle factors are at work during the practice of therapeutic touch.

What are the implications of this study? They are twofold: (1) therapeutic touch can be taught, and (2) its use on people who are ill may affect their respiratory pigment hemoglobin, in a manner as yet unknown. That the final answer is not yet known should deter no one. The imperative to know still exists. The several studies now amassed form a considerable base for the serious attention of other researchers who may wish to explore this singular expression of man for man which incorporates a heretofore poorly probed extension of consciousness.

## Groups and Associations

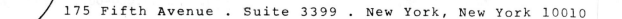

nurse healers
professional associates, inc.
COOPERATIVE
175 Fifth Avenue . Suite 3399 . New York, New York 10010

**(767) NATIONAL SPIRITUALIST ASSOCIATION OF CHURCHES**
General Offices
P.O. Box 128
Cassadaga, FL 32706

(904) 228-2506

*Rev. Joseph H. Merrill, President*

Nationally coordinates Spiritualist Churches and healers who are engaged in spiritual healing and laying on of hands. Also serves as a coordinating and certifying body for individual healers. A *Year Book,* also available from the Association, lists individual members who are certified healers. Founded 1893.

*AFFILIATE AND STATE ASSOCIATIONS*

**SUN SPIRITUALIST CAMP ASSOCIATION**
Star Route, Box 595
Tonopah, AZ 85354

(602) 386-3877

*Atten: Mrs. Susan Hoge, Secretary*

Offers workshops and study groups, spiritual healing, and readings. Recreational facilities available. Member of NSAC.

**SERENITY SPIRITUALIST CAMP ASSOCIATION, INC.**
P.O. Box 137
904 Sir Francis Drake
Kentfield, CA 94904

(415) 924-7475

*Atten: Pauline Leonard, Secretary*

Offers workshops and study groups, spiritual healing, and readings. Recreational facilities available. Member of NSAC.

**CALIFORNIA STATE SPIRITUALIST ASSOCIATION**
7066 Hawthorn Avenue
Los Angeles, CA 90028

(213) 469-1336

*Atten: Catherine Peterson, Secretary*

Disseminates information and coordinates state spiritualist conferences and other activities. Member of NSAC.

**CENTENNIAL STATE SPIRITUALIST ASSOCIATION**
5366 Lynn Drive
Arvada, CO 80002

(303) 420-2507

*Atten: Mrs. Louise Richards, Secretary*

Disseminates information and coordinates state spiritualist conferences and other activities. Member of NSAC.

**STATE SPIRITUALIST ASSOCIATION**
174 Daley Street
Forestville, CT 06010

(203) 582-7385

*Atten: Mary Ann Noddin, Secretary*

Disseminates information and coordinates state spiritualist conferences and other activities. Member of NSAC.

**THE SOUTHERN CASSADAGA SPIRITUALIST CAMP ASSOCIATION**
Cassadaga, FL 32706

*Atten: Duncan Beck, Secretary*

Offers workshops and study groups, spiritual healing, and readings. Recreational facilities available. Member of NSAC.

**SPIRITUALIST BENEVOLENT SOCIETY**
Box 77
Cassadaga, FL 32706

*Atten: Ralph D. Cutlip, Secretary-Treasurer*

Disseminates information and coordinates state spiritualist conferences and other activities. Member of NSAC.

**SPIRITUAL RESEARCH SOCIETY, NSAC**
2500 Curry Ford Road
Orlando, FL 32806

(305) 898-2500

Investigates spiritualistic phenomena. Member of NSAC.

**MISSISSIPPI VALLEY SPIRITUALIST ASSOCIATION (CAMP)**
15 Mt. Pleasant Park
Clinton, IA 52732

(319) 242-0543

*Atten: Mrs. Mabel Leopold*

Offers workshops and study groups, spiritual healing, and readings. Recreational facilities available. Member of NSAC.

**CHERRY VALLEY SPIRITUALIST CAMP**
P.O. Box 114
Cherry Valley, IL 61016

*Atten: Lillian Jones, Secretary*

Offers workshops and study groups, spiritual healing, and readings. Recreational facilities available. Member of NSAC.

**INDIANA STATE ASSOCIATION OF SPIRITUALISTS**
200 Eastern Drive
Chesterfield, IN 46017

(317) 378-0053

*Atten: Lena Walters, Secretary*

Disseminates information and coordinates state spiritualist conferences and other activities. Member of NSAC.

**UNITED MISSIONARY NSAC**
1446 Pattie Street
Wichita, KS 67221

*Atten: Edwin M. Booth, Secretary*

Disseminates information. Member of NSAC.

**MAINE STATE SPIRITUALIST ASSOCIATION OF CHURCHES**
Tasker Road
Augusta, ME 04330

(207) 622-7775

*Atten: Florence Carr, Secretary*

Disseminates information and coordinates state spiritualist conferences and other activities. Member of NSAC.

## ETNA SPIRITUALIST ASSOCIATION, INC. (CAMP)
Etna, ME 04434

(207) 269-2626

*Atten: Wilson C. Gilman, Secretary*

Offers workshops and study groups, spiritual healing, and readings. Recreational facilities available. Member of NSAC.

## SANCTUARY OF TRUTH, SPIRITUALIST, INC.
YWCA Building
210 Forest Spring Lane
Baltimore, MD 21228

*Atten: Mrs. Roberta Miller, Secretary*

Disseminates information on spiritualist activities. Member of NSAC.

## MASSACHUSETTS STATE ASSOCIATION OF SPIRITUALISTS
9 Harbor Street
Danvers, MA 01923

(617) 774-2753

*Atten: Muriel Karolides, Secretary*

Disseminates information and coordinates state spiritualist conferences and other activities. Member of NSAC.

## STATE SPIRITUALIST ASSOCIATION OF MINNESOTA
1545 St. Paul Avenue
St. Paul, MN 55116

(612) 690-2703

*Atten: Ellen L. Manke, Secretary*

Disseminates information and coordinates state spiritualist conferences and other activities. Member of NSAC.

## NORTHERN LAKE MICHIGAN SPIRITUALIST (CAMP)
606 South Main Street
Boyne City, MI 49712

*Atten: Medga Fedley*

Offers workshops and study groups, spiritual healing, and readings. Recreational facilities available. Member of NSAC.

## MICHIGAN STATE SPIRITUALIST ASSOCIATION
89 Delaware Avenue
Detroit, MI 48202

*Atten: Rev. Goldie Dodd, Secretary*

Disseminates information and coordinates state spiritualist conferences and other activities. Member of NSAC.

## SPIRITUALIST RESEARCH SOCIETY OF NEW HAMPSHIRE AND FIRST SPIRITUALIST CHURCH OF DERRY
9 Maple
Hooksett, NH 03106

*Atten: Janet Norton, Secretary*

Disseminates information and coordinates state spiritualist conferences and other activities. Member of NSAC.

## NEW JERSEY STATE ASSOCIATION OF SPIRITUALISTS
793 Eleventh Avenue
Paterson, NJ 07514

(201) 345-0755

*Atten: Diane Trombino, Secretary*

Disseminates information and coordinates state spiritualist conferences and other activities. Member of NSAC.

## CENTRAL NEW YORK SPIRITUALIST ASSOCIATION (CAMP)
Freeville, NY 13068

Offers workshops and study groups, spiritual healing, and readings. Recreational facilities available. Member of NSAC.

## LILLY DALE ASSEMBLY (CAMP)
Lily Dale, NY 14752

(716) 595-3621

*Atten: Julia Goodworth, Secretary*

Offers workshops and study groups, spiritual healing, and readings. Recreational facilities available. Member of NSAC.

## ASHLEY SPIRITUALIST CAMP ASSOCIATION
Wooley Park
Ashley, OH 43003

(614) 747-2800

*Atten: John R. Rowe, Secretary*

Offers workshops and study groups, spiritual healing, and readings. Recreational facilities available. Member of NSAC.

## THE OHIO STATE SPIRITUALIST ASSOCIATION
823 West Maine
Louisville, OH 44641

*Atten: Edward H. Nixon, Secretary*

Disseminates information and coordinates state spiritualist conferences and other activities. Member of NSAC.

## OKLAHOMA STATE SPIRITUALIST ASSOCIATION
4448 Woodedge Drive
Del City, OK 73115

(405) 672-1507

*Atten: Mrs. Alta Scoles, Secretary*

Disseminates information and coordinates state spiritualist conferences and other activities. Member of NSAC.

## PENNSYLVANIA STATE SPIRITUALIST ASSOCIATION
7200 Whitaker Avenue
Philadelphia, PA 19111

(215) 725-5881

*Atten: Rev. Rebecca E. Fasnacht, Secretary*

Disseminates information and coordinates state spiritualist conferences and other activities. Member of NSAC.

## STOW MEMORIAL FOUNDATION
1104 Susan Drive
Edinburg, TX 78539

(512) 383-2510

*Atten: Evelyn Muse, Secretary-Treasurer*

Disseminates information and coordinates state spiritualist conferences and other activities. Member of NSAC.

**MORRIS PRATT INSTITUTE**
11811 Watertown Plank Road
Milwaukee, WI 53226

(414) 774-2994

*Atten: Joseph Sax, Secretary*

The first fully equipped and permanent institution ever established under the auspices of Spiritualism for the training of its ministry. Member of NSAC. Organized December 11, 1901.

**WESTERN WISCONSIN SPIRITUALIST-CAMP ASSOCIATION**
2401 West Plainfield
Milwaukee, WI 53221

*Atten: Pauline Benson, Secretary*

Offers workshops and study groups, spiritual healing, and readings. Recreational facilities available. Member of NSAC.

**(768) SPIRITUAL ADVISORY COUNCIL**
1701 Lake Avenue
Suite 130
Glenview, IL 60025

(312) 729-9490

*Paul V. Johnson, President*

A tax-exempt religious organization dedicated to concerns relating to the metaphysical, psychic and spiritual, with emphasis upon spiritual healing and counseling. Provides for training of healers and certifies them through a course of practical demonstrations. Other services include a bookshop and counseling center. A healing center is in the process of being developed. A bi-monthly newsletter is available to members and other interested people.

**(769) AMERICAN SPIRITUAL HEALING ASSOCIATION**
P.O. Box 1189
6 Bridle Path Circle
Framingham, MA 01701

(617) 485-5114

*Rev. Belding E. Bingham, Founder and President*

Organized to bring credibility to paranormal healing and spiritual healing in particular, and to develop a cooperative relationship with those in the medical arts. Offers training courses, public lectures and demonstrations in spiritual healing. Library facilities and a quarterly newsletter are available to the membership. Founded 1976.

**(770) SPIRITUAL FRONTIERS FELLOWSHIP**
Executive Plaza
10715 Winner Road
Independence, MO 64052

(816) 254-8585

*Robert C. Walker, Executive Director*

A spiritual fellowship dedicated "to sponsor, explore, and interpret the growing interest in psychic phenomena and mystical experience to the traditional churches and others, and relate these experiences to effective prayer, spiritual healing, personal survival and spiritual fulfillment." Provides its members with a free lending library by mail on subjects in psychic, mystical and psychic science. Also

maintains a lending library of cassette tape-recordings of lectures, a mail order book service, and a research program aimed at collecting data about psychical and mystical experiences for further investigation. Founded 1956.

**(771) AMERICAN SOCIETY FOR PSYCHICAL RESEARCH, INC.**
5 West 73rd Street
New York, NY 10023

(212) 799-5050

Nonprofit organization dedicated to understanding the phenomena alleged to be paranormal: telepathy, clairvoyance, precognition, psychokinesis and related fields. This is accomplished through extensive research activities which investigate these various subjects. The Society also publishes a quarterly *Journal*, periodically publishes a *Proceedings*, and maintains a lecture series which includes forums, workshops, and seminars. An annual directory ($2 donation) of university-level study opportunities in parapsychology is available from the above address.

**(772) PARAPSYCHOLOGY FOUNDATION, INC.**
29 West 57th Street
New York, NY 10019

(212) 751-5940

Encourages research in all areas of the paranormal, including ESP, clairvoyance, and telepathy. Sponsors domestic and international conferences and publishes a research series, *Parapsychological Monographs*, and a bi-monthly journal, *Parapsychology Review*. Extensive library facility available to the public.

**(773) NATIONAL FEDERATION OF SPIRITUAL HEALERS**
Shortacres, Church Hill, Loughton
England

Tel: 01-508-8218

*Michael Endacott, Adminstrator*

Dedicated to the encouragement and study of spiritual healing, whether by laying on of hands or at a distance through prayer and meditation. Maintains a trust fund to financially assist healers with claims made against them, and works through political channels to protect the healing movement in general. Educational programs in the form of regular study courses and a summer school are available to members. Membership is open to individual healers, associations of healers, and individuals desiring to support the Spiritual Healing movement. Founded 1955.

## Schools, Centers, and Clinics

**LUKATS' PREVENTION REGENERATION RESORT**/Safford, AZ **(see 164)**

**(774) ESP RESEARCH ASSOCIATES FOUNDATION**
1630 Union National Plaza
Suite 1660
Little Rock, AR 72201

(501) 375-5377

*Harold Sherman, Founder*

Committed to researching ESP and other higher powers of

the mind. Conducts annual workshops which teach people from diverse backgrounds mental and emotional disciplines as aids to mind/body health. Members receive the bimonthly newsletter, written by Harold Sherman. Founded 1964.

**(775) INSTITUTE OF PSYCHIC SCIENCE, INC.**
2015 South Broadway
Little Rock, AR 72206

(501) 372-4278

*Korra L. Deaver, President and Founder*

Aims to unite mind, body and soul through yoga classes, metaphysical philosophy, research for past life causes, and nutrition. Individuals involved with the Institute practice spiritual healing by energy transference, reflexology, and other methods.

**(776) BERKELEY PSYCHIC INSTITUTE**
2545 Regent Street
Berkeley, CA 94705

(415) 548-8020

Offers eight-week courses in psychic healing and psychic meditation. Psychic readings are also offered of aura, chakras, past lives, present goals, and spiritual growth. Specialized readings of female energy are offered by female readers.

**(777) THE NIRVANA FOUNDATION FOR PSYCHIC RESEARCH**
138 West Campbell Avenue
Campbell, CA 95008

(408) 379-1551

*Dal and Sylvia Brown, Founders*

Dedicated to promoting research in and disseminating information on parapsychology. Activities of the Foundation include classes in spiritual healing, psychic diagnosis of many medical problems, individual counseling, and spiritual healing from a distance through a prayer group known as the "Crisis Line." Meditation and hypnosis are sometimes used as adjunctive healing techniques.

**(778) BIOTONICS INSTITUTE**
P.O. Box 342
Corte Madera, CA 94925

(415) 388-8334

*Jonathan Lee Krown, MA, JD, Patricia Riley, Co-Directors*

Utilizes psychic processes to free up tension and "chi" energy blockages, to redefine belief systems, and to effect energy transformations in body and mind. Toward this end the Institute uses workshops, training programs, and private consultations. Founded 1974.

**(779) THE HEALING LIGHT CENTER**
138 North Maryland Avenue
Glendale, CA 91206

(213) 244-8607

*Rosalyn Bruyere, Director and President*

A religious, healing, and educational organization dedicated to the spiritual and religious development of Man.

The Center offers classes, lectures, and seminars in psychic phenomena, natural healing, and spiritualism, performs religious services and healing rituals, and conducts research in a "spiritual, scientific and psychic sense." Natural healing practices are provided "whenever required or requested." Founded 1974.

**BARAKA** (holistic clinic)/Los Angeles, CA **(see 87)**

**(780) CHURCH OF WORLD MESSIANITY—JOHREI**
3068 San Marino Street
Los Angeles, CA 90006

(213) 387-8366

*Mokichi Okada, Founder*

Transmits a spiritual healing technique (*Johrei*, meaning prayer in action) in which the healing energy is focused through the top of the head and passes out through the palms of the hands.

**(781) INNER LIGHT FOUNDATION**
Box 761
Novato, CA 94947

(415) 897-5581

*Betty Bethards, Founder and Director*

Aims to aid people in developing a greater awareness of God through the use of inherent extrasensory faculties. Teaches meditation, holds private counseling sessions, and is planning the development of a center/meeting place for all medical and spiritual healers.

**(782) INSTITUTE FOR MYSTICAL AND PARA-PSYCHOLOGICAL STUDIES**
John F. Kennedy University
12 Altarinda Road
Orinda, CA 94563

(415) 254-0200

*Pascal M. Kaplan, PhD, Director*

Offers courses in alternative healing paradigms, polarity therapy, and the metaphysical basis of healing. Founded 1972; JFKU founded 1964.

**SAN DIEGO NATURAL HEALTH CLINIC**/San Diego, CA **(see 108)**

**EAST-WEST ACADEMY OF HEALING ARTS** (educational center)/San Francisco, CA **(see 110)**

**UNIVERSITY OF CALIFORNIA EXTENSION**/Santa Cruz, CA **(see 115)**

**HUNA INTERNATIONAL** (psychic development workshops)/Santa Monica, CA **(see 591)**

**(783) THE SCHOOL OF ACTUALISM STAR CENTER**
30085 Lilac Road
Valley Center, CA 92082

(714) 749-1863

*Carol Ann Schofield, Staff Director*

Teaches a process of consciousness transformation which makes use of "direct energy flow," developed by Russell

Paul Schofield. In a basic course, students learn to work with a large spectrum of life-light energies. Advanced courses are available for those interested in becoming teachers of Actualism. As part of its basic course, Actualism teaches the "laying on of lighted hands," body work, and acupuncture synthesized with enlightened awareness. Founded 1960.

*AFFILIATED CENTERS*

**ESCONDIDO STAR CENTER**
1130 East Lincoln Avenue
Escondido, CA 92026

(714) 741-8475

**LA JOLLA STAR CENTER**
5653 Desert View
La Jolla, CA 92037

(714) 459-6716

**LOS ANGELES STAR CENTER**
303 South Highland Avenue
Los Angeles, CA 90036

(213) 935-8498

**SAN FRANCISCO STAR CENTER**
312 Gold Mine Drive
San Francisco, CA 94131

(415) 566-9100

**COAST STAR CENTER**
3305 South Timber
Santa Ana, CA 92707

(714) 557-9705

**NEW YORK STAR CENTER**
Olcott Hotel, Apt. 1615
27 West 72nd Street
New York, NY 10023

(212) 877-4200

**DALLAS STAR CENTER**
2530 Electronics, Lane #713
Dallas, TX 75229

(214) 352-5342

**BORDERLAND SCIENCES RESEARCH FOUN-DATION**/Vista, CA **(see 586)**

**STAMFORD CENTER FOR THE HEALING ARTS**
(wholistic clinic in a church)/Stamford, CT **(see 121)**

**(784) NATIONAL SPIRITUAL SCIENCE CENTER**
5605 Sixteenth Street, N.W.
Washington, DC 20011

(202) 723-4510

*Henry J. Nogorka, President*

Provides a four-year progressive course of study in sensitivity and awareness development; spiritual assistance for the hospitalized and imprisoned, and referrals to spiritual healers. Lectures and workshops in spiritual science are offered periodically.

*AFFILIATED CENTERS*

**SPIRITUAL SCIENCE RESEARCH CENTER OF LARGO, MARYLAND**
10305 New Orchard Drive
Upper Marlboro, MD 20780

(301) 336-2041

*Atten: Rev. Thomas Bruck*

Provides spiritual assistance and spiritual healing. Periodically offers workshops and lectures.

**THE GUIDING LIGHT SPIRITUAL SCIENCE CENTER**
2444 Temple Court
Alexandria, VA 22307

(703) 768-9369

*Rev. Katherine Hecox*

Provides spiritual assistance and spiritual healing. Periodically offers workshops and lectures.

**METAPHYSICAL SCIENCES CHURCH OF NORTHERN VIRGINIA**
413 North Irving Street
Arlington, VA 22205

(703) 323-7423

*Rev. Shirley Dee*

Provides spiritual assistance and spiritual healing. Periodically offers workshops and lectures.

**CRYSTAL LIGHT CENTER OF SPIRITUAL SCIENCE**
3878 University Drive
Fairfax, VA 22030

(703) 591-3736

*Rev. Li Baird*

Provides spiritual assistance and spiritual healing. Periodically offers workshops and lectures.

**SPIRITUAL SCIENCE HEALING CENTER**
3600 Old Lee Highway, Route 237
Fairfax, VA 22030

(703) 273-7470

*Rev. Eleanor Courson*

Provides spiritual assistance and spiritual healing. Periodically offers workshops and lectures.

**SPIRITUAL SCIENCE CHURCH AND CENTER**
871 Yorkshire Lane
Manassas, VA 22110

(703) 979-2446

*Rev. Helene Eney*

Provides spiritual assistance and spiritual healing. Periodically offers workshops and lectures.

**SPIRITUAL SCIENCE CENTER FOR METAPHYSICAL STUDIES**
5024 Bruce Street
Norfolk, VA 23153

(804) 857-1610

*Atten: Rev. Shirley Perry*

Provides spiritual assistance and spiritual healing. Periodically offers workshops and lectures.

**PSYCHOPHYSICS FOUNDATION** (workshops)/ Miami, FL **(see 594)**

## (785) THE ROUNDTABLE OF THE LIGHT CENTERS
1801 Southwest 82nd Place
Miami, FL 33155

(305) 264-4118

*Peter M. Creelman, Vice-President*

Serves as an area coordinator of the International Cooperation Council (ICC), and works on developing communication among South Florida groups involved in healing, parapsychology, and spiritual growth. Regular meetings and workshops feature speakers and audio-visual presentations in such areas as ESP, yoga, pyramidology, tarot, dream analysis, astrology, and other aspects of consciousness development. In planning is a holistic health center, which would integrate treatment and educational programs for mental, physical, and spiritual development. Members receive free the monthly Roundtable publication, *The Beacon,* and the monthly ICC publication, *The Spectrum.*

## (786) FLORIDA SOCIETY FOR PSYCHICAL RESEARCH, INC.
4312 46th Avenue South
St. Petersburg, FL 33711

(813) 867-9390

*Laura L. Langan, Executive Director*

Sponsors symposia throughout Florida in "New Dimensions," pertaining to research activities in the fields of parapsychology and medicine. Also sponsors programs for tutorial and professional instruction in psychic self-help, laying on of hands, meditation, reflexology, weight control and thanatology. A newsletter, *New Dimensions,* is circulated among the membership. Founded 1974.

## (787) NEW LIFE CLINIC
Mt. Washington United Methodist Church
5800 Block Falls Road and Smith Avenue
Baltimore, MD 21218

(301) 889-2505

*Olga N. Worrall, PhD, Director*

Conducts healing services and laying on of hands. No fees are charged, and patients must be under competent medical care. Study periods are offered on spiritual healing, constructive thought, power of prayer, and how to hold a healing service.

## (788) PSYCHEGENICS
P.O. Box 332
Gaithersburg, MD 20760

(301) 948-1122

*Win Wenger*

Teaches the individual how to mobilize the survival resources of his own organism—circulation, breath, energy fields, and autonomic processes—by using the principle that breath and mental image together can be used to biofeedback control any autonomic process without machines. Through the use of self-conditioning and distance healing, Psychegenics seeks to decrease the general entropy levels of the organism, and consequently effect a realization of deeper levels of human potential. A book on Psychegenics, *Voyages of Self Discovery,* by Win Wenger, is available from the above address. Founded 1974.

## (789) COSMIC STUDY CENTER
7405 Masters Drive
Potomac, MD 20854

(301) 299-7158

*Cloe Diroll, Director*

Offers workshops and lectures on man's relationship to the "life current of cosmic energy." Employing this principle of relationship, the director, Cloe Diroll, gives Energy Transfusions through the aura and chakras. The process is reported to amplify the life current and release negative energy at the level of the individual's atomic structure.

**INSTITUTE FOR PSYCHOENERGETICS** (psychophysical workshops)/Brookline, MA **(see 128)**

## (790) SIDDHARTHA FOUNDATION, INC.
Siddhartha Health Center
91 Dobbins Street
Waltham, MA 02154

(617) 899-2356

*John Richard Turner, Director*

A center for research, education, and private appointments in auric healing. Auric healing, or aura therapy, is a complimentary aspect of psychotherapy which holds that the aura or bioenergetic field contains all the information upon which the physical, mental, spiritual and emotional aspects of an individual are constructed, and helps people to initiate a self-healing process by focusing on specific points in the energy field. Lectures and workshops in the technique are available for private groups through arrangement with the Director.

**DREAM COUNSELLORS**/Albuquerque, NM **(see 595)**

## (791) NATIONAL SPEAKERS' AND PSYCHICS' REGISTRY
Box 1259
Morristown, NJ 07960

(201) 543-4885

*Mrs. Irene Serra, Director*

Supplies speakers in the field of healing to schools, hospitals, colleges, organizations, and radio and television.

**DREAM DYNAMICS**/Farmingdale, NY **(see 596)**

## (792) CONTACT HEALING SEMINARS
69 Fifth Avenue, Suite 3C
New York, NY 10003

(212) 989-6237

*Joan Ann De Mattia, Director*

Teaches an easy do-it-yourself method of restoring a smooth flow of vital energy throughout the body by gentle pressure of the fingertips on acupuncture points. Workshops also include instruction in herbal medicine, nutrition, and introductory techniques from the School of Actualism.

**(793) GARDEN OF THE EAST, SUFI ORDER**
1 Lighthouse Road
Southhold, NY 11971

(516) 765-1642

*Amir Latif*

Practice group healing rituals of the Sufi Healing Order, founded by Hazrat Inayat Khan. Through prayer, meditation, and "astral massage," the group works on a magnetic cleansing of the aura. Formerly Gandalf Institute.

**(794) THE PSYCHICAL RESEARCH FOUNDATION, INC.**
Duke Station
Durham, NC 27706

(919) 286-0714

*W.G. Roll, Project Director*

A parapsychological research center dedicated especially to the question of whether man survives the death of his body. Areas of study related to this question have included the brain-waves of mediums, out of the body experiences, transpersonal consciousness, ESP, and cases of haunting and poltergeist activity. Research is published in such journals as *Journal of the American Society for Psychical Research* and the *Journal of Parapsychology*. Additionally, the Foundation publishes a quarterly bulletin, *Theta*, maintains a library, and operates a meditation center on the Duke University campus. Founded 1960.

**(795) "ALLETHEIA" PSYCHO-PHYSICAL FOUNDATIONS**
515 Northeast Eighth Street
Grants Pass, OR 97526

(503) 479-4855

*Jack Schwarz, Founder, President*

Offers classes and professional seminars in the voluntary control of internal states, from brain waves, heart rate and body temperature to telekinesis and other paranormal abilities. The techniques, which have been scientifically evaluated by such psychophysiological laboratories as Langley Porter, the Menninger Foundation and the Max Planck Institute, have applications in pain control and medicine. The methods involve an integration of breathing and related exercises and meditative-visualization reveries. Founded 1958.

**(796) ASSOCIATION FOR DOCUMENTATION AND ENLIGHTENMENT, INC.**
314 Arctic Crescent
Virginia Beach, VA 23451

(804) 425-0715

*Jean Campbell, Executive Director*

A state and federally funded nonprofit research organization, dedicated to the study of psychic readings and use of pyschics in healing and medical practice. A large group of MDs, reflexologists, color therapists, astrologers, music therapists and other individuals in the healing arts work with the center in creating a total healing environment. The staff also includes professional counselors, and psychics who give health readings for individuals. Founded 1973.

**ASSOCIATION FOR RESEARCH AND ENLIGHTENMENT** (Cayce)/Virginia Beach, VA **(see 831)**

**(797) FELLOWSHIP OF THE INNER LIGHT**
P.O. Box 206
Virginia Beach, VA 23458

(804) 428-4650

*Paul Solomon, Founder*

Conducts a ten-day training program for inner awakening called "inner light consciousness." The course is given anywhere where twelve people are interested, and is supposed to cultivate capabilities in clairvoyance and spiritual healing. The Inner Light Consciousness course, as well as other workshops offered by the Fellowship, include such areas as prayer, meditation, dreams, diet, exercise, the Akashic records, and Christ consciousness. The content of the courses was developed during trance states of the Fellowship's founder, Paul Solomon. A selection of books and cassette tapes is available by mail. *Reflections*, a newsletter, is printed monthly.

**PAIN AND HEALTH REHABILITATION CENTER/**
La Crosse, WI **(see 157)**

**(798) THE WHITE EAGLE LODGE**
New Lands, Rake
Liss, Hampshire
GU33 7HY England

Tel: LISS (0730 82) 3300

*Geoffrey Dent*

An undenominational Christian church carrying on work in spiritual healing. The healing is of two types: contact healing by the laying on of hands, and healing from a distance through the thought projections of a group prayer meeting. The teachings of spiritual healing practiced by the Lodge are communicated in books and cassette tapes available through the above address. Founded 1936.

**(799) WREKIN TRUST**
Bowers House
Bowers Lane, Bridstow
Ross-on-Wye, Herefordshire, England

*Malcolm Lazarus, Secretary*

While primarily concerned with spiritual education for adults, the Trust occasionally holds conferences and symposia in healing subjects as well as maintaining contact with alternative healing groups throughout Great Britain. Founded 1970.

**WESTBANK HEALING AND TEACHING CENTER**
(laying on of hands)/Fife, Scotland **(see 163)**

## Journals and Publications

**BRAIN/MIND BULLETIN**/Los Angeles, CA **(see 184)**

**(800) THE MOVEMENT NEWSPAPER**
P.O. Box 19458
Los Angeles, CA 90019

(213) 737-1134

*Rick Edelstein, Editor*

Monthly publication of the Church of the Movement of Spiritual Inner Awareness. Articles on prominent spiritual leaders and schools, including methods of psychic healing.

## (801) UNI-COM FOUNDATION
P.O. Box 11716
Palo Alto, CA 94306

(415) 498-2973

*Patricia Wortman, Director*

Publishers of the *Uni-Com Guide*, containing source listings in parapsychology and related fields.

**COMMON GROUND** (multidisciplinary directory San Francisco Bay Area)/San Francisco, CA **(see 187)**

## (802) NEW REALITIES
680 Beach
Suite 408
San Francisco, CA 94109

*James Bolen, Editor-in-Chief*

A holistic magazine for the general public interested in holistic living and being—body, mind, spirit—and straightforward, entertaining material on parapsychology, consciousness research, and the frontiers of human potential and the mind. Formerly *Psychic* magazine.

## (803) FORTEANA—THE PSI-ENTIFIC WORLD
2125 21st Street
Santa Monica, CA 90405

Each monthly issue contains a calendar of human potential activities in Southern California. Also articles pertaining to psychic phenomena and spiritual growth.

## (804) THE JOURNAL OF BORDERLAND RESEARCH
Borderland Sciences Research Foundation
P.O. Box 548
Vista, CA 92083

(714) 724-2043

*Riley Hansard Crabb, Editor*

Bi-monthly journal of the Borderland Sciences Research Foundation **(586)**. Articles in such areas as UFOs, radiesthesia, occult and psychic phenomena, and photography of the invisible.

## (805) SOURCE MAGAZINE
Pathways Foundation
Wrightwood, CA 92397

*Helen and John Wilson*

Dedicated to the spiritual, mental, and physical health of the individual, through love.

## (806) THE PSYCHIC OBSERVER AND CHIMES
Box 8606
Washington, DC 20011

(202) 723-4578

*Henry J. Nagorka, Editor-Publisher*

Open forum magazine with articles on parapsychology, psychic healing, bioenergy, and related subjects.

**ALTERNATIVES JOURNAL** (multidisciplinary new age articles)/Miami, FL **(see 193)**

## (807) THE TRIAD PROGRAM
P.O. Box 15668
Honolulu, HI 96815

(808) 988-6143

Publishes a directory of psychics, healers, and clairvoyants. Write for additional information to the above address.

**EAST WEST JOURNAL** (magazine, multidisciplinary new age articles)/Brookline, MA **(see 195)**

**NEW AGE JOURNAL** (magazine, multidisciplinary)/ Brookline, MA **(see 196)**

**ASPR NEWSLETTER** (American Society for Psychical Research/New York, NY **(see 771)**

**PARAPSYCHOLOGY REVIEW**/New York, NY **(see 772)**

**SCIENCE DIGEST**/New York, NY **(see 602)**

**SEEKERS** (multidisciplinary directory)/New York, NY **(see 202)**

**HUMAN DIMENSIONS** (journal of unusual parapsychology research)/Williamsville, NY **(see 203)**

**JOURNAL OF THE AMERICAN SOCIETY FOR PSYCHICAL RESEARCH**/Durham, NC **(see 794)**

## (808) THE JOURNAL OF PARAPSYCHOLOGY
Parapsychology Press
Box 6847
College Station
Durham, NC 27708

(919) 684-8111

*Louisa E. Rhine and Dorothy H. Pope, Editors*

Quarterly journal with scientific articles of research in ESP, precognition and psychokinesis (PK). Devoted to reporting on cases of individuals able to "interact with their surroundings without the use of their sensory or muscular systems." (Books on parapsychology are also available through the above address.) Founded 1937.

**THETA** (quarterly bulletin on psychic research)/Durham, NC **(see 794)**

## Products and Services

**HEALTH RESEARCH** (books)/Mokelumne Hill, CA **(see 209)**

**BUTTERFLY MEDIA DIMENSIONS** (cassette tapes)/ N. Hollywood, CA **(see 210)**

**NEW DIMENSIONS FOUNDATION** (cassette tapes)/ San Francisco, CA **(see 212)**

**COGNETICS** (cassette tapes)/Saratoga, CA **(see 214)**

**HARTLEY FILM PRODUCTIONS** (multidisciplinary audiovisual)/Cos Cob, CT **(see 219)**

**HERITAGE STORE** (Cayce)/Virginia Beach, VA **(see 230)**

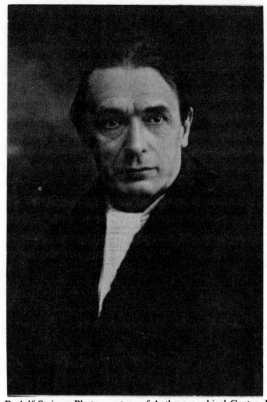

Rudolf Steiner. Photo courtesy of Anthroposophical Center, New York City.

# Anthroposophical Medicine

*Otto Wolff, MD (Translated from German by Herbert J. Fill, MD)*

In anthroposophical medicine the spiritual research of Rudolf Steiner (1861-1925) is brought to bear on the special field of medicine.

The world image on which medical thought and practice are based was once wholistic, but because of necessary specialization it is becoming increasingly narrow. The physician of ancient times, up to the Middle Ages, was at once a natural scientist, botanist, astronomer, and pharmacist. Modern medicine is not only specialized, but also very strongly shaped by natural science. Natural science itself has a completely one-sided orientation. This orientation is pursued consciously; only physical-chemical reactions are grasped, and not what these reactions express in form of forces, orders, and manifestations of a supraordinate world. That world is today viewed as fundamentally unexplorable. It is not generally realized that this separation has been created artificially, arbitrarily, by man's way of viewing nature.

Kepler (1571-1630), for instance, viewed the celestial bodies as still imbued with a "world soul," and he considered the world an animated organism. His works *Mystericum Cosmographicum* and *Harmonices Mundi* proclaim clearly the all-encompassing view which includes soul and spirit (which Kepler distinguished clearly). What is physically calculable in astronomy—the only aspect that counts today—was for him only part of the whole. It was his primary concern to discover the harmony on which the creation of the entire world was founded. By this he understood not only harmonious accord but also the active deeds of concrete spiritual beings.

The intentional, conscious omission—or the denial—of realities creates half-truths that can no longer be assessed objectively, as judgment becomes subject to the prejudices of a world view. That prejudice proclaims that the natural scientific aspect of medicine is the only valid one, the only explorable one, and the only valuable one.

Man is thereby no longer the measure of all things. His spirit and his soul are no longer the foundations of medical action. They pale in the face of the validity ascribed to biomolecular or physical-chemical processes.

Today's medicine, therefore, is founded on a reduced world view that cannot do justice to the complete reality of man. It is widely believed that one can only recognize and accept what can be grasped through natural science. Withal, few will negate the actuality of soul today. But its differentiation from the spirit, for instance, is not recognized. The concrete intervention of soul and spirit in the body, in an organ, in a certain substance in the course of biochemical events, is hardly considered. Their relationship to the being of man, their effect on substance, is not explored.

Since the advent of the natural-scientific age and the discovery of the telescope and microscope, man has continuously sharpened and extended his natural gifts of sensory perception. He has even penetrated the subsensory domains of electricity and magnetism not directly perceptible through our sensory organs. It would be an extraordinary regression were one to renounce these achievements and neglect this world to escape into another.

True evolution can only proceed by adding something to what exists. Thus, it was necessary to indicate that our sensory perception is a natural gift. The current limitation of our world view, however, is not given by nature but created by man himself. A British physicist has commented that man, as a researcher, has made himself into a "one-eyed, color-blind onlooker."

Today, thought itself is being trained and developed one-sidedly as causal-analytical thinking. Here, too, logic cannot be renounced while a more comprehensive mode of thinking is taught. In *every* man there resides a multitude of faculties which for the most part lie fallow today. The more man develops them, the better he can grasp reality.

Consciousness must be expanded to such an extent that it is equal to its object, be it life, soul, or spirit. And this must be done without surrendering the precise thinking for which natural science has been an excellent school. By these means, it is just as possible to cross the border into the suprasensory domain as it is to extend our senses through appropriate instruments. That this, like any kind of study, requires schooling is obvious. Thus, it is possible to take part in the spiritual world only when man makes himself an instrument of cognition.

Man disposes of the soul faculties of thinking, feeling, and will. Of these, it is mainly thinking that is being trained today, and even thinking is being trained only in a very one-sided form—as intellect. Intellect is only a narrow sector within the human ability of thinking. It is capable of grasping only the dead world.

To take hold of the other spheres, even only that of life, it is necessary to enliven one's thinking without surrendering the precision of thought acquired through natural science. In addition, it is necessary to conjoin this thinking with the other soul forces, feeling and will. In this way, thinking moves into the sphere of experience. Experience, as an active force of cognition, is not only neglected today, but considered "subjective" and consciously excluded from research. Active experience, however, can be applied to reality with precision. One can thereby gain a connection to a life process, an animal, a substance, etc., that affords a revelation of its true being that would otherwise be inaccessible. Passive mental behavior allows access to only part of reality.

On the basis of his spiritual research, Rudolf Steiner gave concrete indications as to the relationship of man with the spiritual world and with nature. Stimulated by this comprehensive image of man, physicians asked him for special expositions in the field of medicine. Subsequently, Steiner gave several courses for physicians, from 1920 to 1924, and together with a physician, Dr. Ita Wegman, wrote a book, *Fundamentals of Therapy,* in which they said: "There can be no question of opposition against current medicine that is working with scientific methods. . . . An objection of recognized medicine to what we are presenting cannot be advanced, as we do not refute this medicine. Only he who not only wants approval, but also demands that no knowledge that exceeds his own be pursued, can reject our attempts out of hand.''

In Steiner's works we are not dealing with mere problems of theory of knowledge. We are dealing with concrete insights into the connections of illness and destiny, man and nature. ''Nature reveals itself in its constructive and destructive forces, and now one makes of the art of healing something by which one sees through what it is doing, where one does not apply remedies just because statistics have shown an effect in a number of cases, but out of seeing through man and nature.'' Steiner's fundamental indications have been taken up and extrapolated by scholars of his work. Today physicians practice according to this extended art of healing based on spiritual-scientific knowledge in almost every country of the Western world.

The specific medications that anthroposophically oriented physicians use are applied according to recognized connections between man and nature, so that events within man can be specifically addressed and influenced with the help of a natural process. We are accustomed to classifying illnesses in anatomical-pathological terms. This corresponds to the statistical view. If, however, we start with a comprehensive image of man, if we consider man dynamically, in terms of his own force-effects, it becomes apparent that there are two large groups of illnesses which behave in polarity to each other. These are inflammatory (fever-inducing) illnesses, and their opposite, sclerotic conditions. That these two groups exhibit polar behavior signifies that they can also neutralize each other. This can be illustrated by the behavior of a scale beam. The descent of one side can be caused by excess weight there, or by the fact that a counterweight on the other side is lacking. For this reason, the symptom of an illness can be truly revealing only when one views that illness in the light of its counterpart.

The fact that inflammation and cancer have some mutual relationship has been affirmed from many sides in the past, and this relationship has almost always revealed itself as a form of antagonism. It has been shown that the so-called diathesis inflammatoria is a rarity with cancer patients, that they have a low incidence of infection, that the disposition to cancer creates an immunity against infectious diseases, that the few spontaneous cures of cancer have occurred mostly following highly febrile illnesses, such as erysipelas. That the reciprocal action of inflammation and carcinoma has been known without leading to any significant consequences is because the necessary concept of polarity is missing. In addition, there is no corresponding appreciation of the importance of fever as a life-integrating factor. According to the research of the French Nobel Laureate L. Wolff, defense against viruses depends far more on temperature than on humoral and cellular reactions. The virulence of a strain, therefore, is above all dependent on temperature. Despite many experimental studies along these lines, the importance of fever as a positive factor is rarely acknowledged; on the contrary, in medical practice antipyretics are immediately applied.

Thus, the equilibrium of inflammation and sclerosis is continuously disturbed, without this being recognized. Even less recognized is the great importance of fever as a mechanism of the organism to give the spirit of man, his ego, a chance to connect itself with the body anew, and more correctly. For this reason, with feverish illness, the attentive observer always sees a transformation in patients (especially children), an unfolding of personality. With this view of polarity we can draw fruitful conclusions for pathology and therapy. One is the insight that health does not consist in the absence of inflammatory and sclerotic tendencies in the organism, but in the balance of these two polar forces. We can utilize the indicated dynamics in therapy, taking into account the course of illness and the patient's personality.

Steiner made many new suggestions for the treatment of illnesses and pharmaceutical procedures. For instance, he introduced mistletoe for treatment of cancer. Iscador (the best-known preparation derived from the mistletoe) is already being used successfully in the treatment of cancer by many physicians and hospitals; it is the first preparation to produce a highly cytostatic effect while stimulating the body's own immune system to activate the organism's own defense against cell proliferation.

As conceived by Rudolf Steiner, anthroposophical medicine strives to grasp the whole human being, including his life, soul, and spirit, and to achieve thereby a humanization of medicine so much in demand today.

## Groups and Associations

### (809) ANTHROPOSOPHICAL SOCIETY
211 Madison Avenue
New York, NY 10016

(212) 685-4617

Maintains complete library facilities, information on programs and events sponsored by the various anthroposophical groups, and contact lists of physicians engaged in Anthroposophical Medicine in the United States.

### (810) ANTHROPOSOPHICAL THERAPY AND HYGIENE ASSOCIATION
241 Hungry Hollow Road
Spring Valley, NY 10977

Group of individuals meeting once a month to discuss various aspects of anthroposophical medicine. Also acts as a contact point for the dissemination of information regarding the field.

### (811) THE FELLOWSHIP OF PHYSICIANS
c/o Paul W. Scharff, MD, Secretary
219 Hungry Hollow Road
Spring Valley, NY 10977

(914) 356-8494

A working group of physicians actively supporting anthroposophical medicine.

## Centers and Clinics

### (812) DIAT- UND KNIEPP-SANATORIUM DR. FELBERMAYER
A-6793 Gaschurr
Montafon-Voralberg, Austria

All chronic ailments, specifically digestive disorders, circulation, rheumatism, allergies, eczema, tumors, neurological and post-operative complications. Treatments used include Kniepp gymnastics, healing massage, sauna, physiotherapy, special foot baths, and colonic massage. Founded 1960.

### (813) ITA-WEGMAN-KLINIK
CH-4144
Arlesheim, Pfeffingerweg 1
Switzerland

Tel: (061) 72 10 11

Treats all internal ailments with the exception of TB. Treatment includes mud packs, whirlpool, hydrotherapy, massage, gymnastics, music, art and dance therapy, and a nutritional program. Founded 1921.

### (814) LUKAS KLINIK
CH-4144
Arlesheim, Brachmattstrasse 19
Switzerland

Tel: 061/72 33 33

Treats cancer, tumors and growths by various methods which include hydrotherapy, speech therapy, art, music and dance therapy, and color and light therapies. Vegetarian diet and nutritional program included. Founded 1963.

### (815) SANATORIUM SONNENECK
D-7847 Badenweiler, Kanderner Str. 18,
Switzerland

Tel: (0 76 32) 50 81

Treats all chronic and internal disorders, post operative tumors, and paralysis, if not bedridden. Treatments used include thermal and herb baths, Kniepp, massage, horticulture, art and music therapy, ultraviolet, underwater massage, speech therapy, and raw and vegetarian, salt and sugar free diet. Founded 1939.

### (816) FILDERKLINIK
D-7024 Filderstadt-Bonlanden,
Haberschlaiheide,
West Germany

Tel: (07 11) 7 70 31

An affiliate of the Herdecke clinic (818) Filderklinik specializes in children's and female disorders. Among the treatments included are Kniepp baths, hydrotherapy, whirlpool, underwater massage and hydroelectric and carbon dioxide baths. Founded 1975.

### (817) FRIEDRICH HUSEMANN-KLINIK
D-7801 Buchenbach bei Freiburg im Breisgau,
West Germany

Tel: (076 61) 8 33

Maintains a sanitorium facility. Conditions treated are neurological and organic disorders of the nervous system, emotional disorders and TB. Treatment includes anthroposophical medicine, massage, mud packs, drama, art, music, speech and dance therapy. Also included are gymnastics, arts and crafts, i.e. wood carving and weaving, folk dancing and horticulture therapy. Diet is mixed vegetarian and others. Founded 1925.

### (818) GEMEINNÜTZIGES GEMEINSCHAFTS KRANKENHAUS HERDECKE
Beckweg 4 D-5804 Herdecke (Ruhr)
West Germany

Tel: (0 23 30) 6 21

Multi-therapeutic clinic ranging from births to treating a number of disorders including rheumatism, cancer, cardiovascular disorders, children's disease, neurological disorders, brain, eye, nose, throat, and ear dysfunction. Treatment includes psychotherapy, massage, gymnastics, oilbaths, hydrotherapy, Kniepp baths, and underwater massage, physiotherapy, very hot baths, and deep connective tissue massage. Founded 1969.

### (819) HAUS RAPHAEL
D-5300 Bonn 1,
Rosenburgweg 22,
West Germany

Tel: (0 22 21) 23 35 57

Post-operative recuperation facility treating exhaustion and elderly people who do not wish to be alone. Does not treat major disorders. Treatments include sauna baths. Kniepp, massage, physiotherapy, and art therapy.

### (820) KLINIK ÖSCHELBRONN
D-7532 Niefem-Öschelbronn 2,
Am Eichhof,
West Germany

Tel: (0 72 33) 12 11

Treats cancer and acute and chronic infections, heart and circulatory disorders, digestive dysfunction and ailments of the joints and vertabrae and also various swelling conditions. Treatment consists of movement and rhythm, Kniepp baths, hydrotherapy, massage including rhythm massage, and electronic therapy for circulatory problems. Founded 1975.

### (821) KURHEIM SONNENBLICK
D-7263 Bad Liebenzell Unterlengenhardt,
Johannes-Kepler-Strasse 19,
West Germany

Tel: (0 70 52) 5 87

Converted from a quaint old town and country restaurant in 1975. No major disorders treated, only minor problems requiring a short rest; is not a sanatorium. Treats all manner of physical exhaustion; treatment includes whirlpool and steam baths, physiotherapy, and rhythm massage according to Hauschka.

### (822) PARACELSUS-KRANKENHAUS
D-7263 Bad Liebenzell Unterlengenhardt
West Germany

Tel: (0 70 52) 5 60

Treats all forms of internal disorders, acute and chronic, joint, vertabrae, skin and neurological disorders, except mental disorders and infections. Treatment includes physical therapy, rhythm massage after Wegman-Hauschka, oil dispersion (using etherial oils, i.e. pine and rosemary) and very hot baths, and nutritional counseling. Founded 1970.

### (823) SANATORIUM FÜR DYNAMISCHE THER-APIE STUDENHOF
D-7821 Dachsberg-Urberg,
West Germany

Tel: St. Blasien (0 76 72) 7 39

All internal disorders, tumors, and multiple sclerosis, as long as the patient is not bed-ridden. Therapies include various baths—herbal, salt, hayflower, carbon dioxide and oil dispersion, movement therapy, arts and crafts, spinning and weaving (occupational therapy), and music therapy. Founded 1966.

### (824) SANATORIUM SCHLOSS HAMBORN
D-4791 Borchen 3,
West Germany

Tel: (0 52 51) 3 80 91

Treats all internal disorders; postoperative cancer treatment with Iscador (a special preparation of mistletoe). Does not treat infections or psychiatric disorders. Treatment includes anthroposophical and homeopathic preparations, various types of baths, rhythm massage after Hauska, and art therapy. Diet according to disorder, bakes all their own breads in large wall oven, grows own vegetables, fruits, and has fresh milk and homemade milk products also available. Reconstructed in 1969.

## Products and Services

### (825) RUDOLPH STEINER BOOK SHOP
240 South Normandie
Los Angeles, CA 90004

(213) 382-8847

Books and publications relating to anthroposophy and Rudolph Steiner.

### (826) BEERS BOOK CENTER
c/o Mr. Harvey Shank
1406 "J" Street
Sacramento, CA 95814

(916) 442-9475

Books, publications, and information on anthroposophy and Rudolph Steiner.

### (827) FOUNDATION STUDIES BOOK SERVICE
529 Grant Place
Chicago, IL 60614

(312) 935-2634

Books and publications on anthroposophy and Rudolph Steiner.

### (828) THE GRAIL BOOKSTORE
c/o Karl Schreiber
5 Dwhinda Road
Waban, MA 02168

(617) 244-1804

Books and publications on anthroposophy and Rudolph Steiner.

### (829) THE ANTHROPOSOPHIC PRESS BRANCH BOOKSTORE
211 Madison Avenue
New York, NY 10016

(212) 685-4617

Books and publications on anthroposophy and Rudolph Steiner.

### (830) THE ANTHROPOSOPHIC PRESS
258 Hungry Hollow Road
Spring Valley, NY 10977

(914) 352-2295

Publishes and distributes books on all aspects of the anthroposophic movement.

WELEDA (pharmacy) (homeopathic and anthroposophical medicine)/Spring Valley, NY (see 279)

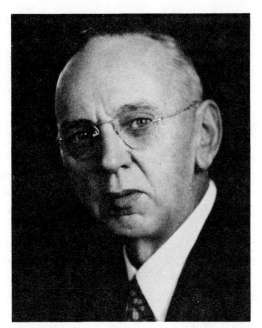

Edgar Cayce. Photo courtesy of A.R.E., Virginia Beach, VA.

# Edgar Cayce And Wholistic Medicine

*William A. McGarey, MD*

*"Prayer is a force as real as terrestrial gravity. As a physician, I have seen men, after all other therapy had failed, lifted out of disease and melancholy by the serene effort of prayer. Only in prayer do we achieve that complete and harmonious assembly of body, mind and spirit which gives the frail human its unshakable strength."*  
*Dr. Alexis Carrel*

Edgar Cayce's psychic work was concerned almost entirely with the concept of holism as it applies to the healing of the human body. Two thirds of his life production of psychic readings gave understanding about the functioning of the human body and suggestions that led toward restoration of a state of health, and they invariably related the body to the mind and to the spirit. These concepts have proved to be viable in the mind of the practitioner and in the experience of the patients who have used them.

Cayce lived in Virginia Beach, Virginia, now the home of the Edgar Cayce Foundation, the Association for Research and Enlightenment (ARE), and the library that houses the legacy of over 14,000 psychic readings Cayce left upon his death in 1945, at the age of 65. Much research has been built on this foundation of information, now indexed and made available for study, and dozens of books have been written about Cayce's work.

The conceptual data found in the readings are thought to have their origin in what have been called the "Akashic Records"; the information about the physical body and its functioning seemed to come from a communication between Cayce's unconscious mind and that of the person for whom he was giving a reading. At times it appeared that Cayce reached out with his mind in a clairvoyant manner to gather factual information from other sources. There were few areas of human endeavor and activity that he did not touch on in the course of 40 years of work.

In the early 1960s, the Edgar Cayce Foundation undertook to make available for the general public the concepts of healing found in the readings. Various research divisions were formed (medical, osteopathic, physical therapy, and chiropractic), and doctors and therapists were informed of this opportunity to participate in the research and the practical use of information from the readings in their own particular area of patient care. The ARE, formed as a membership organization in 1932, immediately made available to its members the lists of those who had signified their interest in using the Cayce material at the clinical level. The number of these "cooperating doctors" has grown over the years and now includes several hundred individuals scattered across the United States and around the world.

During the later sixties, the membership of the ARE grew increasingly interested in healing not only by means of drugs, xray, and surgery but also through using the mind as a constructive force in the healing process and by recognizing the spirit as an integral life-giving energy. As a result of this growth of awareness, the first ARE medical symposium was held in Phoenix early in 1968.

In 1969, the groundwork was laid for the creation of the ARE Clinic in Phoenix. My wife, Gladys McGarey, and I had been in private practice there since 1955, and I had headed up the Medical Research Division of the Foundation since its inception. The clinic was granted the use of the name by the ARE board of trustees that summer and began operating as the ARE Clinic in 1970. It is now a nonprofit Arizona corporation and, as part of its commitment to the Association in Virginia Beach, works to research the physical readings, prepares medical commentaries for the use of the ARE cooperating doctors and the membership, and works with the concepts in the readings at the clinical level. The information thus derived is disseminated to interested persons in the healing professions through publications (such as the *Medical Research Bulletin*), seminars, films, workshops, lectures, and symposia.

Practical use, then, of the information found in the Cayce readings that is helpful in the healing of the human body is gradually gaining wider and wider application and acceptance. As part of its services to its membership, the ARE in Virginia Beach provides circulating files on a number of subjects. Three-fourths of these circulating files are concerned directly with illnesses of the human body and how they might be reversed or corrected—how health might be regained.

Many ARE members began their own exploration of the information in the Cayce readings by using some of the simple information about castor oil packs. I have prescribed these packs for a variety of ailments ranging from appendicitis to cholecystitis and have written a monograph on this particular therapy, exploring theories as to how castor oil applied to the surface of the body could have an effect on the internal portions. Clinical evidence has of course shown this effect, but we wished to understand the mechanisms.

Cayce's readings stated that all substances have a "vibratory" effect on other substances. We concluded that, if applied locally, the oil would have a vibratory effect on tissues similar to (if less than) that which it has when taken internally (where it acts as a cleanser, physiologically a lymphatic function). Thus, when applied as a pack the oil apparently cleanses and eliminates through the lymphatics because of vibratory activity. This concept is not to be found in medical school education, but as information in the Cayce material, it can be related to the nature of atoms and energy as they are understood in the field of physics.

However, the question of healing is far more complicated than a vibratory effect of an oil from the bean of the *Racinus communis*. From the standpoint of the work we have been doing, healing is something that recognizes the work of the spirit in the healing of the mind and body. We have come to look at illness as an adventure in consciousness, and one of Cayce's readings supports that view:

> For all healing comes from the one source, and whether there is the application of foods, exercise, medicine or even the knife—it is to bring [to] the consciousness of the forces within the body that aid in reproducing themselves, the awareness of Creative or God Forces. [2696-1]*

Our approach to healing involves cooperation among the patient, the physician, and the creative forces. Illness is regarded as an opportunity for spiritual development, a true adventure that can lead to a greater awareness and a portion of what could be called enlightenment.

We understand healing to be not merely a process of structural repair, but a process that should lead to the redirection of the entire person, providing a new vision of wholeness and health toward which each of us can strive. The achievement of virtual immunity to disease, as we become attuned, integrated, and centered in our spiritual purpose—that is the goal of this vision.

The concept of wholeness is an integral part of the process of healing. The wholeness must include the concept that man is spiritual in origin and destiny, that mind is the builder and that the physical is the result. This idea grows out of the thousands of readings that Cayce gave over the early years of this

---

*The Edgar Cayce readings are copyrighted by the Edgar Cayce Foundation, reprinted with permission.*

century, and it has become real in the minds of those who have worked with the readings to heal the human body. Our approach is not that something from outside can be applied and make the body better or well, but rather that the forces within the body can be stimulated to bring about that healing process from within. According to another reading:

> Know that all healing forces must be within, not without! The applications from without are to create within a coordinating mental and spiritual force. Set the mind to believe in SOMETHING, and let that be creative—and as we find, as we have indicated, it must be of a spiritual nature. [1196-]*

It seems most reasonable to approach the material we have been working with as a body of information that is valid, practical, usable, and, most importantly, that affords insight to the physician as he or she tries to utilize simple therapies in the practice of medicine—insight into the mental and spiritual nature of man as a whole unit. This information helps us understand why it is important to approach the healing of the body with physical applications, at the same time recognizing the manner in which those simple applications work on the forces of the body, and recognizing that the body is part of the body/mind/spirit wholeness that we call man.

## Groups and Associations

**(831) ASSOCIATION FOR RESEARCH AND ENLIGHTENMENT, INC.**
P.O. Box 595
Virginia Beach, VA 23451

(804) 428-3588

*Charles Thomas Cayce, President*

Established to research and study the 14,256 psychic readings of Edgar Cayce. Included in the readings are thousands of specific treatments for physical diseases, as well as information in such areas as agriculture, world affairs, business, reincarnation, astrology and psychic development. A.R.E. maintains one of the nation's largest libraries for parapsychology and spiritual science, and houses transcipts of all of the Cayce readings. A twenty week conference season features such subjects as dreams, meditation, ESP, healing, mysticism and reincarnation. The Virginia facility also maintains a service to test the individual's ESP, a therapy department implementing health suggestions from the readings, a prayer group, a braille library, and a large bookstore. Membership in the Association entitles one to access to the book and tape library, rights to borrow "circulating files" of readings on specific subjects, and reduced medical expenses at the A.R.E. clinic. Members also receive the *A.R.E. Journal* and the *A.R.E. News*, which include articles on research findings and on A.R.E. activities throughout the world. There is also a summer camp which offers "recreation close to nature for children, youth, and families to awaken interest in things of a spiritual and a psychic nature." Founded 1948.

**(832) EDGAR CAYCE FOUNDATION**
P.O. Box 595
Virginia Beach, VA 23451

(804) 428-3588

Owner-custodian of the Edgar Cayce psychic readings and all of the memorabilia pertaining to Edgar Cayce's life and work (preserved on microfilm). The Foundation organizes and disseminates the Edgar Cayce material in a closely integrated relationship with A.R.E., the Association of Learning (under the charter of Atlantic University), and the A.R.E. Clinic. Preparation of medical data and continuing work with A.R.E. referral doctors has been moving toward the development of a much broader research program. A yearly symposium is sponsored with the A.R.E. Clinic which coordinates all aspects of healing and brings together scientists with a wide variety of interests. The Foundation also sponsors special research projects with other organizations or individuals. Chartered 1948.

## Schools, Centers, and Clinics

**(833) A.R.E. CLINIC**
4018 North 40th Street
Phoenix, AZ 85018

(602) 955-0551

*William A. McGarey, MD, Director*

Offers medical treatment according to the Edgar Cayce readings integrated with modern medical knowledge and treatment. It is also inviolved in medical research of the readings. Findings are published in the clinic's newsletter *Medical Research Bulletin*.

**ATLANTIC UNIVERSITY** (Association of Learning)/ Virginia Beach, VA **(see 154)**

**HOME CENTER** (wholistic clinic and educational center)/Virginia Beach, VA **(see 155)**

**PAIN AND HEALTH REHABILITATION CENTER/** La Crosse, WI **(see 157)**

## Journals and Publications

**MEDICAL RESEARCH BULLETIN** (Cayce)/Phoenix, AZ **(see 833)**

**THE A.R.E. JOURNAL** (Cayce)/Virginia Beach, VA **(see 831)**

## Products and Services

**HERITAGE STORE** (Cayce)/Virginia Beach, VA **(see 230)**

---

*The Edgar Cayce readings are copyrighted by the Edgar Cayce Foundation, reprinted with permission.*

# VII
# PSYCHOPHYSICAL APPROACHES

Introduction To Psychophysical Groups And Centers

Massage

Shiatsu

Polarity Therapy

Sensory Awareness

Alexander: The Use Of The Self

Rolfing

Dance Therapy: The Psychotherapeutic Use Of Movement

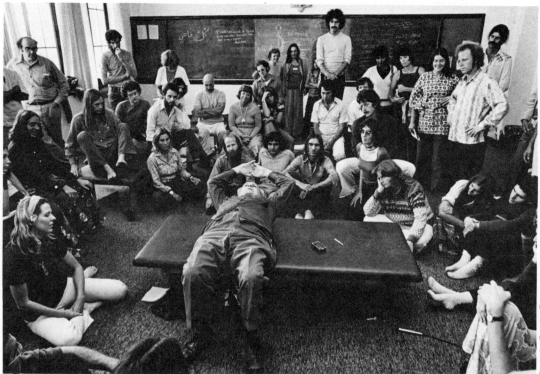

Moshe Feldenkrias, demonstrating his technique.

# Introduction To Psychophysical Groups And Centers

*Robert Masters, PhD*

Except by arbitrary and dangerous division it is not possible to separate the mind from the body. The human being is a psychophysical or bodymind system. Body and mind are so closely interrelated that there is probably no act or process wherein both are not to some degree affected.

Nevertheless, it is possible to behave *as if* the body were one thing and the mind another—to treat patients and educate students as though they were body *or* mind, respectively. The results are unfortunate. The state of the musculoskeletal system, breathing, and the body's positioning with respect to gravity are interactive with our thinking, sensing, and feeling functions. A distorted body image basically affects our perceptions of reality as well as our movements, cognitions, and emotions. Psychophysical reintegration achieved by effecting alterations in the body image and mechanics constitutes expanded awareness.

The approaches described in this section share a common expressed or implied recognition that bodymind should be treated as a whole. In most of these methods the hands of therapist or teacher are used to convey to the nervous system of the patient or student the changes desired in the physical structure. These methods are *communications,* and many or most of the basic changes are made by the student or patient him/herself at an unconscious level in response to what the teacher's or therapist's hands distinctly convey.

## Schools, Centers, and Clinics

**ESALEN INSTITUTE** (multidisciplinary workshops)/Big Sur, CA; also San Francisco, CA **(see 1051)**

**BIOLOGY OF THE MIND/BODY** (workshop)/Davis, CA **(see 80)**

**HUMAN PROCESS INSTITUTE** (group psychotherapy)/Encino, CA **(see 1052)**

**GETTING IN TOUCH** (massage)/Los Gatos, CA **(see 857)**

**(834) SOMA INSTITUTE**
4676 Admiralty Way, Suite 401
Marina Del Rey, CA 90291

(213) 823-7009

*Cindee C. McCallister, BS, RMT, Founder and Director*

Offers a ten-lesson private program in stress-reduction and deep muscular release, known as the "Soma Process," designed to help the person break through conditioned patterns of body tension. This is accomplished with three subprocesses: the "Mind-Body Process" aims at developing a body consciousness to feel how dis-ease is self-created in the body; the "Muscular Release Process" uses deep pressure directly on the muscles to release armoring and relax the body; and the "Self-Help Process," a series of exercises done between sessions to help the individual gain control over the body and reduce tension.

**(835) LOMI SCHOOL**
475 Molino Avenue
Mill Valley, CA 94941
(415) 388-4789

*Robert K. Hall, MD*

Teaches and practices Aikido, manipulative therapy, gestalt, breath awareness, yoga, nutrition, meditative arts, communication, and sexuality. Founded 1970.

**(836) NOVATO INSTITUTE FOR SOMATIC RESEARCH**
1516 Grant Avenue, Suite 220
Novato, CA 94947
(415) 897-0336

*Thomas Hanna, PhD, and Eleanor Criswell, EdD*

Offers individual clinical work and professional training in functional integration, awareness through movement exercises, and biofeedback training. Also conducts research in these fields, the results of which are published in the Institute's journal, *Somatics* **(see 846).**

**AUTOGENIC HEALTH CENTER**/Oakland, CA **(see 98)**

**(837) TOUCH FOR HEALTH FOUNDATION**
1174 North Lake Avenue
P.O. Box 751-C
Pasadena, CA 91104

(213) 794-1181

*John Thie, DC, Director*

Provides instructor training, speakers' bureau, workshops, and symposia in Touch for Health, a method of regaining postural balance. Specific techniques include meridian tracing, neurolymphatic points, neurovascular pulses, acupressure holding points, origin/insertion massage, and nutrition awareness.

**CHILD PSYCHOLOGY INSTITUTE OF SAN DIEGO** (humanistic approach)/San Diego, CA **(see 1058)**

**NATIONAL CENTER FOR THE EXPLORATION OF HUMAN POTENTIAL** (parapsychology workshops)/San Diego, CA **(see 106)**

**(838) AHLEF**
716 Dolores Street, #4
San Francisco, CA 94110

(415) 285-1916

*David Isaacs and Sue Mooney, Founders and Directors*

Offers wholistic approaches to "developing energy and body awareness through massage," and "body/mind integration—the mindgame experience." The first includes work in Esalen and Swedish massage, polarity, and acupressure. The latter is an expansion of work in progressive relaxation, visual imagery, and guided fantasy pioneered by Masters and Houston. Founded in 1975.

**(839) CREATIVE BODYWORK CENTER**
4338 California Street
San Francisco, CA 94118

(415) 221-2683
*Leora Myers, RN, MT, Director*

A New Age education center dedicated to offering experience which develops, explores, and nourishes the individual creative source. This is accomplished through individual bodywork sessions and classes in T'ai Chi, yoga, dance, massage, and psychic development. The bodywork sessions are geared to heighten somatic awareness, to heighten sensitivity, and to relieve tension.

**TOPANGA CENTER FOR HUMAN DEVELOPMENT** (growth center)/Topanga, CA **(see 1070)**

**SCHOOL OF ACTUALISM** (laying on of hands)/Valley Center, also Escondido, La Jolla, Los Angeles, San Francisco, and Santa Ana, CA **(see 783)**

**ENCOUNTERS** (humanistic workshops)/Washington, DC **(see 1078)**

**(840) FLORIDA INSTITUTE OF PSYCHOPHYSICAL INTEGRATION**
5837 Mariner Drive
Tampa, FL 33609

(813) 877-2273

*Joyce K. Johnson, PhD (cand), Director*

Provides dance/movement therapy and deep tissue work, augmented with individual analysis of the whole person. Founded 1976.

**(841) CHICAGO NATIONAL COLLEGE OF NAPRAPATHY**
3330 North Milwaukee Avenue
Chicago, IL 60641

(312) 282-5717

*Norman S. Esserman, JD, DN, Chairperson*

Confers the Doctor of Naprapathy (DN) degree after a three to four year course of study. "Naprapathy is a system of manually applied movements, both passive and active, designed to bring motion, with consequent release of tension, into abnormally tensed and rigid ligaments, muscles and articulations of the human body . . . . Naprapathy contends that a favorable internal environment is essential for growth, development and maintenance of normal health . . . (and) assists the body to maintain this favorable internal environment by releasing points of tension and by the use of rational dietary and hygienic measures." Founded 1907.

**EXPANSION** (family growth center)/Bedford, MA **(see 1090)**

**PSYCHOMOTOR INSTITUTE** (humanistic center)/ Boston, MA **(see 1093)**

**(842) THE JOY OF MOVEMENT CENTER**
536 Massachusetts Avenue
Central Square
Cambridge, MA 02139

(617) 492-4680

Offers courses and workshops in traditional dance forms such as modern, ballet, and jazz; bioenergetics; yoga; massage forms including shiatsu; and mime. Special programs are offered for weight control and for pregnant women.

**(843) NEW ENGLAND CENTER, INC.**
436 Longplain Road
Leverett, MA 01054

(413) 549-0886

*Katie Baker, Exec. Director*

A multimodality therapy center dedicated to the individual's commitment to personal change. Individual work, workshops, and classes are offered in Alexander work, T.A., biofeedback, massage, polarity, gestalt, rebirthing, family and sexual therapies. A catalog of offerings is available on request. Founded 1970.

**SAGARIS-WOMEN'S THERAPY COLLECTIVE** (psychotherapy and body work)/Minneapolis, MN **(see 1109)**

**WOMANKIND** (growth center)/Minneapolis, MN **(see 1110)**

**THE ILANA RUBENFELD CENTER FOR GESTALT SYNERGY**/New York, NY **(see 933)**

**CALIFORNIA BIOENERGETICS SOCIETY** (audiovisuals and books on bioenergetics)/Berkeley-Newport Beach, CA **(see under 844)**

**(844) THE INSTITUTE FOR BIOENERGETIC ANALYSIS**
144 East 36th Street, #1A
New York, NY 10016

(212) 532-7742

*Alexander Lowen, MD, Executive Director*

Promotes research and education in the fields of emotional and physical health. Focus is on the biological energy processes involved in health and illness. Research is directed to the evaluation and development of therapeutic techniques which integrate the fundamental principles of psychoanalysis with a physical therapy based upon the study of the form and motility of the organism. Holds workshops, and has available audiovisual presentations and books on bioenergetics. There is a four-year training program in bioenergetics therapy for professionals. Founded 1956.

*AFFILIATE CENTERS*

**NORTHERN CALIFORNIA BIOENERGETIC SOCIETY**
1307 University Avenue
Berkeley, CA 94702

*Atten: Michael Conant, PhD*

**SOUTHERN CALIFORNIA BIOENERGETIC SOCIETY**
833 Dover Drive, Suite #13
Newport Beach, CA 92660

*Atten: Robert Hilton, PhD and Renato Monaco, MD*

**MID-WESTERN BIOENERGETICS CENTER**
2791 Walton Boulevard
Rochester, MI 48063

*Atten: Jack McIntyre, MD*

**TULSA BIOENERGETIC CENTER**
Tulsa Psychiatric Foundation
1620 East Twelfth Street
Tulsa, OK 74120

*Atten: Frank Hladky, MD, Director*

**NEW YORK STAR CENTER** (Actualism) (laying on of hands)/New York, NY **(see 783)**

**DALLAS STAR CENTER** (Actualism) (laying on of hands)/Dallas, TX **(see 783)**

**PREVENTIVE MEDICINE CLINIC** (holistic)/Bellevue, WA **(see 156)**

**RADIANCE—HERBS AND MASSAGE**/Olympia, WA **(see 864)**

**CAMBRIDGE HOUSE** (humanistic center)/Milwaukee, WI **(see 1129)**

**(845) THE COMPANY OF SOMATOGRAPHERS**
c/o Bryn Jones, MCS
6 Ravenslea Road
London, SW12 8SB, England

Tel: 01-673-3853

Works at analyzing, balancing, and recharging the energic pattern of an individual. Analysis is accomplished with the aid of radiesthetic instrumentation. Balancing techniques include tissue and muscular massage, basic structural adjustments, direct interaction of energy fields, postural exercises, depth relaxation, and various individual breathing, meditation, and contemplation forms. Recharging occurs at three levels: the physical energy body, the mental energy body, and the psychic energy body. The Company is engaged in somatographic research in the following areas: effects of cycles on human life, study of methods of tapping the energy fields of the earth and their relationship to energy bodies of humans, and effects of color and sound on human bodies.

*AFFILIATE CENTER*

**THE COMPANY OF SOMATOGRAPHERS**
George C. King, Jr., MCS
59 East 80th Street
New York, NY 10021

(212) 249-5143

**RIO CALIENTE S.A.** (wholistic resort)/Guadalajara, Mexico **(see 179)**

**KLINIK ÖSCHELBRONN** (anthroposophical clinic) /West Germany **(see 820)**

**SANATORIUM FÜR DYNAMISCHE THERAPIE STUDENHOF** (anthroposophical clinic)/West Germany **(see 823)**

## Journals and Publications

**(846) SOMATICS (Journal)**
1516 Grant Avenue, Suite 220
Novato, CA 94947

*Thomas Hanna, Editor*

Dedicated to publishing quality articles in the area of body-mind interactions. Includes martial arts, Rolfing, Alexander work, and biofeedback. Published twice yearly.

**WELL BEING MAGAZINE** (natural healing)/San Diego, CA **(see 186)**

**COMMON GROUND** (multidisciplinary directory San Francisco Bay Area)/San Francisco, CA **(see 187)**

**ALTERNATIVES JOURNAL** (health related)/Miami, FL **(see 193)**

**EAST WEST JOURNAL** (multidisciplinary)/Brookline, MA **(see 195)**

**NEW AGE JOURNAL** (multidisciplinary)/Brookline, MA **(see 196)**

**SEEKER** (New York area multidisciplinary source listing)/New York, NY **(see 202)**

**HUMAN DIMENSIONS** (multidisciplinary journal)/ Williamsville, NY **(see 208)**

**JOURNAL OF THE RESEARCH SOCIETY FOR NATURAL THERAPEUTICS** (multidisciplinary)/ Dorset, England **(see 70)**

## Products and Services

**LIVING EARTH CRAFTS** (massage tables)/Cotati, CA **(see 887)**

**(847) HAPPINESS PRESS**
160 Wycliff Way
Magdia, CA 95954

(916) 873-0294

Books on "do-in," a Japanese self-massage-energizing series of movements, macrobiotics, acupuncture, and other Oriental systems of medicine.

**CELESTIAL ARTS** (book publishers)/Millbrae, CA **(see 208)**

**BUTTERFLY MEDIA DIMENSIONS** (cassette tapes)/ N. Hollywood, CA **(see 210)**

**CENTER FOR HEALTH EDUCATION** (cassette tapes)/Palos Verde, CA **(see 211)**

**NEW DIMENSIONS FOUNDATION** (cassette tapes)/ San Francisco, CA 94111 **(see 212)**

**COGNETICS** (cassette tapes)/Saratoga, FL **(see 214)**

**BIG SUR RECORDINGS** (multidisciplinary audio-visual)/Sausalito, CA **(see 1135)**

**JAPAN PUBLICATIONS** (book publisher)/Elmsford, NY **(see 872)**

**GREAT EARTH HEALING, INC.** (ma roller)/East Montpelier, VT; Montreal, Canada **(see 229)**

## Reflexology

*The following is a listing of groups, centers and clinics engaged in or making use of reflexology. Reflexology is a manual manipulation technique to designated areas on the body (mainly associated with the feet) which when palpated tend to activate a corresponding organ or system within the body. It is a technique that has been used for many years with a great deal of success indicating a need for further consideration and research.*

## Groups and Associations

**(848) NATIONAL INSTITUTE OF REFLEXOLOGY**
Box 948
Rochester, NY 14603

(716) 244-2016
*Eusebia B. Messenger, RN, Co-director*
Box 1575
St. Petersburg, FL 33731
(813) 347-6016

*Dwight C. Byers, RMT, Co-director*
Professional organization devoted to the promotion of and

instruction in foot reflexology, a science dealing with the principle that there are reflexes in the feet relative to each and every organ or area in the body. Presents complete book review seminars with theory and demonstration in the Ingham Method of foot reflexology, developed by Eunice D. Ingham Stopfel. Ms. Stopfel's books on reflexology are available through the Institute.

## Schools, Centers, and Clinics

**BERKELEY HOLISTIC HEALTH CENTER** (educational workshops)/Berkeley, CA **(see 76)**

**NURSE CONSULTANTS AND HEALTH COUN-SELORS** (workshops)/San Francisco, CA **(see 112)**

**GARDEN OF SANJIVANI** (herbal school, workshops in bodywork)/Santa Cruz, CA **(see 543)**

**BOULDER SCHOOL OF MASSAGE THERAPY**/Boulder, CO **(see 861)**

**INTEGRAL HEALTH SERVICES** (holistic clinic)/Putnam, CT **(see 120)**

**STAMFORD CENTER FOR THE HEALING ARTS** (wholistic clinic in a church)/Stamford, CT **(see 121)**

**(849) REFLEXOLOGY CENTER**
1307 Avenue J
Brooklyn, NY 11230

(212) 951-6482

*Joseph Bonfiglio, Director*

Teaches a comprehensive self-help course in reflexology, acupressure, iridology, nutrition and muscle testing.

**EAST-WEST ACADEMY OF HEALTH PRACTICES** (acupuncture and acupressure training)/Portland, OR **(see 644)**

**ESOTERIC PHILOSOPHY CENTER** (community education)/Houston, TX **(see 151)**

**ASSOCIATION FOR DOCUMENTATION AND EN-LIGHTENMENT, INC.** (psychic investigation and workshops)/Virginia Beach, VA **(see 796)**

**HOME CENTER** (educational and workshops)/Virginia Beach, VA **(see 155)**

**PREVENTIVE MEDICINE CLINIC**/Bellevue, WA **(see 156)**

**SERENITY HEALTH EDUCATION CENTRE** (workshops, nutrition and bodywork)/Vancouver, BC, Canada **(see 159)**

## Journals and Publications

**WELL BEING MAGAZINE** (natural health)/San Diego, CA **(see 186)**

**COMMON GROUND** (multidisciplinary source listings Bay area)/San Francisco, CA **(see 187)**

**EAST WEST JOURNAL** (multidisciplinary)/Brookline, MA **(see 195)**

**SEEKER** (New York area multidisciplinary source listing)/New York, NY **(see 202)**

## Products and Services

**QUINTESSENCE UNLIMITED** (consciousness tools)/Boulder, CO **(see 215)**

**(850) BEN AKERLEY ENTERPRISES**
574 Ninth Avenue
New York, NY 10036

(212) 594-8363

Distributor of the Raymax Foot Exercise Mat.

**(851) STIRLING ENTERPRISES, INC.**
P.O. Box 216
Cottage Grove, OR 97424

(503) 948-4622

Manufacturers manual instruments to assist with reflexology of the hands and feet. Also distributes body lotions and reflexology charts and books.

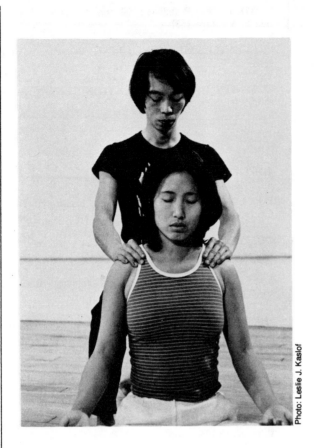

Photo: Leslie J. Kaslof

# Massage
*Katsusuke Serizawa, MD*

Even without medical knowledge, human beings naturally tend to resort to some kind of massage for relief from muscular pain or numbness. Even instinctive massage will calm hyperactive nerves and relieve muscle cramps. Massage of this kind, though not organized into a therapeutic system, has been practiced since earliest times.

Though the word *massage* is French, it is derived from the Arabian *massa,* which means "to press" and the Greek *massein,* "to knead." Interestingly, in China and Japan, the ancient words used for massage also derive from terms meaning "to press" or "to knead." The principle on which massage operates is the application of dynamic pressure to the surface of the skin to stimulate physical reactions to correct disorders, to prevent sickness, and to promote good health. Disorders in the internal organs, acting through the intervention of related nerves, cause pain, numbness, chilling, and stiffness in the skin and muscles. By relieving these symptoms the internal organs can return to sound condition. The scientific validity of the massage method in producing this effect has been proved on the basis of the influence of hormone secretions and what is called the "neurohumoral function."

In the fifth century B.C. the Greek, Hippocrates, advocated that anyone wanting to be a doctor must master massage among other medical therapies. During the first century A.D. the Roman physician Celsus studied massage, and Galen wrote a book on the subject. Later, however, massage fell from grace in the world of Western medical therapy, but remained alive in the form of a folk cure. It was not until the second half of the sixteenth century, with the detailed explanations written by Ambroise Paré, that massage once again found favor as a clinical therapeutic technique in Western medicine. In the eighteenth and nineteenth centuries, the Swede Peter Ling proposed a system of therapeutic calisthenics, which, used in connection with massage, gradually spread into Germany, France, and Holland. In Amsterdam, the Dutchman Megger and his student Berghmar introduced a specialized therapeutic system based on the physiological study of the effects of massage. In the late nineteenth century massage received great attention in conjunction with plastic surgery, which was then developing rapidly. At this time the Medical School of the University of Sweden employed massage as a clinical technique in physical therapy. As time passed, massage increased in popularity. Such giants in the field as Albert Reibmayr, Anton Hoffa, Anton Bum, and Johannes Miller pursued study in the physics of massage, attempted to improve techniques, and established the modern system of massage as applied to internal medicine, surgery, and plastic surgery.

In Japan, Oriental massage *(amma)*, which originated in China and reached the Japanese islands by way of the Korean Peninsula, continued to grow and develop until the middle of the nineteenth century. The introduction of Western massage in 1880 had a tremendous influence on traditional amma massage. Western massage and amma were entirely different in terms of origins, courses of development, and therapeutic principles. Whereas amma massage is based on the theory of *tsubo* (vital points on the body) and the *keiraku* (meridians) connecting them, and prescribes massage moving from the center of the body outward to the limbs, Western massage stresses motion towards the heart. Moreover, the two kinds of massage have different areas of effectiveness. Amma massage brings relief from fatigue, sluggishness, stiff shoulders, headaches, chilling in the hands and feet, and swelling. Western massage, on the other hand, acts on the nerves, joints, muscles, and endocrine system to bring relief in cases of apoplexy, infantile paralysis, stiffness in the muscles caused by age, numbness and pain in the arms, pain in the stomach and intestines, and chronic constipation.

At the time European massage was introduced, Japanese specialists studied the imported theories and techniques, and ultimately developed a system combining them with amma massage to evolve a distinctive Japanese massage system unlike any other in the world. When it became obvious that massage was effective in surgery and plastic surgery, medical institutions started using it as a clinical procedure. Its popularity with the general public grew, as did the demand for masseurs.

There are six basic massage techniques:

1. *Light Pressure:* Suitable light pressure applied to the area being massaged improves the circulation of blood and lymph, and provides stimulation to the nerves, muscles, and internal organs. This, in turn, regulates the sensitivity of the skin and invigorates dermal breathing and the functioning of the sweat and sebaceous glands, thus nourishing and rejuvenating the skin itself. The effect of such massage on the abdomen is to regulate the functioning of the stomach and intestines, to facilitate digestion and absorption of food, and to remove the causes of constipation. Light pressure of this kind on the affected place removes such symptoms as chilling caused in the feet and hands by paralysis and numbness, and swelling caused by obstructions in the circulatory system.

2. *Rubbing and Kneading:* This technique is used mostly on muscles. The muscle, held firmly but lightly, is moved in circular patterns by the palm or the balls of the fingers. Improving the circulation and metabolism helps the muscles recover from fatigue, strengthens them, and improves their powers of contraction and their resilience. It strengthens the arms and legs of children who are thin or afflicted with paralysis, removes fat from the elderly, strengthens the stomach and intestines, and relieves constipation.

3. *Pressing:* In this method, one presses on the surface of the body with the palms, thumbs, or four fingers, with the aim of calming hyperfunctioning of the nerves and muscles, and moderating excitement. It is excellent for treating neuralgia or muscular aches and tensions. Light pressure on the abdomen regulates the functioning of the stomach and intestines.

4. *Vibration:* The masseur holds the muscle and shakes it lightly. This is especially helpful in paralytic numbing in small muscles—fingers and toes—and in the fine branchings of the nervous system.

5. *Tapping:* Tapping with both hands improves blood circulation and the motor nerves in skin and muscles, and in this way relieves fatigue and stimulates the metabolism. Used on the chest, it can relieve

asthma. On the abdomen, it strengthens the stomach and intestines, and relieves gastroatony and gastroptosis.

6. *Circular Pressure:* In this rubbing and kneading method, pressure is applied in decreasing concentric circles around the affected part. It is good for breaking up and stimulating the absorption of pathological deposits in joints. It is effective when joints remain rigid and painful even after fever and swelling have ceased and when joints do not bend properly after partial paralysis or apoplexy. It works well against the severe pain and grating that sometimes develop in the joints of people over 50.

The complications and tensions of modern living affect all of us. Many of the sicknesses and nervous symptoms prevalent today cannot be solved or cured by medical science. This is, of course, something for the medical profession to think about.

One of the steps that ought to be taken is to synthesize the good aspects of both Western and Eastern medical traditions—including both kinds of massage—for the production of a clinical science suited to our times.

## Groups and Associations

(853) **THE ALLIANCE OF STUDENTS AND PRACTITIONERS OF MEDICAL MASSAGE AND RELATED THERAPIES**
c/o The Swedish Institute
875 Avenue of the Americas
New York, NY 10001

(212) 855-1720

*Mary Lou Clairmont, President*
Serves to bring together students and practitioners of massage in mutual support for intertherapy, information exchange, and collective economic strength. The alliance circulates to its members a newsletter and announcements, a calendar of New York City events, copies of current and proposed legislation, and annotated reading lists. Economically, the group is involved in group advertising, group rates for liability insurance, a supplies co-op, and workshops and seminars with reduced rates for members. Workshops cover such areas as herbology, polarity and other forms of massage, medical systems review, and psychic and bioenergetic aspects of massage.

(854) **NEW YORK STATE SOCIETY OF MEDICAL MASSEURS**
P.O. Box 219
Pearl River, NY 10965

(212) 288-6962

*Otto Kellberg, President*
Dedicated to promoting the benefits of massage, maintaining professional and ethical standards, developing continuing education, and fostering professional interests and protecting the legal rights of those engaged in the massage profession. Membership consists of licensed New York masseurs and masseuses, students of massage, and members of allied health professions. Founded 1927.

(855) **AMERICAN MASSAGE AND THERAPY ASSOCIATION, INC.**
152 West Wisconsin Avenue
Milwaukee, WI 53203

(414) 271-1475

A nonprofit organization with chapters and individual members in the U.S. and Canada. List of individual massage therapists available.

## Schools, Centers, and Clinics

**HEALTH AWARENESS INSTITUTE** (clinic)/Phoenix, AZ **(see 74)**

**BERKELEY HOLISTIC HEALTH CENTER** (educational)/Berkeley, CA **(see 76)**

**METAMORPHOSIS** (growth center)/Berkeley, CA **(see 1048)**

**ESALEN INSTITUTE** (educational workshops)/Big Sur; San Francisco, CA **(see 1051)**

**CENTER FOR FAMILY GROWTH** (birth)/Cotati, CA **(see 8)**

**HIDDEN VALLEY HEALTH RANCH** (resort, fasting)/Escondido, CA **(see 166)**

**ASHTON SCHOOL OF PHYSIOHYDROTHERAPY**/Los Angeles, CA **(see 235)**

**BARAKA** (holistic clinic)/Los Angeles, CA **(see 87)**

**HOLISTIC HEALTH CENTER** (treatment and education)/Los Angeles, CA **(see 90)**

**MONOVIN** (touch, silent communication)/Los Angeles, CA **(see 889)**

(856) **VINCENT SCHOOL AND INSTITUTE**
6230 Wilshire Boulevard
Los Angeles, CA 90048

(213) 937-3510

*Ernest V. Athenour, DC, Director*

A California Department of Education approved school of massage therapy. Presently developing a holistic system of therapy called "kinesiotherapy," involving work at three levels of psychophysical function: (1) spiritual/mental, (2) nutritional/biochemical, and (3) mechanical/Kinesiotherapeutic.

**(857) GETTING IN TOUCH**
Box 1225
Los Gatos, CA 95030

(408) 354-3433

Offers workshops in massage, centering, breathing, and other body awareness techniques. Emphasis is on the value of touch in human relationships. Training programs are offered for helping professionals.

**WHITE CROSS SOCIETY** (workshops)/Lucerne Valley, CA **(see 93)**

**SOMA INSTITUTE** (workshops)/Marina Del Rey, CA **(see 1034)**

**McCORNACK CENTER FOR THE HEALING ARTS** (multidisciplinary clinic)/Mendocino, CA **(see 95)**

**WELLNESS RESOURCE CENTER** (prevention)/Mill Valley, CA **(see 96)**

**(858) MASSAGE CENTER**
300 Bryant
Palo Alto, CA 94301

(415) 321-7133

*Bonnie R. Richardson*

Seven partners dedicated to giving and teaching sensitive, therapeutic massage. Massage techniques are drawn primarily from the Swedish and Esalen style, but also incorporate elements of shiatsu, polarity, and Rolfing. Classes and workshops are given on both beginning and advanced levels, and include work with breathing, movement, anatomy, and exploration of non-verbal experience. Founded 1971.

**SAN ANDREAS HEALTH CENTER** (multidisciplinary therapy center)/Palo Alto, CA **(see 101)**

**HUMAN POTENTIAL CAMP** (holistic resort)/Point Arena, CA **(see 169)**

**AGE OF ENLIGHTENMENT CENTER FOR HOLISTIC HEALTH** (Transcendental Meditation and therapy)/San Diego, CA **(see 104)**

**AHLEF** (massage center)/San Francisco, CA **(see 838)**

**(859) AU-MAKUA SCHOOL OF PRACTICAL MASSAGE**
95 Grand View Avenue
San Francisco, CA 94114

(415) 826-8233

*Maureen Barber, Founder and Director*

Provides students with training to qualify as professional massage technicians. Areas of study include anatomy, relaxation techniques, sensitivity through touch, body movement, and at least 100 hours of practical instruction in acu-

pressure and Swedish massage.

**CHURCH OF GENTLE BROTHERS AND SISTERS** (educational)/San Francisco, CA **(see 109)**

**EAST-WEST ACADEMY OF HEALING ARTS** (educational)/San Francisco, CA **(see 110)**

**FAMILY SAUNA SHOP** (bath facilities)/San Francisco, CA **(see 236)**

**(860) THE MASSAGE INSTITUTE**
3119 Clement Street
San Francisco, CA 94121

(415) 668-0550

*Carole F. Turman, Director*

Offers massage utilizing principles of breathing awareness, sensory awareness, postural efficiency, anatomy and physiology.

**NURSE CONSULTANTS AND HEALTH COUNSELORS** (educational)/San Francisco, CA **(see 112)**

**ORR SPRINGS ASSOCIATION** (resort and spa)/Ukiah, CA **(see 170)**

**STEWART MINERAL SPRINGS** (resort spa type facilities)/Weed, CA **(see 171)**

**WILBUR HOT SPRINGS** (bath facility)/Wilbur Springs, CA **(see 1071)**

**(861) BOULDER SCHOOL OF MASSAGE THERAPY**
2855 Walnut Street
Boulder, CO 80301

(303) 443-5131

*Honora Lee Wolfe, Director*

Prepares students for careers as massage technicians. Offers a 1000-hour program of study in nutrition, anatomy and physiology, acupressure, Swedish, polarity, Reichian, and reflexology massage, hydrotherapy, and massage ethics and business practices.

**COMMUNITY FREE SCHOOL** (educational)/Boulder, CO **(see 119)**

**NEW HAVEN CENTER FOR HUMAN RELATIONS**/New Haven, CT **(see 1077)**

**INTEGRAL HEALTH SERVICES** (holistic clinic and educational facility)/Putnam, CT **(see 120)**

**CENTERS FOR HEALTH AND LIFE** (wholistic treatment facility)/Des Moines, IA **(see 126)**

**MARTIN BUBER INSTITUTE** (wholistic, educational and treatment)/Columbia, MD **(see 127)**

**INSTITUTE FOR HUMANISTIC AND TRANSPERSONAL EDUCATION**/Amherst, MA **(see 1147)**

**COMPREHENSIVE THERAPIES** (family and group)/Brookline, MA **(see 1097)**

**PSYCHOPHYSICAL APPROACHES**

**INSTITUTE FOR PSYCHOENERGETICS** (psychophysical workshops)/Brookline, MA **(see 128)**

**NEW ENGLAND CENTER** (body workshops)/Leverett, MA **(see 843)**

**SAGARIS-WOMEN'S THERAPY COLLECTIVE** (psychotherapy and body work)/Minneapolis, MN **(see 1109)**

**INSTITUTE FOR SELF DEVELOPMENT** (body workshops and treatment)/Manhasset, NY **(see 137)**

**NEW AGE HEALTH FARM** (wholistic resort and rest home)/Neversink, NY **(see 172)**

**REILLY'S ON 34th ST** (physiotherapy)/New York, NY **(see 141)**

**(862) SERENITY**
Natural Living Center
310 East 72nd Street
New York, NY 10021

(212) 988-9320

Facilities include massage, sauna, yoga meditation, and an herb and spice shop.

**(863) SWEDISH INSTITUTE**
875 Avenue of the Americas
New York, NY 10001

(212) 695-3964

*Sydney Zarinsky*

Workshops and classes in Swedish massage, Oriental medicine, herbology, and related subjects.

**PSI CENTER** (wholistic clinic and educational facility)/Cincinnati, OH **(see 145)**

**EUGENE CENTER FOR THE HEALING ARTS** (educational)/Eugene, OR **(see 148)**

**EAST-WEST ACADEMY OF HEALTH PRACTICES** (educational)/Portland, OR **(see 644)**

**INSTITUTE OF PREVENTIVE MEDICINE**/Portland, OR **(see 149)**

**CLYMER HEALTH CLINIC** (wholistic clinic)/Quakertown, PA **(see 150)**

**ESOTERIC PHILOSOPHY CENTER** (community education)/Houston, TX **(see 151)**

**THE COMMUNITY HEALTH CENTER** (wholistic clinic)/Burlington, VT **(see 152)**

**HOME CENTER** (wholistic clinic and educational center)/Virginia Beach, VA **(see 155)**

**PREVENTIVE MEDICINE CLINIC**/Bellevue, WA **(see 156)**

**(864) RADIANCE—HERBS AND MASSAGE**
218½ West Fourth Street
Olympia, WA 98501

(206) 357-9470

A therapeutic massage studio teaching and practicing Swedish and Esalen massage, with additional work offered in reflexology, polarity, acupressure, kinesiology and iridology. There is also a retail shop which sells herbs and herbal products, oils, and books on herbs and massage. Founded 1975.

**DIAT- UND KNIEPP-SANATORIUM DR. FELBERMAYER** (wholistic spa: anthroposophical)/Austria **(see 812)**

**(865) SMAE INSTITUTE**
New Hall
Maidenhead, Berkshire
England

Tel: Maidenhead 21100

*D.M. Eames, Principal*

Offers a correspondence course in Swedish Massage and physiotherapy. Graduates are eligible to become Associates of the Institute of Swedish Massage; further study confers eligibility to become Members. The SMAE journal is available to both Associates and Members. Founded 1919.

**TYRINGHAM NATUROPATHIC CLINIC** (wholistic spa)/Bucks, England **(see 177)**

**COMPANY OF SOMOTAGRAPHERS** (body work)/London, England **(see 845)**

**ROYAL PUMP ROOM** (physiotherapy)/Warwickshire, England **(see 237)**

**ITA-WEGMAN-KLINIK** (anthroposophical clinic)/Arlesheim, Switzerland **(see 813)**

**SANATORIUM SONNENECK** (anthroposophical clinic)/Arlesheim, Switzerland **(see 815)**

**FILDERKLINIK** (anthroposophical hospital)/West Germany **(see 816)**

**FRIEDRICH HUSEMANN-KLINIK** (anthroposophical clinic)/West Germany **(see 817)**

**GEMEINÜTZIGES GEMEINSCHAFTSKRANKENHAUS HERDECKE** (anthroposophical hospital)/West Germany **(see 818)**

**KLINIK ÖSCHELBRONN** (anthroposophical clinic)/West Germany **(see 820)**

**OTTO BUCHINGER CLINIC** (wholistic resort)/West Germany **(see 181)**

**PARACELSUS-KRANKENHAUS** (rest home)/West Germany **(see 822)**

**SANATORIUM SCHLOSS HAMBORN** (anthroposophical clinic)/West Germany **(see 824)**

## Journals and Publications

**WELL-BEING MAGAZINE** (multidisciplinary)/San Diego, CA **(see 186)**

**COMMON GROUND** (multidisciplinary directory, San Francisco Bay Area)/San Francisco, CA **(see 187)**

**ALTERNATIVES JOURNAL** (multidisciplinary new age articles)/Miami, FL **(see 193)**

**EAST WEST JOURNAL** (magazine) (multidisciplinary new age articles)/Brookline, MA **(see 195)**

**NEW AGE JOURNAL** (magazine) (multidisciplinary)/Brookline, MA **(see 196)**

**SEEKER** (multidisciplinary newsletter directory NY area)/New York, NY **(see 202)**

## Products and Services

**LIVING EARTH CRAFTS** (massage tables)/Cotati, CA **(see 887)**

**ELECTROPEDIC PROFESSIONAL MASSAGERS**/Los Angeles, CA **(see 423)**

**HEALTH RESEARCH** (books)/Mokelumne Hill, CA **(see 209)**

**QUINTESSENCE UNLIMITED** (consciousness tools)/Boulder, CO **(see 215)**

**J.A. PRESTON CORPORATION** (massage unit)/New York, NY **(see 432)**

**GREAT EARTH HEALING, INC.** (ma roller)/East Montpelier, VT; Montreal, Canada **(see 229)**

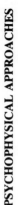

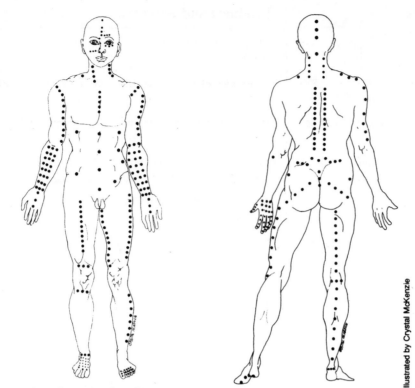

Illustrated by Crystal McKenzie

Anterior and posterior view of the shiatsu pressure points.

# Shiatsu
*Shizuto Masunaga*

Some Japanese words like *Zen, judo,* and *tofu* have already been accepted into other languages unaltered because the things they stand for are so characteristically Japanese and reflect so distinctive a Japanese cultural and spiritual element that they are extremely difficult to translate. The same thing is true of the word *shiatsu.* Though this word can be literally translated as finger *(shi)* pressure *(atsu)* and though these English words give a vague idea of the techniques used in shiatsu, such terms by no means convey the depth of experience which shiatsu produces through contact with the human skin. This is one of the reasons for the rapid growth in popularity of shiatsu both in Japan and in other countries today.

Manipulation with the hands for therapeutic purposes is as old as mankind. In the ancient past the Indians and the Chinese placed special emphasis on massage. Under the name of *amma,* massage was introduced into Japan with other aspects of Chinese medicine, in the eighth century. But by the Edo period (1600–1867), it had fallen from esteem. Because of its relaxing effects amma came to be thought of more as a pleasure than as a therapy. Later many different people developed many different amma massage techniques which were given various names. In the late Meiji period (1868–1911), a law was passed regarding amma. A reevaluation was made of a book on amma *(Amma Zukai),* published in the early nineteenth century, and based on the methods shown in that book, shiatsu, as a system of manual massage therapy, was legally born in 1955—after a 2,000-year gestation as an Oriental medical tradition.

Japanese law now recognizes three therapeutic systems in which the practitioner applies manual pressure to the surface of the patient's body: amma massage, Western-style massage, and shiatsu. Shiatsu differs from the rhythmical, varied and very complicated amma and Western-massage systems in that it is a simple, basic application of pressure on the body to one point at a time. The three principles of shiatsu are pressure applied in a direction perpendicular to the patient's body, prolonged pressure, and spiritual concentration. The characteristics that truly set shiatsu off from the other systems are prolonged pressure and spiritual concentration. Shiatsu is so simple and so easily accepted and passed on by ordinary people that there are those who insist that it has broken from the subordinate position in therapeutic treatment and that its very motions themselves produce healing effects.

In recent times, with the growing popularity of acupuncture, the tsubo and meridians *(keiraku),* are seen to represent elements of primary importance to this treatment method. The theories of tsubo and meridians are fundamental to Oriental medical thought. Greater emphasis on the validity of these theories resulted in a greater recognition of the effectiveness of shiatsu, which is, in effect, nothing but stimulus applied to the tsubo.

Because documents on the meridians relate largely to acupuncture, theories connected with them have developed mainly in connection with that branch of therapy. The tsubo, located along the various meridians, are the places at which the acupuncture needle is inserted. Much study has been devoted to determining which tsubo are related to which sickness. Shiatsu has adopted the same system of meridians, and shiatsu pressure is applied on the same tsubo. In the distant past, however, according to Chinese medical documents, manual manipulation (massage) was regarded as of the utmost importance in diagnosing diseases and in ascertaining the locations of the tsubo for the insertion of the acupuncture needle.

I began to study the actual nature of the meridians without relying on ancient Chinese documents. However, I was more fully able to clarify the basic concept of the meridians when I saw that the Chinese method of manipulating for diagnosis was the origin of prolonged pressure applications. Since then modern charts of meridians have been simplified for easy understanding in acupuncture and moxa therapy.

The theory of meridians must be recognized on the basis of traditional Oriental medical theory by means of the principles of manual therapy. To this end it is necessary that shiatsu techniques be correctly carried out and that continued research be performed in order to prove the validity of this kind of treatment. In pathological cases, the areas around the affected tsubo on the meridians harden. Pressure applied to them calls into play the entire cooperative organization of the body and stimulates flow in the meridians, restoring health.

Dr. Katsusuke Serizawa proved that ordinary massage has the effect of increasing heartbeat and pulse waves, and, in this way, of stimulating the circulation. Using the same experimental system in a follow-up test on shiatsu, I showed that its effect is exactly the opposite. Whereas ordinary massage stimulates the sympathetic nervous system to encourage circulation, shiatsu operates on the parasympathetic nervous system, which tends to retard circulation. Thus, shiatsu treatment produces a state of muscular relaxation of both mind and body. Though the pressure stimulates the skin, which activates the sympathetic nervous system, because the pressure is steady and prolonged, it suppresses the working of these nerves. Furthermore, since the pressure is applied in a direction perpendicular to the skin and towards the deep inner organs, it stimulates these organs and leads the body into a condition in which the parasympathetic nervous system becomes activated.

To exert this kind of prolonged pressure, the practitioner and his movements must be stable. He must not press with hands and fingers only but must lean his entire body on the body of the patient. He must have the feeling that the body of the patient is supporting his own. The action of the cerebral marginal systems of both patient and practitioner will be stimulated, and this in turn will stimulate the operation of the old layer of the cerebral cortex, thus creating a communal sense of primitive life. The human rapport established between the two people awakens the patient's innate curative powers and increases the therapeutic effects of treatment.

To effect flow in the meridians, pressure on one point alone is insufficient. Instead, the practitioner must use both hands, one on each of two points. Ancient documents show that people of the past employed this method, which I have systemized and popularized in recent years. This system, which might be called "meridian shiatsu," is based on the kind of duality that runs through Oriental thought as the theory of yin and yang, or negative and positive elements. The power of yin and yang makes possible mystical operations. The yin elements are difficult to see, but their concealed actions help life assume its proper forms. The yang elements are visible. In pathological incidents, the disordered part is the yang element, but it is the operation of the yin, or concealed elements, that brings about the cure.

Ordinary shiatsu and ordinary acupuncture and moxa correspond almost exactly to yin and yang, but two-hand shiatsu encompasses in itself both yin and yang and therefore constitutes a complete therapy. For this reason, it can be of especially great value to people living in modern society.

## Schools, Centers, and Clinics

**BERKELEY HOLISTIC HEALTH CENTER** (educational center)/Berkeley, CA (see 76)

**(866) ACUPRESSURE WORKSHOP**
1872 Sepulveda Boulevard
Los Angeles, CA 90025

(213) 478-7828

*Iona and Ron Teeguarden*

Offers a series of lectures and workshops on Jin Shin Jyutsu, a form of acupressure massage. Personal treatments in Jin Shin are also available. Additional course offerings include yoga, T'ai Chi, cooking, anatomy, and physiology.

**HOLISTIC HEALTH CENTER** (educational center)/Los Angeles, CA (see 90)

**KHALSA MEDICAL AND COUNSELING ASSOCIATES** (wholistic clinic)/Los Angeles, CA (see 92)

**INSTITUTE FOR CREATIVE AGING** (growth center)/Malibu, CA (see 94)

**McCORNACK CENTER FOR THE HEALING ARTS** (wholistic clinic and school)/Mendocino, CA (see 95)

**GEORGE OHSAWA MACROBIOTIC FOUNDATION**/Oroville, CA (see 535)

**(867) SHIATSU THERAPY CENTER**
924 29th Street
Sacramento, CA 95816

(916) 441-5011

A center staffed by certified shiatsu (acupressure) therapists, for individual treatment.

**AGE OF ENLIGHTENMENT CENTER FOR HOLISTIC HEALTH** (clinic)/San Diego, CA (see 104)

**SAN DIEGO NATURAL HEALTH CLINIC**/San Diego, CA (see 108)

**AHLEF** (massage center)/San Francisco, CA (see 838)

**NURSE CONSULTANTS AND HEALTH COUNSELORS** (holistic clinic)/San Francisco, CA (see 112)

**GARDEN OF SANJIVANI** (herb school)/Santa Cruz, CA (see 543)

**UNIVERSITY OF CALIFORNIA EXTENSION** (holistic health program)/Santa Cruz, CA (see 115)

**BOULDER SCHOOL OF MASSAGE THERAPY**/Boulder, CO (see 861)

**INTEGRAL HEALTH SERVICES** (wholistic clinic and workshops)/Putnam, CT (see 120)

**CORNUCOPIA CENTERS** (holistic school)/Miami, FL (see 124)

**EAST WEST FOUNDATION** (macrobiotics)/Boston, MA (see 536)

**CONTACT HEALING SEMINARS** (acupressure)/New York, NY (see 792)

**(868) SHIATSU DOJO OF NEW YORK**
52 West 55th Street, 2nd Floor
New York, NY 10019

(212) 582-3424

*W. Ohashi, Director*

Offers ongoing workshops as well as treatment in shiatsu.

**EAST-WEST ACADEMY OF HEALTH PRACTICES** (acupuncture center and clinic)/Portland, OR (see 644)

**HOME CENTER** (educational center)/Virginia Beach, VA (see 155)

**(869) THE TORONTO SHIATSU CENTER**
177 College Street
Toronto, Ontario, Canada

(416) 979-2824

*T. Saito*

Offers ongoing workshops as well as treatment in shiatsu.

**(870) IOGAI SHIATSU CENTER**
7-3-6 Ginza
Chuo, Tokyo, Japan

Tel: 03-573-3169

Offers ongoing workshops and treatment in shiatsu.

**(871) IOKAI SHIATSU CENTER**
1-8-9 Higashi Ueno
Taito Ward
Tokyo, Japan

Tel: 03-832-2983

Offers ongoing workshops and treatments in shiatsu.

## Journals and Publications

**WELL-BEING MAGAZINE** (natural health articles)/San Diego, CA **(see 186)**

**COMMON GROUND** (multidisciplinary directory San Francisco Bay Area)/San Francisco, CA **(see 187)**

**ALTERNATIVES JOURNAL** (multidisciplinary new age articles)/Miami, FL **(see 193)**

**EAST WEST JOURNAL** (magazine) (multidisciplinary new age articles)/Brookline, MA **(see 195)**

**NEW AGE JOURNAL** (magazine) (multidisciplinary)/Brookline, MA **(see 196)**

**SEEKER** (multidisciplinary newsletter directory NY area)/New York, NY **(see 202)**

## Products and Services

**LIVING EARTH CRAFTS** (shiatsu massage tables)/Cotati, CA **(see 887)**

(872) **JAPAN PUBLICATIONS TRADING CO., LTD.**
200 Clearbrook Road
Elmsford, NY 10523

*Masakatsu Mochizuki, President*

1225 Howard Street
San Francisco, CA 94103

P.O. Box 5030 Tokyo International
Tokyo 101-31
Japan

In recent years has begun to develop a line of books on wholistic medicine from a Japanese perspective. The books have covered such areas as acupuncture, shiatsu, Oki-yoga, ki development, and biorhythms.

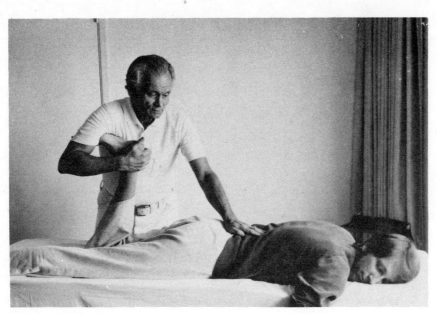

Photo courtesy of Pierre Pannetier

# Polarity Therapy
*Pierre Pannetier*

In recent years science has examined the existence of energy fields within the human body. The knowledge of energy currents and their integral relationship throughout the body has opened up opportunities for the reevaluation of health maintenance. Polarity therapy is a comprehensive and practical system of health developed by Dr. Randolph Stone. Drawn from his 60 years of the practice and study of Western and Oriental medicine and philosophy, polarity therapy coordinates diet, exercise, and techniques of body manipulation to increase and balance the flow of vital energy for the physical, emotional, and mental well-being of the individual. According to Dr. Stone, the vital energy of the body follows certain channels which interlink and reflect the condition of particular parts of the body all along the energy channels. Moving between the positive and negative poles—the head and feet, respectively—the energy channels sweep through all the vital organs and glands.

All of nature reflects the forces of positive, neutral, and negative energy, whether it is in the structure of the atom, the human cell and its division, or the magnetic lines of our planet. The polarity of these three forces is nature's means of balancing its diverse elements; the alignment of forces creates harmony, while their disorientation produces confusion. The health of the individual is a subtle balance of the mental, emotional, and physical forces, and their disruption appears in disease or "imbalance"—a block in the flow of the energy along the channels of the body. By means of external and internal treatment of the body, following the principles of polarity therapy, there is a strengthening and balancing of the energy systems producing a state of relaxation, calm, and health.

Polarity therapy attempts to restore balance to the body-mind of an individual by a four-point program of good clear thinking, manipulation, exercise, and correct diet.

*Right Thinking* is the basis of good health. As we think, so we are. The philosophy of polarity therapy advances the concept that self-improvement is a must, and that people should never limit themselves. This positive attitude is all-important because self-confidence is the primordial factor for success. But although polarity therapists support a right attitude, they do not force anything on anyone, not even themselves. In this, they follow the wisdom of Nature, which does not force but builds slowly and steadily.

*Manipulations* balance the flow of vital energy, causing relaxation and the return of normal function to all organs. In polarity therapy manipulations are carried out with gentle body contacts which alleviate tensions and blocks by application of both hands to specific pressure points on the body.

*Exercise*, as used in polarity therapy, is known as "polarity yoga" and comprises postures and movements chosen to give immediate results when practiced even for only a few minutes daily. This group of easy stretching postures was developed for self-help, to release energy blocks, and balance the energy flow.

*Diet*, as defined by polarity therapy, is based on a cleansing and purifying process, emphasizing the value of fresh fruits and vegetables combined with other natural foods. Persons seeking help from polarity therapists are also instructed about the effects of the emotions on eating and digestion. When this interaction is rightly understood, the person desiring total health learns to eat only when feeling calm and happy.

Polarity therapy is a simple and direct approach, easily comprehended by anyone interested in self-improvement and in helping others. Love and understanding are the chief qualifications for applying the art of polarity therapy. Teachers see themselves as mere channels; everyone has the power to heal himself or herself.

In *Energy, the Vital Polarity in the Healing Art*, Dr. Stone writes: "In this age of overspecialization, with emphasis on chemistry, bacteriology, and mechanical and surgical research, we have lost sight of the overall picture of man as a living being with lines of force working in fields of finer energies. These lines of force constitute his real being, and operate in and through the body in a continual exchange of new energy."

The ideal of a subtle invisible energy that is everywhere and sustains all life has been put forth by all the major religions of mankind. And in our time science calls it different names—"bioplasma," "L-fields," "psychoenergetics," and "orgone." Energy exists in space and courses around and through the individual, beginning with the growth of the fetus and withdrawing at the moment of death. Polarity therapy recognizes the integral nature of the body and mind and that health forms a demonstrable bond between them. This wholistic health model adds a dimension beyond the interrelated material systems of the blood, muscle, and bone. Whether it is for the body or mind, the balm of life has come through the transforming agent of energy. It is energy that restores the spent corporeal resources, balances the strained mind, and ultimately lifts the spirits so that man feels whole again.

## Schools, Centers and Clinics

**BERKELEY HOLISTIC HEALTH CENTER**
(workshops)/Berkeley, CA **(see 76)**

(873) **POLARITY CENTER OF BERKELEY**
2054 University Avenue, Room 607
Berkeley, CA 94704

(415) 848-6460

*Atten: Ray and Sandra Castellino*

Offers treatment and training workshops in polarity therapy.

(874) **THE POLARITY HEALTH INSTITUTE**
Fall River Mills, CA 96028

(916) 336-5141

*Jefferson and Sharon Campbell, Directors*

Offers treatment and training workshops in polarity therapy.

**MEADOWLARK** (holistic resort)/Hemet, CA **(see 167)**

(875) **THE POLARITY CENTER**
620 Palomar
La Jolla, CA 92037

(714) 459-0967

*Atten: Plum Tree*

Offers treatment and training workshops in polarity therapy.

(876) **POLARITY HEALTH CENTER OF MILL VALLEY**
9 Bernard Street
Mill Valley, CA 94941

(415) 383-4833

*Atten: Peter Pick and Steven Shimm*

Offers treatment and training workshops in polarity therapy.

(877) **PIERRE PANNETIER POLARITY CENTER**
401 North Glassell Street
Orange, CA 92666

(714) 532-3035

*Pierre Pannetier, Director*

Offers treatment and training workshops in polarity therapy.

INSTITUTE FOR MYSTICAL AND PARAPSY-CHOLOGICAL STUDIES (workshops)/Orinda, CA (see 782)

(878) POLARITY THERAPY CENTER OF PALO ALTO
748 Bryant Street
Palo Alto, CA 94301

(415) 326-4270

*Atten: Harold and Nancy Boritz*

Offers treatment and training workshops in polarity therapy.

(879) POLARITY CENTER
1620 Sacramento Street
Redding, CA 96001

*Atten: Jeffrey McMeans*

Offers treatment and training workshops in polarity therapy.

AHLEF (massage center)/San Francisco, CA (see 838)

(880) POLARITY HEALTH CENTER OF SAN FRANCISCO
649 Irving Street
San Francisco, CA 94122

(415) 661-1884

*Atten: James Feil*

Offers treatment and training workshops in polarity therapy.

(881) POLARITY CENTER OF SAN JOSE
165 North Redwood Avenue
San Jose, CA 95128

(408) 984-0774

*Atten: Rune Moeller*

Offers treatment and workshops in polarity therapy.

GARDEN OF SANJIVANI (herb school)/Santa Cruz, CA (see 543)

STEWART HOT SPRINGS (resort)/Weed, CA (see 171)

(882) POLARITY HEALTH & WELL BEING CENTER OF MENDOCINO COUNTY
P.O. Box 1129
Willits, CA 95490

*Atten: Diane Dickey*

Offers treatment and workshop training in polarity therapy.

(883) POLARITY THERAPY
2011 Bluff
Boulder, CO 80302

(303) 449-7938

*Atten: Joe Raffaelo*

Offers treatment and training workshops in polarity therapy.

BOULDER SCHOOL OF MASSAGE THERAPY/Boulder, CO (see 861)

INTEGRAL HEALTH SERVICES (holistic clinic and school)/Putnam, CT (see 120)

NEW ENGLAND CENTER (massage)/Leverett, MA (see 843)

(884) DUTTON POLARITY THERAPY
3083 Glencreek Court
Caledonia, MI 49316

*Atten: Grant and Violet Dutton*

Offers treatment and training workshops in polarity therapy.

DESERT LIGHT FOUNDATION (holistic clinic and school)/Albuquerque, NM (see 134)

EUGENE CENTER FOR THE HEALING ARTS (educational center)/Eugene, OR (see 148)

(885) POLARITY HEALTH STUDIO
755½ West Tenth
Eugene, OR 97402

(503) 895-2863

*Atten: Gene Bicksler*

Offers treatment and training workshops in polarity therapy.

EAST-WEST ACADEMY OF HEALTH PRACTICES (acupuncture, acupressure center and clinic)/Portland, OR (see 644)

INSTITUTE OF PREVENTIVE MEDICINE (holistic clinic and school)/Portland, OR (see 149)

(886) POLARITY CENTER OF SEATTLE
1107 Eighteenth Avenue
Seattle, WA 98144

(206) 324-1937

*Atten: David Mohler*

Offers treatment and training workshops in polarity therapy.

## Journals and Publications

WELL-BEING MAGAZINE (natural health)/San Diego, CA (see 186)

COMMON GROUND (multidisciplinary directory San Francisco Bay Area)/San Francisco, CA (see 187)

ALTERNATIVES JOURNAL (multidisciplinary new age articles)/Miami, FL (see 193)

SEEKER (New York area multidisciplinary source listing)/New York, NY (see 202)

## Products and Services

(887) LIVING EARTH CRAFTS
10028 C Minnesota Avenue
Cotati, CA 94928

(707) 795-4226

Professionally made, easily adjustable massage tables for Rolfing, shiatsu, physical therapy, polarity and acupuncture.

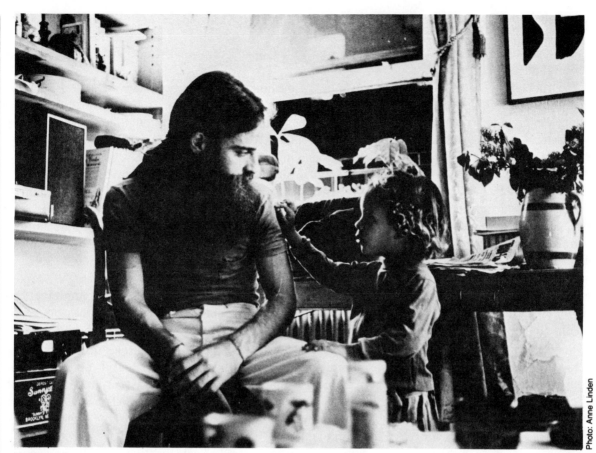

Father and Son

Photo: Anne Linden

# Sensory Awareness
*Charles V. W. Brooks*

The function of Sensory Awareness is nothing less than to breathe life into everything we do. We address ourselves to the whole spectrum of living. In our classes we allow time, over and over again, to become quiet in our minds and awake in our perceptions—exploring activities that may at first glance seem novel, even bizarre, but are essentially the raw material of daily living itself. Our classwork consists in practicing an ever fuller attention to whatever we are doing. We gradually come to discover how and where our habits of mind and the efforts we have learned to make, both in their conscious thought forms and in their incarnation as nerve and muscle syndromes, inhibit us from the total organismic functioning that is natural to us.

There is no way to understand Sensory Awareness other than through the down-to-earth experience of attending a workshop. The workshops, like religious or psychedelic experience, open the door on a new and wonderfully richer world, confirming the intuition we had forgotten, but never lost; that living can be its own reward.

For professionals, such an experience can cast a new light on therapy. They may no longer view themselves as "therapists" who, with techniques and learning, heal "patients." Rather, the healing situation becomes one in which people with varying experience explore together the hindrances to fuller living, and then that fuller living itself.

The "technique" is finding a means to quiet the compulsive intellectual processes—the evaluations, the rationalizations, the fantasies—so that messages from the whole sensory nervous apparatus can come through to consciousness and bring about, through the entire person, appropriate readjustments to any actual situation. The impetus to total functioning is no longer a "struggle for survival," but *joie de vivre, élan vital*—the indefinable impulse of living itself.

What actually happens in a Sensory Awareness workshop that can—and often does—bring about such far-reaching consequences?

In an actual class we might spend twenty minutes at a time sensing how we relate to the floor under our feet—perhaps shifting weight gently from side to side, perhaps just exploring balance. Or, standing or lying, we might move our arms and legs, taking time to feel the movement through, to allow the sensory nerves that accompany all our muscular constellations to rediscover their voice and speak to us. We might explore sound for a while or spend a few minutes playing ball, or a couple of seconds jumping or running.

Sensory awareness has nothing to do with speed or slowness; it has to do only with the time people need to "come to their senses" and really experience the activity they have undertaken, so that it may be unimpeded and fully conscious. The crucial factor is *taking time*—finding in ourselves ever more patience to permit the recognition of what is merely learned exercise in our movements, what is only our *image* of grace or strength or limberness or relaxation. Gradually we begin to discard such foreign elements, acquired from others, and sense the gradual but unmistakable reappearance of authentic movement that owes no allegiance to any of our ideals but springs directly from our nature. We explore touching ourselves and others, taking time to sense our urgencies and our timidities, permitting them slowly to dissolve, sensing our anticipations, our covetousness, our unease, permitting these to recede, feeling little by little how the warmth and aliveness of our tissues communicates involuntarily.

Sensory awareness means the awakening of all the nerves and joints and muscles involved in every act—for instance, shaking hands, smiling, or frowning. Instead of leading to greater "self-consciousness" or self-concern, it helps us discard acquired attitudes from the past, making way for what is called for in the uniqueness of the present. A number of therapies offer methods for *achieving* this result; we explore the ways in which it happens by itself. It can only come about through practice, and practice is what work in Sensory Awareness provides.

We are concerned perhaps above all with our conditioning in the basic function of breathing and with release from that conditioning. Conditioning of breathing comes equally from the anxieties inherent in being born and growing up, and from the methods of teachers and gurus designed to counteract anxiety. Such methods may derive from health manuals or high school calisthenics or from very ancient traditions. This is sensitive territory; it has become the sacred turf of numerous disciplines. There is certainly nothing easy about the separation of natural from conditioned breathing, and the control of one's own nature can be very tempting. But anyone who has ever experienced a sigh of relief or listened to someone breathing peacefully in sleep has an idea of the values at stake.

We also work a good deal on *seeing*. Our "five senses"—that is, the senses relating to the external world—are vital to us; less appreciated, but equally vital, are our inner, or proprioceptive, senses. All living is the interaction of inner and outer worlds; peaceful, attuned living (like that enjoyed by Buddhist practitioners and young children) occurs when these worlds merge to the point where the distinction disappears. But one of our senses, that of sight, has been emphasized (and distorted) out of all proportion to the others. Forgetting that the function of the eye is to perceive, we assign it the intellectual function of making judgments. We say, for instance, "I see it's no use." We speak of "foresight" and "hindsight." We "look inward." We say that God is "watching" us. Nothing so divides us into the observer and observed, the "higher" and "lower," as this venerable confusion of the function of seeing with the functions of definition and evaluation. We forget that the eye is only a window through which, in a thousand ways, we reach out to the world or let it in.

The work sketched here is only a hint of the territory covered. Elsa Gindler of Berlin, who originated the approach sixty years ago, called it "Work on the Human Being." Charlotte Selver, who brought it to this country, named it "Sensory Awareness." Encapsulated in "techniques," it may be of little value, but assimilated through practice, it can open up new worlds of experience.

## Groups and Associations

**(888) THE CHARLOTTE SELVER FOUNDATION, INC.**
32 Cedars Road
Caldwell, NJ 07006

(201) 226-2202

*Mary Alice Roche, Managing Secretary*

A nonprofit, educational corporation dedicated to supporting "the work known as sensory awareness as it is taught by Charlotte Selver, and making it better known in its general content." A list of teachers of sensory awareness is available. Information on sensory awareness is disseminated by the Foundation in the form of workshops, tape recordings of these workshops, and books and publications. A *Bulletin* and notices of workshops and classes are available to financial contributors to the Foundation. Founded 1971.

## Schools and Centers

**(889) MONOVIN (Mostly Non-Verbal Institute)**
1872 South Sepulveda Boulevard
Los Angeles, CA 90025

(213) 479-7110

The Institute offers a variety of programs for individuals, couples, and disabled persons, in massage, sensory awareness, and related techniques. The basic theory and practice at the Institute is the development of human potential through nonverbal forms of interaction.

**PSYCHOTHERAPY AND GROWTH CENTER**/San Jose, CA **(see 1066)**

**BOULDER WORKSHOP** (growth center)/Boulder, CO **(see 1073)**

**SARGASSO: CENTER FOR GROWTH AND DEVELOPMENT** (humanistic approach)/Silver Spring, MD **(see 1088)**

**CAMBRIDGE HOUSE** (humanistic center)/Milwaukee, WI **(see 1129)**

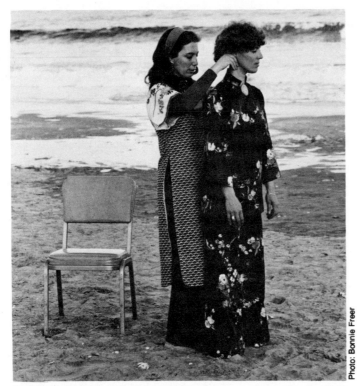

Photo: Bonnie Freer

Ilana Rubenfeld doing Alexander at the Association for Humanistic Psychology Convention, Atlantic City 1976.

# Alexander: The Use Of The Self

*Ilana Rubenfeld*

Born in Australia in 1869, F. M. Alexander came to create his system of body awareness through a problem he encountered in his own life. As a Shakespearean actor he kept losing his voice and finally sought help. "Stop talking and your voice will come back," he was told. He tried this several times, regaining his voice only to lose it again.

Determined to solve his problem, he began observing how he was speaking by using a set of mirrors. Monitoring every subtle movement in the act of speaking, he noticed that the second he began to "think" about a movement, the muscles in his body were already preparing for that movement. In addition, he realized that certain movements were not reflexes, as he once thought, but learned habits. Alexander concluded that if these movements had been learned, they could also be unlearned.

Witnessing his own activity, Alexander discovered that a set of complex actions precedes the beginning speech process and that these actions were contributing to the loss of his voice. Whether he was talking or performing, the pattern of pulling his head back, depressing his larynx, and sucking in breath persisted. After several months Alexander ascertained that he could neither directly control the sucking of breath, nor the depression of his larynx. He could, however, consciously control pulling his head back and down, which had previously shortened the muscles in his neck and depressed his chest.

He began to comprehend that his throat problem was not local, but one that concerned his entire organism. The movements of his head and torso were integrally connected. After dealing with the dynamic relationship among head, neck, and torso, he observed their interconnection with the use of his limbs, the position of his pelvis, and the relationship of his feet to the ground.

The knowledge of this relationship led him to examine his total posture. Once he became aware of how he misused his body, his next task was to discover how to alter old habit patterns and consciously choose a more economical way of using himself. Alexander continued to experiment for over 10 years, and then he returned to the stage. His extraordinary breath control was greatly admired, and subsequently he began teaching other actors how to use themselves properly. In America he taught and befriended John Dewey, who supported his work vigorously. George Bernard Shaw, George Coghill, Sir Charles Sherrington, and Aldous Huxley were among his students, and in 1973 Nikolaas Tinbergan praised his work at a speech he delivered on receiving the Nobel Prize.

Until his death at age 86, Alexander continued developing and refining a method encompassing body-mind awareness, conscious control, and organismic thinking. His remarkable journey helped to underscore an essential aspect of man; the body ''in concert'' with the mind. The Alexander Technique encompasses certain basic principles:

1. Without awareness, we cannot change.
2. In performing an action, the minute you ''think,'' the muscles begin to move.
3. The posture that seems ''right'' may not be. Thus, you could unknowingly be hurting yourself.
4. Habit patterns, in general, are not reflexes, but learned.
5. The use of one part of your body affects the whole body.
6. ''Conscious control'' can be exerted over habit patterns.
7. You have the ability to ''inhibit'' habit patterns and choose an alternate route. Paying attention to ''how'' you get to your goal means staying with your process rather than focusing on the goal itself.
   Alexander termed process as ''means-whereby'' and goals as ''end-gain.''

To understand these principles on only a conceptual level is not enough. To change, a kinesthetic experience must accompany the concept. The following instructions are often used in the process of reeducation:

1. Become aware of what you do, how you think, how you habitually act.
2. Do nothing. Suspend judgment and be willing to leave yourself alone.
3. Imagine other actions, alternatives.
4. Give yourself the ''directions'' (directions are specific sets of words through which guided physical experiences come to have kinesthetic meaning).

To use the directions, the student needs a kinesthetic education. For example, many people think they are moving their neck when, if they looked in the mirror, they would see they are moving their head. Also, people think they are relaxed and when touched by a skilled hand are surprised to discover the opposite.

The following are some of the basic Alexander Directions to which I have added my own comments:

1. *Let the neck be free and move back.* Think about the neck moving back in space. Then ''allow'' it to move back.
2. *Let the head go forward and up.* Think of nodding yes. This motion gives you an idea of forward. Then, think of moving up from the top of your head as though it were a helium balloon. These two directions are interdependent. When the neck is free and moves back in space, and the head goes forward and up, the spine has room to lengthen.
3. *Let the torso lengthen and widen.* This is the opposite of shortening the spine and arching at the lower back.

Misunderstanding these directions may lead to further misuse of the self. Thus, the teacher guides students forward toward discovering the relationship of each part of the body-mind, separately and together, so that they come to experience themselves integrally. In body-mind awareness we discover that nothing is local. What is fundamental is the practice of psychophysical ecology—the full awareness of the synergistic interdependence of body-mind usage in daily functioning.

Initially, there are two main tools used to teach the technique—one is a chair. Observing a student in the activity of getting in and out of a chair provides the teacher with valuable information about the student's habit patterns. Before introducing any directions, the teacher usually requests the students to sit down and get up in their own habitual patterns, making sure that the students notice *how* they use their bodies. In this way the idea is introduced that the process of getting into a chair is as important as the goal of sitting itself. As the use of the entire body comes more and more into the foreground, the act of sitting recedes into the background.

PSYCHOPHYSICAL APPROACHES

Then the teacher begins to guide the student in and out of the chair with words *and* touch. The instructions aid in the integration of the complex relationship of the head, neck, and torso, and eventually include other parts of the body. The word "inhibit" is used here to mean the ability to stop using the old habit patterns, a willingness to leave oneself alone, and subsequently to experience a different total pattern.

At the beginning the student may also lie down on a table and experience a maximum degree of release from tension because of the added support. This is in contrast to doing the same activity while sitting, standing, or walking. Teachers concern themselves not only with the head, neck, and torso relationship but also with the interrelationship of each part of the body with gravity. Activities are individually tailored to the student so that they can become more closely allied with how they use themselves in everyday life.

In this work, touching is a special skill. It is a unique kind of touching—teachers wait to see "where the person is." They do not push through resistances, rather, they wait until the person gives them permission to enter and consents to change. The responsibility for change rests within the person. The will to change is communicated internally, moving outward toward the teacher while the teacher's touch, from the outside, moves inward to meet the person.

The collaborative effort is as necessary for change in body alignment as is the therapeutic alliance in psychotherapy. To a casual observer, it may seem that teachers are doing something "to" students as they move limbs and muscles, but it is the students who release and allow teachers to move them. I call this kind of touching "open hands" since the teacher can sense nonverbally what is occurring in the student's thought, musculature, and skeletal systems. The open hand is not pushy or tense; rather, it is a hand that allows space between the teacher and student for movement and change.

The application of Alexander's work—the concept of inhibition, or the unlearning of uneconomical habits—is far-reaching. Each of us, regardless of occupation, could learn to use our bodies better by applying these principles in daily functions. Alexander's principles have consistently been helpful to those who use their bodies in particular ways. Musicians, dancers, actors, typists, psychotherapists, and architects are among those who seek to apply these principles in their work. Certainly we would benefit if we understood better that we function wholistically. Nikolaas Tinbergan wrote that a "biologically interesting aspect of . . . Alexander . . . is that every session clearly demonstrates that the innumerable muscles of the body are continuously operating as an intricately linked web."

## Groups and Associations

**(890) THE AMERICAN CENTER FOR THE ALEXANDER TECHNIQUE, INC.**
142 West End Avenue
New York, NY 10023

(212) 799-0468

931 Elizabeth Street
San Francisco, CA 94114

(415) 282-8967

812 Seventeenth Street
Santa Monica, CA 90403

(213) 451-3641

Teaches and coordinates training programs in the Alexander Technique, a system of mental concentration designed to realign the body and correct improper habits of posture and movement. A program for the training of Alexander teachers is housed in the New York office.

## Schools, Centers, and Clinics

**HEART HAUS CENTER** (holistic center)/Mill Valley, CA **(see 1056)**

**SAN ANDREAS HEALTH CENTER** (holistic clinic and school)/Palo Alto, CA **(see 101)**

**ASSOCIATES FOR HUMAN RESOURCES** (growth center)/Concord, MA **(see 1101)**

**NEW ENGLAND CENTER** (massage)/Leverett, MA **(see 843)**

**THE ILANA RUBENFELD CENTER FOR GESTALT SYNERGY**/New York, NY **(see 933)**

**SHALIMAR HEALTH HOME** (wholistic resort)/Essex, England **(see 178)**

**RAMANA HEALTH CENTRE** (wholistic center and clinic)/Hants, England **(see 161)**

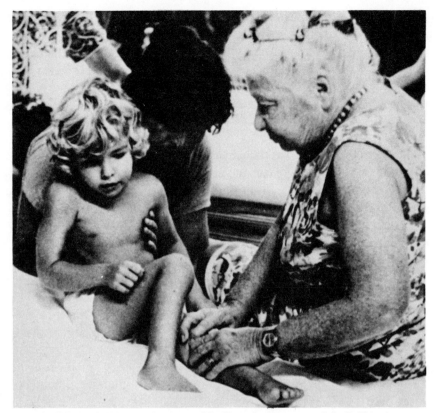

Ida P. Rolf, PhD, founder and developer of Rolfing; photo courtesy of the Rolf Institute.

# Rolfing
*Ida P. Rolf, PhD*

In general people have subscribed to the idea that even though they must acknowlege their apparent animal origin and relation, they nevertheless feel themselves unique in being, as they think, "upright." (Indeed, this idea of "upright" extends to the mental and emotional makeup as well.) However, no reliable methods have been developed for the establishment of the upright stance other than the time-honored formula of "shoulders back, guts in, head up." Unfortunately, as a method for the establishment of a truly upright stance, these directions are a snare and a delusion. In the average body, any effort to take the shoulders back will actually force the spine forward; an effort to bring the gut in gives rise to structural aberration of the pelvis; and the direction "head up" elicits almost as many postural misalignments as there are people who try it, and each variation clearly underlines the structural aberrations of the particular physical individual making the "effort."

For the fact is, verticality of the person can only be attained by the organization of his or her basic structure, the establishment of deep-lying structural relationships appropriate to the inherent design of humans—or, in other words, the establishment of an order that is expressed outwardly in balance and symmetry. Such balance can be seen in the outer contour of the individual and shows up clearly in photographs, especially lateral photographs.

All schools of body mechanics, from the most to the least orthodox, agree on the importance of verticality in human structure. Measurements accompanied by pictures have been made within the past few years demonstrating the improved energy patterns of the muscular system as bodies have been aligned and verticaled by the Rolf System of Structural Integration. Valerie Hunt of the Movement Behavior

Laboratory of the University of California, Los Angeles has demonstrated clearly the improved functioning of the myofascial system as the body structurally approaches the vertical. J. Silverman, in a pilot project on the effect of structural integration, demonstrated significant changes in the blood chemistry, especially of substances known to be associated with changes in emotional levels. All schools of body mechanics define the vertical in one, and only one, fashion. In a structurally balanced body the knees are vertically over the ankles, the hip joints vertically over the knees, shoulders vertically above the hip joints (and if this is so, the lumbar vertebrae are normally "back"), and, finally, ears vertically above the shoulders.

Fifty years ago radical restructuring of the posture was thought impossible because the body was viewed as a "unit." The body is *not* a unit, and for that very reason it can be changed. A body is an aggregate of large segments (head, thorax, pelvis, legs) each having significant weight, and "straightening" a body depends on changing the relationships between those segments.

The body is truly a "plastic medium." A substance is called plastic if it may be deformed under pressure but can revert to its original shape under the application of appropriately directed energy. The various body units are joined by ligaments, tendons, and fascial sheets of connective tissue—in other words, by collagen structures. Collagen is a protein unusually well adapted for this role. Like all proteins, it forms a colloidal suspension—not a true solution—in water, and, like all colloidal suspensions, changes its characteristics in response to its energy level. The addition of energy by whatever means moves it along its spectrum from the more solid "gel" to a more fluid "sol" phase. Energy may be added as heat, as chemical energy (i.e., change in the oxygen content), or mechanical energy (the pressure of the rolfer's fingers or arms). As the collagen is energized (i.e., moved towards its sol stage), the body loses its stiffness and is able to move more freely, to move more truly with respect to its joint structure, thereby showing a wider and at the same time a more subtle range of movement. Therefore, the body is more comfortable and feels more competent as well as more graceful. On the other hand, as energy is withdrawn (for example, in a lower temperature or following a traumatic accident), there is a more random, less appropriate joint organization, and the colloid reverts to the more solid gel state.

As a body departs from the vertical, the energy contributed by gravity is withdrawn. The structure itself, in consequence, shows a lessened energy; take, for example, the changes that we think of and label as "old age." This restricted movement registers with the individual as "incoordination." The body slows down in its movement, feels itself as rigid, unmoving, awkward.

Through the years, these effects have always been so apparent that a vertical stance has always been valued. The directive "stand straight" is among the traditional "horrors" remembered from childhood. It was not widely recognized that the child whose basic structure was badly organized is required to put out an "effort" which defeats the goal—that neither physical pleasure nor graceful movement can result from the "shoulders back, guts in, head up" system. However, the value of verticality as such seemed beyond question, and the more metaphysically minded postulated many esoteric causative factors for this value.

Among the many voices raised in praise of the vertical stance, no voice proclaimed the self-evident fact that when a body is truly vertical, the energy of the gravitational field, itself a "vertical" energy in relation to the horizontality of the earth's surface, would not and could not tear the body down. It could only flow through that vertical body and in so doing add an energy increment, thus augmenting and supporting it. But if one views a body not as a unit but as the manifestation, the expression of a basic energy field, and recognizes that this energy field exists within the much larger earth field, gravity, then it becomes all too apparent that gravity can literally cancel, in whole or in part, the smaller energy field that is expressed as the individual. It becomes clear that this smaller field, verbally referred to as "a human," may be conscious of itself as augmented by the supportive presence of the larger field flowing through it, or diminished if its own energy is partly canceled. In human terms, the field of gravity, under conditions in which it can support and augment the human field, acts as a "therapist."

Structural integration is a system for aligning the random body into an orderly balanced energy system that can operate within the field of gravity, accepting and transforming energy from this larger field. In this way, the human's potential is expanded. Gravity is the therapist; the rolfer (through manipulation, verbal direction, and understanding) merely helps rolfees use their bodies in all situations in a way that allows gravity to contribute energy. In short, the Rolf System of Structural Integration consciously and deliberately utilizes gravity as a tool in the enhancement of human potential. Clearly this potential is not limited to the physical body alone but is expressed through the mental and emotional manifestations of the individual because of the chemical changes induced by the rolfing. Silverman has shown that every trauma, whatever its origin, expresses itself and perpetrates itself in hook-ups in the physical body. It can only be released totally when and as the physical body, the outward manifestation of the energy field, attains the degree of balance and order that can be designated not as average but as normal.

In the earlier stages of integration, body changes are induced by manipulation in which muscles that have deviated from normal positions are brought nearer to their optimal location and then required to move in that less energy-demanding position. The body, unless too severely traumatized, responds quickly and "gladly" to this demand for normalization. The system is designed to raise the general level of functioning and competence of the individual. It is not designed as a therapy nor a system to relieve certain symptoms. However, as rolfees experience predictable and reliable improvements in their general level, symptoms are apt to disappear. However, a rolfer regards such improvements as the work of the great therapist, gravity. Rolfers see themselves as merely teachers, stressing their students' responsibility to understand body movement and its effect on well-being, and to invoke the energy of the earth to enhance their own potential.

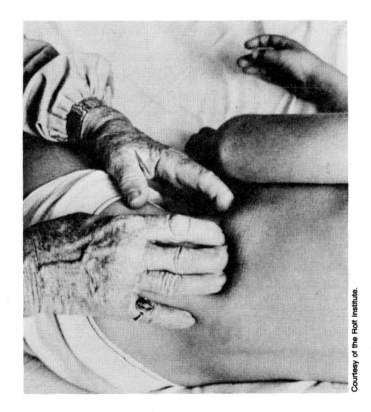

Courtesy of the Rolf Institute.

## Groups and Associations

(891) **ROLF INSTITUTE**
P.O. Box 1868
Boulder, CO 80302

(303) 449-5903

*Richard A. Stenstadvold, Executive Director*

Trains and certifies Rolfers and informs the public of the benefits of Rolfing and Aston (structural) Patterning. Information on Rolfing and Aston (structural) Patterning, the Rolf Institute's training program, and a list of Rolfers is available from the above address.

## Schools, Centers, and Clinics

**ESALEN** (multidisciplinary growth center)/Big Sur, CA **(see 1051)**

**SAN ANDREAS HEALTH CENTER** (holistic clinic and school)/Palo Alto, CA **(see 101)**

(892) **ASTON PATTERNING INSTITUTE**
P.O. Box 114
Tiburon, CA 94920

(415) 435-0433

*Judith Aston, Director*

Aston patterning (formerly called structural patterning) was developed by Judith Aston. Patterning is a step by step process of becoming aware of "holding" patterns in order to learn about "letting go." The patterner is trained to recognize that there are many ways we hold. For example holding onto beliefs, holding back feelings, holding down exuberance: "It is these patterns that begin to shape us into a more stressful body than we really are." Patterning has evolved as a comprehensive framework for reeducating an individual about his/her body and movement. It is compatible with and beneficial to all improvement and especially body disciplines, and enhances those disciplines by providing a framework in which to understand and apply the concepts involved. Further information, as well as a list of "Patterners" may be obtained by writing to the Institute.

**COMMUNITY FREE SCHOOL** (multidisciplinary)/ Boulder, CO **(see 119)**

**INSTITUTE FOR PSYCHOENERGETICS** (psychophysical workshops)/Brookline, MA **(see 128)**

(893) **THE NEW YORK CENTER FOR STRUCTURAL INTEGRATION AND STRUCTURAL PATTERNING**
165 West 91st Street, #8E
New York, NY 10024

(212) 724-6677

Treatment and training workshops in Aston patterning.

## Products and Services

**LIVING EARTH CRAFTS** (Rolfing massage tables)/ Cotati, CA **(see 887)**

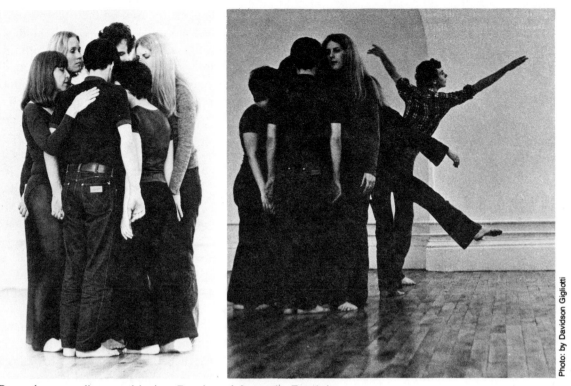

Dance therapy, audience participation, Experimental Intermedia Foundation, New York City, 1975. Alexandra Ogsbury dancing with the audience; photo courtesy of Elaine Summers.

# Dance Therapy: The Psychotherapeutic Use Of Movement

*Claire Schmais, MA, DTR*

The dance therapist walks slowly with the group into the center of the circle and out again, meeting each patient's eyes and greeting them with subtle changes in the body. As a simple phrase is repeated again and again, a common rhythm emerges. The dance therapy session has begun.

Prior to this the patients were scattered throughout the ward. One was stalking ferociously up and down the room, another was curled in the corner gesturing away his ghosts, yet another was rocking back and forth with enormous intensity. The rest were either dozing off or staring blankly at the television.

Now they are moving as a group, not necessarily looking at or talking to one another, but connected by a kinetic bond through the sound of the music and the movements of the therapist. This cohesion, stemming from common rhythmic action, nurtures new roles and supports spontaneous dance dramas. Latent fears, angers, and sorrows become visible within the confines of this magical circle, and the group, like a Greek chorus, encourages the development of the dance.

Rhythmic group action as a healing ritual has its roots in antiquity. For centuries people have danced to express their ecstasy, to conquer their pain, to exorcise their devils, and to communicate with their demons. Through dancing, they have acquired skills, marked stages in their development, and gained solace and strength.

Dance as therapy is American in origin. Early modern dancer/choreographers searched their psyches to create dances based on personal struggles and emotional experiences. Concurrently, growing government support, the development of tranquilizers, and an interest in group activities changed the climate of the mental health field. The new dance form and the changed attitude of mental health practitioners converged to make dance therapy possible in post-World War II America.

In the forties and fifties a number of accomplished modern dancers focused on their feelings as the primary source of their work. Combining self-knowledge and personal analysis with studies in psychotherapy, they rediscovered dance as a healing art. Using dance as the core concept, they incorporated the psychoanalytic theories of Adler, Jung, Freud, and Sullivan into their practice of therapy. Pioneers such as Mary Whitehouse, Blanche Evans, Trudi Schoop, and Liljan Espenak found that basic elements in the dance such as rhythm, synchrony, and creativity had curative possibilities. They recognized that giving support to expressive actions in a safe environment had a salutary effect on students who tended to suppress, deny, or distance their feelings.

Dance therapy received official recognition when Marian Chace, a Denishawn dancer and teacher, was employed at St. Elizabeth Hospital in Washington, D.C. She was asked to work there by local psychiatrists who had heard of her from their private patients. These nonprofessional dancers were drawn to the Chace dance studio as a place where their uniqueness was valued, their expressions were welcomed, and their needs were met. Members of the psychiatric community hoped that Chace's experiences with her students could be duplicated with mental patients.

Chace was indeed able to reach out to the chronic regressed patients on the back, back wards. She awakened movements in catatonics and made contact with mutes. By reflecting a patient's pain, conflicts, and protective mechanisms in her body, she would expand these patients' awareness of self and give them space in which to move and to grow.

A basic premise underlying dance therapy is that there is an isomorphic relationship between mind and body. All movement behaviors are considered meaningful, reflecting both intrapsychic dynamics and interpersonal functioning. Each body is sculpted over time by experiences and perceptions. For example, therapists recognize patterns of muscular tension molded by inhibitions and reinforced by repression, body parts distorted or disconnected to deny sexual feelings, and body textures frozen or flaccid to mask anger or fear. Movement behavior is both the cause and effect of these body configurations. A person's movement repertoire is an amalgam of his or her hereditary makeup and his or her experience as a member of a family, a culture, and a society. These movements are the content of the dance therapy session.

Chace's method of group dance therapy assumes that the movement relationship between therapist and patients enables and supports behavioral change. Music is used as a catalytic agent awakening motor responses and reinforcing rhythmic unity. The initial phase of the session is concerned with meetings and greetings. After initiating a simple movement in a circle formation, the therapist responds to each person's variations. These variations, which encompass the patient's past history and present needs, are accepted and validated by the therapist's verbal and movement responses. Through this interplay the therapist senses the tenor of the individuals and the group. The therapist acknowledges emerging themes and chooses to clarify, intensify, or expand on those issues which the group is ready and willing to support. Frequently, themes of depression uncover anger and themes of assertion lead to moments of gently sharing and touching. Barely recognizable feelings are brought to fruition by the therapist's reaction and the group's reinforcing responses. Powerful emotions are vented with movements, sounds, and words. Patients feel safe making strong statements when they are part of a group dance contained in rhythm and structured in space. Fragments of expression evolve into actions and then into interactions. Closing fingers may change to a fist and then to a punch, leading the patient toward the source of his or her anger.

In the dance therapy session people are able to express their feelings and to recapture a sense of liveliness and joy. They can literally and symbolically lean and be leaned on, they can give and take, and they can share or control their feelings. As they expand their capacity to move, they find there are choices available to them. For example, they can choose to take a stand or to shrug something off. Movement interactions in the group setting help them realize their potential on a psychomotor level. They learn a new, integrated vocabulary of behaviors.

Today the majority of dance therapists work in public facilities with the most abandoned segment of our population, the mentally ill poor. They use their skill to maximize whatever potential these people have.

230

Some of these patients may never leave the hospital, and for them the hour of dance may bring comfort and contact. Others may begin to feel integrated and to act appropriately, so that eventually they can leave the hospital and return to their communities.

Dance therapists have found ways of building a sense of community among other isolated populations such as the blind, the deaf, the aged, and the autistic. They adapt their tools and techniques to accommodate the special concerns of each group. A small number of dance therapists are working in pain clinics and with postoperative patients to restore an awareness of body and a sense of self. Dance therapists also work with children who are retarded, handicapped, or disturbed. Through movement and dance activities these children are able to recapitulate developmental stages, to learn new skills, to be playful and to be creative.

A growing number of dance therapists work with neurotic clients, individually, in families, and in small groups. They may move with their patients or they may direct, guide, comment on, or interpret the observable movement behaviors. Employing movement and dance as well as massage, hypnosis, dream work, and other related modalities, they enable their clients to shed those defensive patterns which prevent them from acting with ease, authenticity, and spontaneity.

The dance therapist initially trains as a dancer and while learning the art and craft of dance discovers the body's potentials and limitations. Exploring the range of motion in muscle and joints during hours of disciplined practice, the dancer creates shapes that are distorted or aligned, motions that are smooth or jarring, and rhythms that are easy or agitated. While rehearsing leaps, falls, and turns, the dancer becomes conscious of the play between tension and relaxation, and learns what it feels like to be alone on a stage or to be part of a performing group.

The intrinsic knowledge acquired in the dance studio is made explicit in the formal training of dance therapists. They study human anatomy, kinesiology, and movement observation, as well as normal and abnormal human development and group process. Dance therapists are also educated in a wide range of related disciplines concerned with breathing, posture, relaxation, etc., and learn to recognize when their patients might benefit from work in these areas. Some choose to study these related fields further in order to broaden their scope and to enhance their work.

The work of the dance therapist branches out to intersect many other disciplines. But in performing a modern version of an ancient ritual, the dance therapist is primarily a clinician/dancer using movement to effect therapeutic change.

## Groups and Associations

(894) **AMERICAN DANCE THERAPY ASSOCIATION**
2000 Century Plaza, Suite 230
Columbia, MD 21044

(301) 997-4040

Dedicated to establishing and maintaining high standards of education and professional competence in dance therapy, ". . . the psychotherapeutic use of movement as a process which furthers the emotional and physical integration of the individual." ADTA stimulates communication among dance therapists and members of allied professions through publication of a national newsletter (**1078**), printing of current and relevant papers, monographs, bibliographies, and annual conference proceedings. In addition, the Association holds an annual conference and supports formation of regional groups, conferences, seminars, workshops, and meetings throughout the year. Founded 1966.

*CONTACTS FOR REGIONAL AND LOCAL ACTIVITIES*

**AMERICAN DANCE THERAPY ASSOCIATION**
Erma Alperson, DTR, Coordinator
1202 Raintree Circle
Culver City, CA 90230

**SOUTHERN CALIFORNIA CHAPTER**
c/o Kathleen C. Mason
4141 Edenhurst Avenue
Los Angeles, CA 90039

**NORTHERN CALIFORNIA CHAPTER**
c/o Barbara Kirsch, DTR
928 Laurel Avenue
Menlo Park, CA 94025

(415) 329-8190

**NEW ENGLAND/CANADA CHAPTER**
c/o Jennifer Hill, DTR
Elmcrest Psychiatric Institute
25 Marlborough Street
Portland, CT 06480

(203) 342-0480

**WASHINGTON/MARYLAND/VIRGINIA CHAPTER**
c/o Karen Ruback
2147 "O" Street, N.W.
Washington, DC 20037

(202) 659-3926

**MID-WEST CHAPTER**
c/o SuEllen Fried
4003 Homestead Drive
Shawnee Mission, KS 66208

(913) 367-2227

**ST. LOUIS MISSOURI GROUP (CHAPTER)**
c/o Helen Haskins
6029 Carlsbad
St. Louis, MO 63116

**NEW JERSEY CHAPTER**
c/o Summemann Dance Therapy Training Program
758 West Eighth Street
Plainfield, NJ 07060

**NEW YORK CITY (CHAPTER)**
c/o Linni Silberman, DTR
526 West 113th Street, #4
New York, NY 10025

(212) 666-7790

**GENESEE VALLEY, NY DANCE THERAPY GROUP**
c/o Carolee Powers
159 Booklawn Drive
Rochester, NY 14618

**PHILADELPHIA (CHAPTER)**
c/o Emily Samuelson
233 South Melville Street
Philadelphia, PA 19139

**SOUTH CENTRAL STUDY GROUP**
c/o Wynelle Delaney, DTR
2416 Yorktown, #349
Houston, TX 77056

(713) 627-7655

## Schools, Centers, and Clinics

**(895) OPEN SPACE STUDIO**
2118 Vine Street
Berkeley, CA 94709

*Lorle Kranzler-Kennedy, MA*

Offers ongoing courses and workshops; write for schedules and details.

**(896) UNIVERSITY OF CALIFORNIA EXTENSION**
2223 Fulton Street
Berkeley, CA 94720

(415) 642-4111

*Joanna Harris, Lorle Kranzler-Kennedy, Gloria Rubin*

Offers ongoing courses and workshops; write for schedules and details.

**(897) GERIATRIC-CALISTHENICS**
c/o Eva Desca Garnet, MS, DTR
1227 South Curson Avenue
Los Angeles, CA 90019

(213) 933-5162

Offers ongoing courses and workshops; write for schedules and details.

**HOLISTIC HEALTH CENTER** (clinic and school)/Los Angeles, CA **(see 90)**

**SAN ANDREAS HEALTH CENTER** (clinic and workshops)/Palo Alto, CA **(see 101)**

**(898) SAN FRANCISCO DANCE/MOVEMENT THERAPY CENTER**
442 Shotwell Street
San Francisco, CA 94110

(415) 989-8802

P.O. Box 15206
San Francisco, CA 94115

A nonprofit collective of professionals in dance/movement and recreation therapy. Focus is on the importance of the body in therapy and the use of movement as a unifying force in personal development. This includes body image and awareness, movement exploration, nonverbal communication, personal growth, and expression through movement and exploration. The Center offers professional training, dance/movement therapy groups, workshops for children, movement exploration for pleasure, and special events.

**UNIVERSITY OF CALIFORNIA EXTENSION**/Santa Cruz, CA **(see 115)**

**(899) MOVEMENT FOR LIVING CENTER**
Box 39
Smartsville, CA 95977

(916) 742-5766

*Gloria Simcha Ruben, DTR*

Offers ongoing courses and workshops; write for schedules and details.

**NEW HAVEN CENTER FOR HUMAN RELATIONS** (growth center)/New Haven, CT **(see 1077)**

**FLORIDA INSTITUTE OF PSYCHOPHYSICAL INTEGRATION**/Tampa, FL **(see 840)**

**(900) HUMAN RESOURCE INSTITUTE**
227 Babcock Street
Brookline, MA 02146

(617) 731-3200

*Naomi Leaf Halpern, DTR*

Offers ongoing courses and workshops; write for schedules and details.

(901) **HELION CENTER**
Cayuga Trail
Oak Ridge, NJ 07438

(201) 697-6592

*Pat Sonen Paulsen, MA, DTR, and Shirley J. Weiner, DTR*

Sixteen-week preparatory course (50 clinical hours); 80 classwork hours followed by three months full-time internship; supervised home study; private consultations. Program emphasizes Marian Chace group and individual methodology. Also: one-day workshops for professionals.

(902) **SUMMEMANN DANCE THERAPY TRAINING PROGRAM**
758 West Eighth Street
Plainfield, NJ 07060

*Jane Kettering, DTR, and Harold Kettering*

BA degree through University Without Walls; MA degree through Goddard College (Field Study Center); internship possible. Courses in dance therapy training.

(903) **CANTALICIAN CENTER FOR LEARNING**
Creative Arts Program
3233 Main Street
Buffalo, NY 14214

(716) 833-5353

*Crystal L. Kinda*

Opportunity for fieldwork in creative arts in a therapeutic environment for trainable mentally retarded, autistic, physically/multiply handicapped children and young adults. Flexible program; can be coordinated with academic courses.

(904) **INSTITUTE FOR SOCIOTHERAPY**
39 East Twentieth Street
New York, NY 10003

(212) 260-3860

*Fran Levy, MA, MSW, DTR*

Experiential workshops and professional training; covers a period of one and a half years. Five seminars precede interning. Admission to program: prerequisites include experiential workshops and interview.

**TURTLE BAY MUSIC SCHOOL** (music and dance programs)/New York, NY **(see 991)**

(905) **HUDSON RIVER PSYCHIATRIC CENTER**
North Road
Poughkeepsie, NY 12601

(914) 452-8000

*Robin Engel and Pei Fin Chin Kupferman*

Ongoing dance therapy session in a state research hospital; uses a multitude of techniques within a team setting; coordinates with an assortment of state civil service courses offered at the hospital and many courses offered at nearby colleges (Vassar, New Paltz, Bard, Milbrook).

**ITA-WEGMAN-KLINIK** (anthroposophical)/Arlesheim, Switzerland **(see 813)**

**FRIEDRICH HUSEMANN-KLINIK** (anthroposophical)/West Germany **(see 817)**

**LUKAS KLINIK** (anthroposophical)/West Germany **(see 814)**

## Schools (Universities)

(906) **CABRILLO COLLEGE**
Dance Department
6500 Soquel Drive
Aptos, CA 95003

(408) 425-6000

*Roberta Le Gear Bristol, Chairperson*

A small (5-10 student) special training program for undergraduate dance majors. Opportunities for leadership in community health programs.

(907) **IMMACULATE HEART COLLEGE**
2021 North Western Avenue
Los Angeles, CA 90027

(213) 462-1301

*Beth Kalish, DTR, Director*

Offers Master of Arts degree in dance therapy and art therapy.

(908) **UNIVERSITY OF CALIFORNIA, LOS ANGELES**
405 Hilgard Avenue
Los Angeles, CA 90024

*Alma H. Hawkins, EdD, DTR*

Offers MA degree in dance; 2-year program; includes study or research in a hospital or clinic.

(909) **LONE MOUNTAIN COLLEGE**
2800 Turk Boulevard
San Francisco, CA 94118

(415) 752-7000

*Joanna G. Harris, PhD, DTR, Director, Creative Arts Therapy Program*

Offers Master of Creative Arts Therapy degree with specialization in art, music, or dance therapy; 36-unit three-quarter semester program; opportunities for interdisciplinary study; fieldwork; internships required.

(910) **AMERICAN DANCE FESTIVAL, CONNECTICUT COLLEGE**
New London, CT 06320

(203) 447-2077

*Linni Silberman, MA, DTR, Director, Dance Therapy Intensive*

Graduate or undergraduate credit (4 credit hours); two 3-week dance therapy courses June through August. Chace Dance Therapy, Effort/Shape Movement Analysis, group process and dynamics, leadership techniques.

**(911) COLUMBIA COLLEGE**
4730 Sheridan Road North
Chicago, IL 60640

(312) 663-1600

*Jane Ganet, MA, CSW, DTR*

Offers Introduction to Dance/Movement Therapy; 16-week, 2-unit course. Dance/Movement Therapy II; 16-week, 2-unit course. Credit applied to BA or MA degree.

**UNIVERSITY OF LOUISVILLE** (art and dance therapy)/Louisville, KY **(see 959)**

**(912) GOUCHER COLLEGE**
Towson, MD 21204

(301) 825-3300

*Ms. C. Bond, Director of Dance*

Since September 1976, the Department of Performing Arts at Goucher College has offered three undergraduate courses in dance therapy. Courses are taught by Arlynne Stark, DTR.

**(913) UNIVERSITY OF MASSACHUSETTS**
Department of Preparation for Physical Education and Dance
North Physical Education Building
Amherst, MA 01002

(413) 545-0111

*Daniel Peterson, DTR*

Dance concentration with BS in Physical Education. One course in Theories of Therapeutic Dance.

**LESLEY COLLEGE** (art and dance therapy program)/Cambridge, MA **(see 962)**

**COLLEGE OF SAINT THERESA** (music, art, and dance therapy programs)/Winona, MN **(see 1008)**

**(914) UNIVERSITY OF DETROIT**
Marygrove College
8425 West McNichols Road
Detroit, MI 48221

(313) 862-8000

*Stephanie S. Katz, DTR, Dance Therapy Coordinator*

BA in Dance with dance therapy specialization. Ms. Katz also supervises 6-month internship at Detroit Psychiatric Institute.

**(915) WASHINGTON UNIVERSITY**
Lindell and Skinker Boulevards
St. Louis, MO 63130

(314) 863-0100

*Becky Egle Engler, MA, Department of Dance*

Introduction to Dance Therapy offered to senior dance majors.

**(916) ANTIOCH GRADUATE SCHOOL**
Dance Movement Therapy Program
Department of Counseling
1 Elm Street
Keene, NH 03431

*Penny Bernstein, MA, DTR, and Mara Capy, MA, DTR, Co-Coordinators*

Offers MEd degree; 15-18 month, 60-credit program; interning, 6-9 months; program stresses variety of theoretical approaches. Master of Arts in Movement Therapy (MAMT) degree as an alternative to MEd in process.

**(917) HUNTER COLLEGE**
695 Park Avenue
Box 1425
New York, NY 10021

(212) 360-2415

*Claire Schmais, DTR, Director*

Offers MA degree in dance; 45-credit, 2-year program; 6 months are devoted to full time internships.

**(918) THE INTERNATIONAL GRADUATE UNIVERSITY AT THE AMERICAN COLLEGE OF SWITZERLAND**
Director of Admissions
U.S. Office
205 West End Avenue, Suite 1P
New York, NY 10023

(212) 799-3535

*Dianne Dulicai, MA, DTR, Coordinator*

Offers continuing education courses leading to a doctorate in dance/movement therapy.

**(919) NEW YORK MEDICAL COLLEGE, MENTAL RETARDATION CLINIC**
Fifth Avenue at 106th Street
New York, NY 10029

(212) 860-7041

*Liljan Espenak, MA, DTR, Director, Dance Therapy Program*

Offers postgraduate certification in Psychomotor Therapy. September to June, 20 hours weekly.

**(920) NEW YORK UNIVERSITY**
School of Education
Division of Creative Arts
675 D Education Building
Washington Square
New York, NY 10003

(212) 598-3481

*Marcia Leventhal, DTR*

Offers MA degree; 37 units; interning; program blends theorizing, experiencing, and application of dance therapy techniques and methods.

**(921) STATE UNIVERSITY OF NEW YORK/ COLLEGE AT PURCHASE**
Office of Continuing Education
Purchase, NY 10577

(914) 253-5000

*Claire Schmais, MA, DTR*

Offers course work: "Understanding Body Movement and Language"; lecture and studio experience.

**HANNEMANN MEDICAL COLLEGE** (art, dance, and movement therapy)/Philadelphia, PA **(see 974)**

**(922) TEMPLE UNIVERSITY**
Department of Dance
Broad and Montgomery Avenues
Philadelphia, PA 19122

(215) 787-7000

*Bonnie Shuman, Instructor*

Offers course work as extension of dance program. Ms. Shuman also offers a practicum, 20 hours per week in methodology with emotionally disturbed and retarded populations.

**(923) GODDARD COLLEGE**
Admissions Office
Graduate Program Division
Plainfield, VT 05667

(802) 454-8311

*Atten: Eunice Gray*

Offers a student-designed external program with a fieldwork supervisor for advanced, self-directed students.

**(924) UNIVERSITY OF WISCONSIN**
1050 University Avenue
Madison, WI 53706

(608) 262-1234

*Deborah Thomas, MA, Dance Therapy Program—Women's Physical Education*

Offers 3-year program including theory, studio work, fieldwork, and supervised practicum; BS degree.

**(925) YORK UNIVERSITY**
Faculty of Fine Arts
Dance Department
4700 Keele Street
Downsview, Ontario
Canada M3J 1P3

(416) 667-3237

*Julianna Lau, DTR, Director, Dance Therapy*

Offers BA degree program for dance majors requiring three years of study. Training based on Laban's effort/shape theories; field placement.

**HERTFORDSHIRE COLLEGE OF ART AND DESIGN** (therapy)/Hertfordshire, England **(see 979)**

## Journals and Publications

**(926) ADTA NEWSLETTER**
American Dance Therapy Association, Inc.
2000 Century Plaza, Suite 230
Columbia, MD 21044

(301) 997-4040

*Linni Silberman, Editor*

Six issues yearly. Contains communications from ADTA president and membership, regional news, film and book reviews, student section, theory and philosophy, listing of courses and workshops available.

# VIII
# HUMANISTIC AND TRANSPERSONAL PSYCHOTHERAPIES

---

Gestalt

Art Therapy As A Means Of Wholistic
Individuation Through Creative Expression

Drama Therapy

Music Therapy/Guided Imagery

Hypnosis/Active Imagination

Humanistic Psychology

Psychosynthesis

Transpersonal Psychology

Life After Life

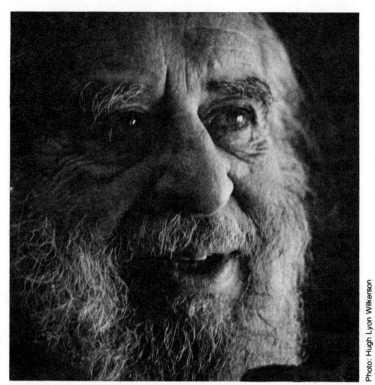

Photo: Hugh Lyon Wilkerson

Fritz Perls, pioneer and developer of gestalt therapy; courtesy of Ilana Rubenfeld

# Gestalt

*Laura Perls, DSc*

The German word *gestalt* covers a multitude of related concepts such as countenance, shape, form, figure, configuration, structural entity, a whole that is more than (or different from) the sum of its parts. A gestalt stands out from the background, it "exists," and the relationship of a figure to its ground is called "meaning." If this relationship is tenuous or nonexistent, or if it is not recognized and understood, it does not "make sense"; it is meaningless.

Gestalt therapy is an existential, experiential, and experimental approach. As an existential approach it takes its being from what is, rather than from what has been or what should be. The past is present in the form of memory with all its emotional ramifications, particularly in the futile repetitive attempts to resolve unfinished situations. It is present in the fixed attitudes and habit patterns originally developed as support that have now (like most "fixed gestalten") become blocks in the ongoing life process. The future is present here and now as anticipation, expectation and hope, fear and despair, and in the fixed habits of impatience, avoidance, and withdrawal, ignoring or bypassing and belittling the actual present as "too obvious."

Gestalt therapy deals with the obvious, with what is or can be made immediately available and accessible in the awareness of client or therapist and can be shared in the ongoing therapeutic situation. The actual experience of any present situation does not need to be explained or interpreted; it can be directly contacted, felt, and described here and now. Gestalt therapy facilitates the awareness continuum, the freely ongoing gestalt formation, by deautomatizing those fixed habit patterns which have become blocks (the muscular tensions and resulting desensitization and immobilization, the rationalizations, use and misuse of language, the fixed ideas, ideals, and ideologies); it does so by bringing these patterns into the foreground where they can be fully experienced again as active interferences rather than merely as afflictions, inhibitions, symptoms, and anxieties. Only in any present moment can the experienced and recognized activity be changed. We can explore every available detail and experiment with alternatives.

But a new contact is possible only to the extent that support for it is available. Support is everything that facilitates the assimilation and integration of experience, thus building up the background against which the new experience makes sense. Support starts with primary physiology (breathing, digestion, circulation, etc.) and proper care of the embryo and infant, who must develop from a state of complete dependence and confluence with the environment to the state of an independent, responsible adult who, with fully developed awareness, makes contact with the facts and possibilities of any present situation. Further essential support develops with upright posture and coordination, sensitivity and mobility, language, habits and customs, social manners and relationships, and everything else that has been learned, experienced, and assimilated during a lifetime.

Contact is the boundary phenomenon between organism and environment, the locus of the egofunctions of identification and alienation, the sphere of excitation, interest, and concern—or if support is lacking, of unease and anxiety.

Fixed boundaries characterize the obsessional personality and most social organizations and institutions (family, church, bureaucracy, etc.). They support stability and tradition but also develop rigidity, isolation, boredom, and resentment. Aggressiveness shows in hostility against everything different and new, in the growing polarity of authoritarianism and submission, or if retroflexed, in self-reproach, guilt feelings, even suicide.

Broken or blurred boundaries open the door for projection and introjection, the confusion and confluence of self and others. Paradoxically, it is only *within* the fixed boundaries of social institutions (marriage, family, school, church) that not only does confluence happen but also complete identification is actively supported and even taken for granted. Since the abilities for making real contact (for recognizing and coping with the other as the other) are underdeveloped, only more or less complete alienation—a breaking of boundaries, getting out of bounds—remains as a means of saving the individual or group identity from the tyranny of the confluence code (in youth movements, revolution, desertion, delinquency, schizophrenia).

The *elasticity of the boundary* equals the *awareness continuum*. How we go about reorganizing bound-up energies and reowning alienated parts of the personality, building up support for being on the contact boundary depends on the individual resources of therapists and clients. In gestalt therapy there are no strictly prescribed techniques or experiments. Therapists use themselves and whatever skills and experiences they have coupled with the fullest possible awareness of what is available and what is lacking in the client. Gestalt therapists develop different styles rather than using specific, potentially mechanistic techniques (fixed gestalten). Thus, many other modalities (movement and art therapies, bioenergetics, primal and transactional methods) have been and are being integrated into different styles of gestalt therapy. Gestalt therapy itself is not a fixed gestalt but an ongoing innovative process on the boundary of actual and potential experience.

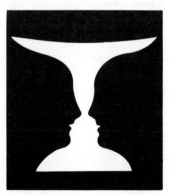 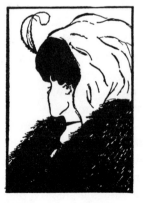

The following two diagrams are visual examples of the natural process of Gestalt information. As one looks at each diagram note the spontaneous interchangeability of each figure with its background. From *Gestalt Therapy*. By Perls, Hefferline, and Goodman. Courtesy of Julian Press, New York, 1975.

## Groups and Associations

**NATIONAL INSTITUTE FOR PSYCHOTHERA-PIES**/New York, NY **(see 1045)**

## Schools, Centers, and Clinics

**METAMORPHOSIS** (growth center)/Berkeley, CA **(see 1048)**

**CENTER FOR FAMILY GROWTH** (birth)/Cotati, CA **(see 1048)**

**HUMAN PROCESS INSTITUTE** (group pyschotherapy)/Encino, CA **(see 1052)**

**(927) GESTALT INSTITUTE OF SAN DIEGO**
P.O. Box 1084
La Jolla, CA 92037

(714) 459-2693

Offers gestalt therapy, education, and training at both the individual and group levels. A Monday night clinic makes sessions available for a nominal fee. Other activities include weekend workshops held three to four times a year, classes in female sexuality, and sexuality counseling for both couples and individuals. Founded 1964.

**PSYCHOTHERAPY CENTER**/Los Angeles, CA **(see 1054)**

**HEART HAUS CENTER** (holistic center)/Mill Valley, CA **(see 1056)**

**WELLNESS RESOURCE CENTER** (preventive)/Mill Valley, CA **(see 96)**

**SAN ANDREAS HEALTH CENTER** (holistic clinic and school)/Palo Alto, CA **(see 101)**

**CHURCH OF GENTLE BROTHERS AND SISTERS** (workshops)/San Francisco, CA **(see 109)**

**FAMILY GROUP INSTITUTE** (humanistic growth center)/San Francisco, CA **(see 1060)**

**TOPANGA CENTER FOR HUMAN DEVELOPMENT** (humanistic workshops)/Topanga, CA **(see 1070)**

**WILBUR HOT SPRINGS** (psychotherapy center)/Wilbur Springs, CA **(see 1071)**

**ASPEN CENTER FOR HUMAN GROWTH** (humanistic workshops)/Aspen, CO **(see 1072)**

**BOULDER WORKSHOP** (growth center)/Boulder, CO **(see 1073)**

**NEW HAVEN CENTER FOR HUMAN RELATIONS** (growth center)/New Haven, CT **(see 1077)**

**ENCOUNTERS** (humanistic growth center)/Washington, DC **(see 1078)**

**SISYPHUS HUMANISTIC INSTITUTE OF FLORIDA** (workshops and training)/Merrit Island, FL **(see 1079)**

**(928) GESTALT INSTITUTE OF THE CHICAGO CENTER FOR BEHAVIOUR MODIFICATION**
310 South Michigan Avenue
Chicago, IL 60604

(312) 922-5500

Gestalt psychotherapy.

**(929) GESTALT INSTITUTE OF CHICAGO**
609 Davis Street
Evanston, IL 60201

*Charlotte Rosner, Chairperson, Postgraduate Training Faculty*

Includes postgraduate training in art therapy.

**MARTIN BUBER INSTITUTE** (multidisciplinary workshops)/Columbia, MD **(see 127)**

**SARGASSO: CENTER FOR GROWTH AND DEVELOPMENT** (gestalt workshops)/Silver Spring, MD **(see 1088)**

**NEW ENGLAND CENTER FOR PERSONAL AND ORGANIZATIONAL DEVELOPMENT** (humanistic workshops)/Amherst, MA **(see 1089)**

**COMPREHENSIVE THERAPIES** (family and group)/Brookline, MA **(see 1097)**

**ASSOCIATES FOR HUMAN RESOURCES** (humanistic behavior therapy)/Concord, MA **(see 1101)**

**NEW ENGLAND CENTER** (psychophysical approaches)/Leverett, MA **(see 843)**

**WALNUT HOUSE ASSOCIATES** (workshops—family, groups)/Lincoln, MA **(see 1103)**

**ASSOCIATES FOR CREATIVE THERAPY** (training and psychotherapy)/Newtonville, MA **(see 1105)**

**SARGARIS-WOMEN'S THERAPY COLLECTIVE** (psychotherapy and gestalt)/Minneapolis, MN **(see 1109)**

**WOMANKIND** (growth center)/Minneapolis, MN **(see 1110)**

**ENTAYANT INSTITUTE** (humanistic center)/Centerport, NY **(see 1114)**

**(930) GESTALT CENTER FOR PSYCHOTHERAPY AND TRAINING**
150 East 52nd Street, Suite 401
New York, NY 10022

(212) 752-1932

*Marilyn B. Rosanes-Berrett, PhD, Founder and Executive Director*

Provides outpatient psychotherapeutic treatment for neurotics, situational disturbances, personality disorders, and psychotics. Psychotherapy is totally within a gestalt framework; both individual and group sessions are offered.

The Center qualifies as a state-certified mental health program. Also the Center is a postgraduate educational institute chartered by the State of New York to grant a certificate to licensable professionals who have completed an extensive training program.

### (931) THE GESTALT PSYCHOTHERAPY ASSOCIATES
211 Central Park West
New York, NY 10025

(212) 362-1212

Gestalt psychotherapy and training.

### (932) THE GESTALT THERAPY INSTITUTE OF NEW YORK
7 West 96th Street
New York, NY 10025

(212) 850-5080

Gestalt psychotherapy and training with Laura Perls.

### (933) THE ILANA RUBENFELD CENTER FOR GESTALT SYNERGY
115 Waverly Place
New York, NY 10011

(212) 254-5100

*Ilana Rubenfeld, Director*

Gestalt Synergy is a new therapeutic approach encompassing the principals of the gestalt therapy of Fritz and Laura Perls and the bodymind work of F.M. Alexander and Moshe Felderkrais; it is based on the belief that each person is an inseparable unity of body, mind, and spirit. Memories and emotions are stored in the body as well as in the mind, with the result that each person's body posture reflects his or her attitude towards life, including past experiences and traumas. Gestalt Synergy uses a variety of techniques to open the gateways to deep feelings which, to be successfully integrated into a person's everyday life, must not only be contacted and expressed but also worked through. To achieve this goal, neither intellectual insight nor emotional catharsis alone suffices; both are necessary. Thus, Gestalt Synergy relies on verbal expression, physical movement, and the special use of touch. Breathing patterns, body posture, sound, and kinesthetic sense are also stressed. Clients learn to increase their awareness of their own bodymind process, to accept responsibility for their actions, and to make new choices. The Center offers workshops in the Alexander technique, gestalt theory and practice, as well as intensive weekends to train professionals in Gestalt Synergy. Individual treatment is given by trained Gestalt Synergists.

### (934) NEW INSTITUTE FOR GESTALT THERAPY
251 West 92nd Street
New York, NY 10025

(212) 799-3142

Offers a three-year program in gestalt therapy leading to a certificate on completion of requirements. Program is open to psychiatrists, social workers, psychologists, and other qualified psychotherapists.

**WAINWRIGHT HOUSE** (humanistic center)/Rye, NY **(see 1122)**

**CENTER FOR HUMAN DEVELOPMENT** (growth center)/Pittsburgh, PA **(see 1128)**

### (935) GESTALT INSTITUTE OF DALLAS
8616 Northwest Plaza Drive
Dallas, TX 75225

(214) 363-7581

*Ben Goodwin, MD, President*

Promotes education, research, training, and innovation in gestalt theory and method. The Institute holds professional training seminars, individual and group therapy, and weekend marathons. Founded 1971.

**ESOTERIC PHILOSOPHY CENTER** (wholistic workshops)/Houston, TX **(see 151)**

**CAMBRIDGE HOUSE** (humanistic center)/Milwaukee, WI **(see 1129)**

**COLD MOUNTAIN INSTITUTE** (humanistic school)/Vancouver, British Columbia, Canada **(see 1130)**

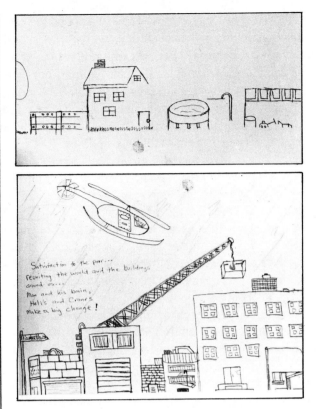

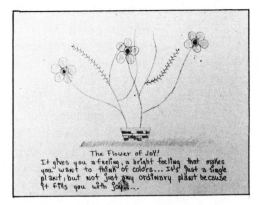

The Flower of Joy!
It gives you a feeling, a bright feeling that makes you want to think of colors... It's just a single plant, but not just any ordinary plant because it fills you with joy...

This sequence of drawings are from an Art Therapist's case book and shows how a predelinquent boy with a negative self-image was able, with the help of his art therapist, to move toward the incorporation of a positive self-image.

Lester's Art, courtesy of Robert Wolf, Director Art Therapy, The Henry Street School, New York City.

# Art Therapy as a Means of Wholistic Individuation through Creative Expression

*Josef E. Garai, PhD, ATR*

Art, music, and dance are the three universal languages of mankind. Through the use of these expressive modalities, people from widely divergent countries, cultures, and ethnic backgrounds can experience a spontaneous exchange of intimate feelings, moods, impressions, sensations, ideas, and thoughts. We perceive the world as a kaleidescope of images, pictorial impressions, and dreamlike shifts as if in all our thinking, planning, reminiscing, and meanderings of mind our "inner eye" were watching a motion picture composed of stimulating and often confusing scenarios. There is a continuous interplay between our inner vision and our perception of external "reality" or our view of the world at large.

Art therapy is characterized by the use of symbolic communication presented by graphic, pictorial, sculpted, modeled, collage-composed, or other art media. Modern technocratic societies tend to overemphasize the importance of verbal expression and logical or rational thought. Words can be used to hide and conceal as well as to disclose and reveal feelings, attitudes, ideas, and thoughts. Networks of verbal communication are subject to the sending and receiving of confusing "double-bind" messages. Therapeutic techniques based on verbal communication tend to reinforce an eloquent client's resistance to development of insight into compulsive repetition of self-destructive patterns of behavior. Spontaneous artistic creativity frequently helps to break down the barriers of a person's defensive structure to reveal the underlying primary processes of the id. Repressed anger, frustrated sexual desires, and feelings of loneliness, isolation, and despair may surge forth in paintings, drawings, sculptures, collages, clay modelings, weavings, sandplay, prints, etc. The client may learn to interpret the symbolic meanings of these creative products and the processes of creative expression under the sympathetic guidance of the trained art therapist, who will thus enable him or her to move toward increased self-awareness and discovery of the roots of intrapsychic and interpersonal conflicts.

241

Art therapy can be most effectively utilized with those types of patients who fail to respond to verbal methods. Autistic children, brain-damaged individuals, persons with speech defects, the deaf and the blind, stutterers, mute or noncommunicative schizophrenics, depressed patients who refuse to talk, and patients who suffer from partial or total amnesia have learned to communicate their feelings, conflicts, anxieties, and problems through drawings, clay modelings, collages, sculptures, weaving, bead stringing, fingerpainting, and other media. The spoken or graphically depicted stories they make up in response to these pictures reveal their genuine feelings of loneliness, abandonment, despair, and alienation, their inner sufferings caused by feelings of hurt and rejection from parents, siblings, spouses, and other significant persons, and their repressed longings for nurturance, love, recognition, and self-actualization.

Group art therapy techniques include a wide variety of styles, approaches, and philosophies. Groups range in size from four to twenty, with a preferred range of six to ten members. They engage in the drawing of group murals with crayons, luma paints, collages, etc., based on "theme-choice" derived from the group members' discussion of potential group themes, developing a group process of conflict, consensus, and increased group interaction clarifying mutual relationships. In the earlier stages, with less group-oriented members, participants are permitted to contribute whatever they want at whatever moment in time to a rather undefined large white sheet of mural paper so as to enable them to develop trust and a relaxation of defensive structures at their own convenience. In recent years, art therapists have begun to integrate music, dance, and movement approaches into their group mural work. Group art therapy assists many isolated clients to learn to accept friendly and also critical interaction with other group members to create a more realistic basis for genuinely trusting interpersonal relationship.

Group art projective techniques can be derived from diagnostic drawing tests administered on a group basis. In addition, the "theme-centered" mural may reveal deep intrapsychic and interpersonal conflict areas. Thus, for instance, the theme might be chosen by the clients themselves to discover what their most urgent concerns at a certain time might be. The therapists may themselves select a relevant theme to break through defenses that prevent movement toward conflict resolution.

Art therapy is also particularly effective in work with schizophrenic and hysteric families. Conjoint family art psychotherapy can uncover primary process material, break down resistances in an atmosphere of minimal threat, and promote more spontaneous and honest patterns of communication among family members, based on the expression of genuine needs and feelings rather than on expected role performance and projections. Repressed feelings related to aggressive, sexual, creative, and competitive drives frequently emerge quite spontaneously in the symbolic expressions of the family members.

A variety of theoretical frameworks integrate art therapy techniques. In the United States, the earliest influence was exerted by Margaret Naumburg, whose numerous writings follow the traditional psychoanalytic approach. Spontaneous art expression releases the unconscious. It has its roots in the transference relations between therapist and patient, and in the encouragement of free association, developing the patient's own interpretations of his or her symbolic design. Naumberg defines this type of communication as "symbolic speech." She regards the introduction of painting and clay modeling into analytically oriented psychotherapy as an adjunct method accelerating the therapeutic process rather than as an independent therapeutic method in its own right. She describes the following four advantages of this "adjunct" technique over traditional verbal analysis:

1. It permits direct expression of dreams, fantasies, and other inner experiences that occur as pictures rather than words.
2. Pictured projections of unconscious material escape censorship more easily than do verbal expressions; thus, the therapeutic process is speeded up.
3. The productions are durable and unchanging, their content cannot be erased by forgetting, and their authorship is hard to deny.
4. The resolution of the transference is made easier because the autonomy of patients is encouraged by their growing ability to contribute to the interpretation of their own creations. They are enabled gradually to substitute a narcissistic cathexis to their own art for their dependence on the art therapist.

I have developed a humanistic approach to art therapy. Based on a variety of recently emerging wholistic theoretical models and reflecting an effort to broaden and deepen the scope of interaction between "inner space," or experience, and "outer space," or "external reality," it relies on the following assumptions:

1. Rather than being classified as "mentally ill," people are seen as encountering difficult problems in their efforts to cope with life. Treatment must therefore be directed toward reinforcing the will to live and developing the ability to find meaning and identity in as fully creative a lifestyle as possible.
2. The inability to cope with the vicissitudes of life or to find satisfactory avenues toward self-actualization, meaning, and identity is a common phenomenon affecting people not only during adolescence but at different crucial junctures in their lives. Problems and lifestyles tend to change continually. Humanistic art therapists assist clients to accept life as an ever-ongoing process requiring continuous change, growth, and development. Instead of waiting to "cure" people when periods of tension and "identity crises" occur, they help clients to integrate the various "identity crises" into creative-expressive lifestyles and to prepare movement toward further experiences of change. Life experiences that enhance curiosity, excitement, self-expression, and intimacy are encouraged.
3. Self-actualization remains basically sterile unless the self-disclosing and genuinely open person is able to formulate a *self-transcendent* goal which makes life more meaningful, adding a "spiritual" dimension to it. This requires a conscious commitment to relate one's own self-actualizing needs to those of the community at large, both through the attainment of genuine interpersonal intimacy and through increasing openness and honesty in relations with others in efforts to improve and expand the opportunities in the life space of the community.

These three principles can be summarized as follows: (1) emphasis on life problem solving, (2) encouragement of self-actualization through creative expression, and (3) emphasis on relating self-actualization to intimacy and trust in interpersonal relations, and the search for self-transcendent life goals.

The wholistic-humanistic orientation in art therapy and creativity development encourages the creation of an atmosphere of total absence of moralistic judgmental attitudes, guiding the person toward the development of the rhythmically balanced personality that can establish a flow between the polarities of love and anger, weakness and strength, privacy and intimacy, cooperation and competition, dependency and independence, dominance and submission, hope and despair, life and death. Once people are aware of these conflicting polarities, they can give up perfectionistic standards of performance and behavior, and proceed toward self-actualizing choices and commitments rather than self-destructive ones. In humanistic art therapy the client, together with the therapist, embarks on a journey of exploration of inner images, fantasies, dreams, myths, fairy tales, ghosts, and archetypes. This adventure into the depths of the unconscious psyche enables both to crystallize blocked or unexplored facets of the inner experience to bring about enhanced awareness of deep feelings, anxieties, and hopes. Thus, wholistic art therapy can become the royal road toward the emergence of the *creative person* who is no longer alienated from the inexhaustible wellsprings of the vital inner energies revealed in dreams, images, myths, fantasies, and intuitive perceptions.

Otto Rank has pointed out that art is the true way of education, or the "drawing out" of inner experience. It is the task of every person to become an "artist-in-life" by integrating experiences into a particular lifestyle. Art therapy is not a means to "adjust" the individual to society; it is, rather, a way of living fully and creatively for the purpose of forging one's own peculiar existence. The goal of therapy is not to transform individuals into cogs of a smoothly functioning machine; it consists in the achievement of genuine individuation and self-transcendence.

Creative work is self-transcending and task-oriented. Art expression involves a confrontation with the psychic images of the realm of inner perception. It is an experience leading to symbol-making, symbol-digesting, and symbol-integrating processes. It is mediated by the self which is the creator within.

Art products, like symbols, are derived from the unconscious, the preconscious, and the conscious components of creative expression. They are therefore understandable and compatible with the forms of logic and consciousness located in the left cerebral hemisphere of the brain. But they are also partly obscure, ghostly, mysterious, and ambiguous, because they contain elements of unfathomable illumination from the realms of "inner space" located in the right cerebral hemisphere, which can transform the life-germinating chaos and turmoil into inchoate flows of energy reflected by meaningful symbolic imagery.

Those art therapists who follow the wholistic-humanistic approach are developing a specific philosophical orientation which perceives therapy as a continuous process leading to change and individuation through the harmonious integration of the basic faculties of sensing, feeling, thinking, and intuiting to achieve a rhythmically balanced personality. They encourage their clients to set out on the journey toward a more compassionate and community-involved lifestyle based on the vision of the "whole" person whose thinking is no longer imbued with cold logic and dehumanized "rationality," whose thoughts and ideas have become infused with feelings of tenderness, compassion, and reliance on the faculties of empathetic sensitivity and imaginative intuition. The compassionate, integrated, individuated, and self-transcendent person is the genuine artist-in-life.

## Groups and Associations

**(936) AMERICAN ART THERAPY ASSOCIATION**
c/o Kay Martinez, Corresponding Secretary
1412 Morgan
Parsons, KS 67357

(316) 421-0024

Dedicated to the progressive development of the therapeutic use of art, the advancement of research, the improvement of standards of practice, the development of criteria for training art therapists, the encouragement of the development of professional training opportunities, and the provision of vehicles for the exchange of information through the means of publications, meetings, and seminars. The Association publishes a *Guidelines for Art Therapy Training* and a biannual *Membership Directory* to assist in the location of art therapists. AATA members meeting certain professional standards may apply to the Association for a certificate of registration, entitling the applicants to use the initials "ATR."

**(937) NEW YORK ART THERAPIST ASSOCIATION**
c/o Janet Lewis, Secretary
226 West Eleventh Street
New York, NY 10014

(212) 675-5618

Conducts periodic workshops and conventions for an exchange of professional experiences, both theoretical and practical. Lines of communication are maintained with the American Art Therapy Association. The NYATA also keeps a roster of art therapists, maintains a listing of available educational programs, and keeps abreast of legislation which would affect the practice of art therapy.

## Schools, Centers, and Clinics

**WHOLISTIC MEDICINE AND PERSONAL GROWTH CENTER**/Hawthorne, CA **(see 84)**

**HOLISTIC HEALTH CENTER** (clinic and school)/Los Angeles, CA **(see 90)**

**INSTITUTE FOR CREATIVE AGING** (clinic)/Malibu, CA **(see 94)**

**AUTOGENIC HEALTH CENTER** (clinic and school)/ Oakland, CA **(see 98)**

**(938) THE ART AND GROWTH STUDIO**
3827 California Street
San Francisco, CA 94118

(415) 387-1993

*Rochelle Myers, MA, MS, Founder and Director*

Structures art experiences in "visual evolution" for adults who feel disconnected from a creative life. The process begins with a dot and extends into line, shape, texture, space, and color. Music, relaxation, discussion, and mandala painting all enhance the philosophy that the purpose of life is to grow. Founded 1971.

**(939) SAINT ELIZABETHS HOSPITAL**
Washington, DC 20032

(202) 562-4000

*Anne K. Bushart, Chief, Recreational Therapy Section*

Clinical Experience at undergraduate and graduate levels provided through accredited colleges.

**GESTALT INSTITUTE OF CHICAGO** (art therapy)/ Evanston, IL **(see 929)**

**EXPANSION** (family-oriented art therapy)/Bedford, MA **(see 1090)**

**INTERFACE** (art therapy and workshops)/Newton, MA **(see 131)**

**WOMANKIND** (growth center)/Minneapolis, MN **(see 1110)**

**(940) ESSEX COUNTY HOSPITAL CENTER**
Department of Music and Creative Art Therapies
Box 500
Cedar Grove, NJ 07009

(201) 239-1900

*Sandra C. Golden, RMT, Director, Music and Creative Art Therapies*

Offers a certificate in art or music with a six-month affiliation.

**(941) CREATIVE ARTS THERAPIES ASSOCIATION TRAINING INSTITUTE**
54 West Ninth Street
New York, NY 10011

(212) 533-3237

*Steve Ross, ATR*

Offers a certificate of completion of a two-year program.

**TURTLE BAY MUSIC SCHOOL** (training in art therapy)/New York, NY **(see 991)**

**(942) HIGHLAND VIEW HOSPITAL—ART STUDIO**
3901 Ireland Drive
Cleveland, OH 44122

(216) 464-9600

*Ms. Mickie McGraw, Director*

Offers clinical experience at undergraduate and graduate levels through accredited colleges.

**(943) THE ART PSYCHOTHERAPY INSTITUTE OF CLEVELAND**
(Formerly The Cleveland Institute of Art Psychotherapy)
2800 Mayfield Road, #202
Cleveland Heights, OH 44118

(216) 932-0120

*Pamela Diamond, ATR, Director*

Offers a certificate for a one-year program in art psychotherapy.

**(944) HARDING HOSPITAL CLINICAL INTERNSHIP PROGRAM**
445 East Granville Road
Worthington, OH 43085

(614) 885-5381

*Donald Jones, ATR*

Offers a certificate and Ohio registration for nine months, full time, ATR-supervised training.

**(945) BETHESDA HOSPITAL**
2951 Maple Avenue
Zanesville, OH 43701

(614) 454-4000

*Bernard O. Stone, ATR, MFA, Director, Art Psychotherapy Department*

Offers eight-week graduate interims; spring, summer, fall, and winter.

**(946) NORTHWESTERN INSTITUTE OF PSYCHIATRY**
Lafayette Avenue and Bethlehem Pike
Fort Washington, PA 19034

(215) 542-8820

*Lea Camero, Department of Adjunctive Therapy*

Offers a six-month practicum.

**(947) HOME FOR CRIPPLED CHILDREN: REGIONAL COMPREHENSIVE REHABILITATION CENTER FOR CHILDREN AND YOUTH**
1426 Denniston Avenue
Pittsburgh, PA 15217

(412) 521-9000

*Roberta Davis, ATR*

Offers art therapy treatment and program.

**(948) EASTERN VIRGINIA MEDICAL SCHOOL**
c/o Ronald E. Hays, ATR
Director of Adjunctive Therapies
Norfolk Community Mental Health Center
721 Fairfax Avenue
Norfolk, VA 23507

(804) 627-0211

Offers a certificate of completion in art therapy.

**(949) MILWAUKEE PSYCHIATRIC HOSPITAL**
1220 Dewey Avenue
Wauwatosa, WI 53213

(414) 258-2600

*Bill Smith, Director, Education, Vocation, and Recreation*

Offers a certificate for a six-month internship.

**COLD MOUNTAIN INSTITUTE** (humanistic workshops)/Vancouver, British Columbia, Canada **(see 1130)**

**(950) TORONTO ART THERAPY INSTITUTE**
216 St. Clair Avenue, West
Toronto, Ontario, Canada

(416) 921-4374

*Martin A. Fischer, MD, DPsych, Executive Director*

Offers courses in art therapy and closely related subjects.

**(951) MIDDELOO TRAINING SCHOOL FOR CREATIVE ACTIVITIES AND GROUP WORK**
Koningin Wilhelminalaan 1
Amersfoort, The Netherlands

*M.M. Brom, Director*

Four-year courses are offered. Group work and use of creative activities in institutional settings. Creative therapy with specializations in dramatics, manual expression, and music.

**ITA-WEGMAN-KLINIK** (anthroposophical clinic)/ Arlesheim, Switzerland **(see 813)**

**SANATORIUM SONNENECK** (anthroposophical clinic)/Arlesheim, Switzerland **(see 815)**

**FRIEDRICH HUSEMANN-KLINIK** (anthroposophical clinic)/West Germany **(see 817)**

**LUKAS KLINIK** (anthroposophical clinic)/West Germany **(see 814)**

**SANATORIUM SCHLOSS HAMBORN** (anthroposophical clinic)/West Germany **(see 824)**

## Schools (Universities)

**(952) CALIFORNIA STATE UNIVERSITY, SACRAMENTO**
6000 "J" Street
Sacramento, CA 95819

(916) 454-6166

*Donald M. Uhlin, EdD, ATR, Department of Art*

Master of Arts in art with emphasis in art therapy.

**LONE MOUNTAIN COLLEGE** (graduate program in art, music and dance therapies)/San Francisco, CA **(see 909)**

**(953) JUNIOR COLLEGE OF CONNECTICUT**
University of Connecticut
Bridgeport, CT 06602

(203) 516-4131

*Susan Mann, Mental Health Program*

Offers Associate in Arts degree in mental health with a specialty in art therapy.

**(954) ALBERTUS MAGNUS COLLEGE**
New Haven, CT 06511

(203) 777-6631

Offers major in art or psychology with an emphasis in art therapy.

**(955) THE GEORGE WASHINGTON UNIVERSITY**
Graduate School of Arts and Sciences
Bacon Hall #201
Washington, DC 20052

(202) 676-6210

Offers Master of Arts in art therapy.

**(956) UNIVERSITY OF EVANSVILLE**
P.O. Box 329
Evansville, IN 44702

*Leslie Miley, Jr., Chairman, Department of Art*

Offers BS degree in art and associated studies with a major in art therapy.

**(957) EMPORIA KANSAS STATE COLLEGE**
1200 Commercial Street
Emporia, KS 66081

(316) 343-1200

*Dal H. Cass, Chairman, Psychology Department*

Offers Master of Science in psychology with a major in art therapy.

**(958) KANSAS STATE COLLEGE OF PITTSBURG**
Pittsburg, KS 66762

(316) 231-7000

Offers Bachelor of Science degree in education with a major in art therapy.

**(959) UNIVERSITY OF LOUISVILLE**
Institute of the Expressive Therapies
Louisville, KY 40202

(502) 588-5265

*Sandra L. Kagin, ATR, Director*

Offers a Master of Arts in art therapy, dance therapy, and drama therapy.

**(960) UNIVERSITY OF MARYLAND**
Crafts Department
College of Human Ecology
College Park, MD 20742

(301) 454-0100

*Harold McWhinnie*

Offers field work and internships in conjunction with art education and crafts courses.

**(961) MASSACHUSETTS COLLEGE OF ART**
364 Brookline Avenue
Boston, MA 02215

(617) 731-2340

*Dorothy Simpson, PhD, Director, Graduate and Continuing Education*

Offers Master of Science in art education with a major in art therapy.

**(962) LESLEY COLLEGE**
Institute for the Arts and Human Development
9 Mellon Street
Cambridge, MA 02138

(617) 868-9600

*Shaun A. McNiff, Coordinator, Graduate School of Education*

Offers Master of Education; major emphasis is expressive: art therapy, dance therapy, and other creative therapies.

**(963) DEAN JUNIOR COLLEGE**
Franklin, MA 02038

(617) 528-9100

Offers Associate in Science degree with a major in art therapy.

**(964) WILLIAM WOODS COLLEGE**
Fulton, MO 65251

(314) 642-2251

*George E. Tutt, Chairman, Department of Art*

Special education/art therapy, leading to state certification in special education. Major in art with concentration in art therapy.

(965) **LINDENWOOD 4, THE LINDENWOOD COL-LEGES**
4635 Maryland Avenue
St. Louis, MO 63108

(314) 361-1404

*Atten: P. Glick, MA, ATR*

Offers Master of Arts in art therapy through individualized study programs in St. Louis, MO, St. Charles, MO, Washington, DC, and Santa Monica, CA.

(966) **TRENTON STATE COLLEGE**
Trenton, NJ 08625

(609) 771-1855

*Mark Wilensky, Director of Art Therapy*

Offers undergraduate program in art therapy.

(967) **MONTCLAIR STATE COLLEGE**
Upper Montclair, NJ 07043

(201) 893-4000

*Susan E. Gonick-Barris, ATR, Director, Graduate Studies in Art Therapy*

Offers Master of Art in art education with option in art therapy techniques.

(968) **PRATT INSTITUTE**
125 Higgins Hall
Brooklyn, NY 11205

(212) 636-3600

Master of Professional Studies in Art Therapy and creativity development.

(969) **COLLEGE OF NEW ROCHELLE**
New Rochelle, NY 10801

(914) 632-5300

Offers Master of Arts in art education with option in art therapy techniques.

(970) **NEW YORK UNIVERSITY**
80 Washington Square East
New York, NY 10003

(212) 598-1212

*Barbara Polny, Advisor, Department of Art Education*

Offers undergraduate program in art education with major in art therapy techniques as well as Master of Arts in art therapy.

(971) **CAPITAL UNIVERSITY**
2199 East Main Street
Columbus, OH 43209

(614) 236-6011

*Richard Phipps, Chairman, Art Department*

Offers undergraduate degree in art with emphasis on psychology as well as internship in art therapy. Nine months clinical and practicum during senior year.

(972) **WRIGHT STATE UNIVERSITY**
c/o Gary Barlow, ATR
Professor and Coordinator, Art Education
326 Creative Arts Building
Dayton, OH 45431

(513) 873-8333

Offers Master's degree in art education with a major in art therapy.

(973) **MOUNT ALOYSIUS JUNIOR COLLEGE**
Cresson, PA 16630

(814) 886-4131

*Hettie Osborne, Chairman, Art Department*

Offers Associate of Arts degree program in art therapy.

(974) **HAHNEMANN MEDICAL COLLEGE**
Department of Mental Health Sciences
New College Building
230 North Broad Street
Philadelphia, PA 19102

(215) 448-7000

*Myra Levick, MEd, ATR, Director, Adjunctive Therapies Education*

Offers Master of Creative Arts in Therapy (MCAT) with specializations in Art Therapy, Movement Therapy, and Music Therapy.

(975) **PHILADELPHIA COLLEGE OF ART**
Broad and Pine Streets
Philadelphia, PA 19102

(215) 893-3100

*Dolores Francine, Art Therapy Advisor*

Offers major in any department with concentration in art therapy.

(976) **TEMPLE UNIVERSITY**
Department of Recreation and Leisure Studies
College of HPERD
c/o Bonnie Klein
Temple University Hospital
Psychiatric In-Patient Unit
2 Main South
Broad and Ontario Streets
Philadelphia, PA 19140

(215) 221-2000

Offers Master of Arts in therapeutic activities and art therapy.

(977) **GODDARD COLLEGE**
Plainfield, VT 05667

(802) 454-8311

*Gladys L. Agell, ATR, Program Director*

Offers a 15-month program with two summers on campus, nine months in the field, for a Master of Arts degree in art therapy.

(977.1) **MOUNT MARY COLLEGE**
2900 North Menomonee River Parkway
Milwaukee, WI 53222

(414) 258-4810

*Sr. M. Regine Collins, Chairperson, Art Department*

Offers undergraduate program in art therapy.

**(978) CITY OF BIRMINGHAM POLYTECHNIC**
School of Art Education
26 Priory Road
Birmingham, BS 7UQ, England

*Michael Edwards*

Offers an MA in art education, with special reference to therapeutic and remedial situations. One-year program plus dissertation.

**(979) HERTFORDSHIRE COLLEGE OF ART AND DESIGN**
7 Hatfield Road
St. Albans
Hertfordshire, England

*J.P. Evans, Head of Remedial Art Department*

Offers a certificate in remedial art. One-year postgraduate course providing a qualification for art therapists in health and social services departments. Accredited programs in music therapy and movement therapy also offered.

## Journals and Publications

**(980) AMERICAN JOURNAL OF ART THERAPY: ART IN EDUCATION, REHABILITATION, AND PSYCHOTHERAPY**
6010 Broad Branch Road, N.W.
Washington, DC 20015

*Elinor Ulman, Publisher*

Published in affiliation with the American Art Therapy Association. Contains articles in the field of art therapy.

**(981) ART PSYCHOTHERAPY: AN INTERNATIONAL JOURNAL**
Pergamon Press, Inc.
Maxwell House
Fairview Park
Elmsford, NY 10523

(914) 592-7700

Contains articles and research on an international scope, relating to the use of art in psychotherapy.

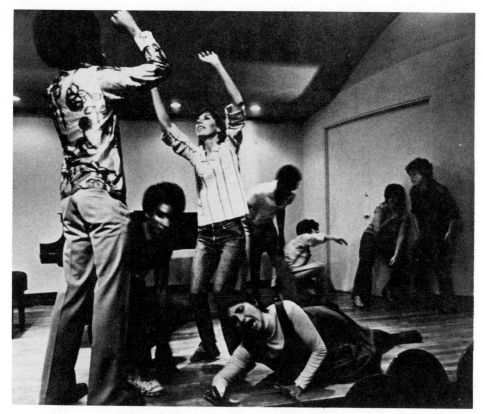

Drama therapy at Turtle Bay School of Music, New York City; photo courtesy of Gertrude Schattner.

# Drama Therapy
*Richard Courtney*

Drama therapy uses spontaneous enactment to help people to become "better." This ranges from general education, through the helping professions, to psychotherapy with the disturbed. Techniques vary from creative drama, through all types of improvisation, dramatic games, and role playing, to specific clinical techniques.

Originating from the works of the nineteenth-century thinkers (e.g., Rousseau, Spencer, Froebel) who advocated natural play for both learning and psychological health, drama came to be used thus for the first time early in this century, and in two contexts: in British education by Caldwell Cook, and with the disturbed by Jacob L. Moreno in Austria and America. From the 1930s on, British education increased creative drama activities with a variety of techniques; recent developments can be seen in the films of Dorothy Heathcote. In psychotherapy Moreno's techniques of psychodrama and sociodrama have continued, while other spontaneous drama techniques have evolved through gestalt therapy, transactional analysis, and other modes. Other than in education and work with the disturbed, spontaneous drama has been used throughout the "helping professions"; with prisoners and criminals, the perceptually and physically handicapped, with the retarded, the aged, the hospitalized, and with deprived groups of all kinds.

The goals are to develop ego strength, perceptual awareness, empathetic response, communication techniques, social and human skills, and all types of learning. Because drama is a representation, an expression, of the *whole* self, it naturally evolves into a myriad of other modes—music, visual and plastic arts, word, dance, the creation of environments, group discussion and decision-making, etc. Modern techniques transmute across all applied fields but are fundamentally based upon improvisation.

## Schools, Centers, and Clinics

**(982) PRECISION PSYCHODRAMA INSTITUTE**
3960 Ingraham Street
Los Angeles, CA 90005

(213) 387-9164

*Laurence O. Anderson, DC, ND, Director*

Conducts private psychodrama groups for problem-solving and consciousness enhancement. The precision psychodrama technique involves three stages: (1) the release of unexpressed feelings; (2) actual training in a new behavior pattern; and (3) development of a self-selected, new belief system based on actual "feeling" experience. Public demonstrations are held both at the Institute and elsewhere by arrangement. The Institute also provides training for individuals wishing to become directors.

**HIGH POINT FOUNDATION** (psychosynthesis)/ Pasadena, Fresno and Oakland, CA; Edmonds, WA **(see 1136)**

**CHILD PSYCHOLOGY INSTITUTE OF SAN DIEGO**/San Diego, CA **(see 1058)**

**UNIVERSITY OF LOUISVILLE** (art and drama workshops)/Louisville, KY **(see 959)**

**SARGASSO: CENTER FOR GROWTH AND DEVELOPMENT** (psychodrama workshops)/Silver Spring, MD **(see 1088)**

**(983) PSYCHODRAMA INSTITUTE OF BOSTON, INC.**
3 Franklin Place
Cambridge, MA 02139

(617) 547-7846

*Bob and Ildri Ginn, Executive Co-Directors*

Devoted to the practice and teaching of psychodrama and developing applications to other fields of mental health. The Institute is also concerned with all current action and expressive techniques of psychotherapy, especially bioenergetics. Offers intensive psychodrama groups, workshops, and training sessions in the Boston area and in Scandinavia.

**WALNUT HOUSE ASSOCIATES** (humanistic workshops)/Lincoln, MA **(see 1103)**

**(984) TURTLE BAY SCHOOL OF MUSIC**
Arts Therapy Program
244 East 52nd Street
New York, NY 10022

(212) 753-8811

*Gertrude Schattner, Instructor*

Explores the varied use of drama therapy techniques, providing participants with the means to help both children and adults who have neurological, psychological, or sociological handicaps.

**WAINWRIGHT HOUSE** (humanistic workshops)/Rye, NY **(see 1122)**

**CENTER FOR HUMAN DEVELOPMENT** (growth center)/Pittsburgh, PA **(see 1128)**

**YORK UNIVERSITY** (transpersonal workshops)/ Downsville, Ontario, Canada **(see 68)**

**MIDDELOO TRAINING SCHOOL FOR CREATIVE ACTIVITIES AND GROUP WORK**/Amersfoort, The Netherlands **(see 951)**

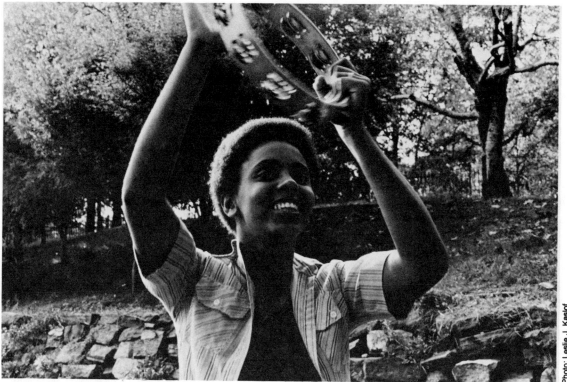

Photo: Leslie J. Kaslof

# Music Therapy/Guided Imagery

*Helen L. Bonny, PhD, RMT*

*"Music has power to ease tension within the heart and to loosen the grip of obscure emotions. The enthusiasm of the heart expresses itself involuntarily in a burst of song, in dance and rhythmic movement of the body. From immemorial times, the inspiring effects of the invisible sound that moves all hearts and draws them together has mystified mankind."*

*I Ching*

Mystified and awed as mankind has been about the effects of music, every effort has been made to use it to correct human suffering and, through its aesthetic appeal, to add dimensions of joy and beauty to both performer and listener. In order to meet these needs, melodies have been composed, from the simplest folk and children's songs to complex symphonies and ragas. In all ages and in all cultures music has been a part of human life.

Music therapy is the application of music to influence changes in behavior. In other words, music is used functionally: it is a means to a goal, a catalyst to affect people psychologically, physically, and emotionally. Viewed as a functional entity, music has a number of qualities that facilitate its action:

1. Music is a nonverbal communication: it is music's wordless meaning that gives it its potency and value.
2. Music is adaptable or flexible: it can be used in many ways, by solo artists as well as retarded children who play rhythm instruments in happy community, or by geriatric or terminal patients.
3. Music is a socializing agent: it encourages group interaction and communication.
4. Moods of music seem to be derived from the tender emotions; themes such as love of family, religion, patriotism, and loyalty abound in musical composition.
5. Music provides structured reality for patients who are in conflict and need positive support.
6. Music provides instant gratification: it can lower anxiety levels and give one a feeling of accomplishment.
7. In both individual and group therapies, music can facilitate emotional catharsis leading to insight and to a healing of the personality.

251

Music therapy has been used in a variety of situations: in hospitals for the mentally retarded and mentally ill, with physically handicapped individuals, with geriatric patients, in community recreation centers, in penal institutions, with special education students in public schools, as music-assisted psychotherapy in crisis counseling centers, and in private practice. Activities range from use of rhythm bands, group singing, teaching of recreational-type instruments, to specialized listening procedures, research into the influence of music on behavior, individual lessons on piano, strings, woodwinds, to learning through music, expression through music, catharsis through music, physical activity with music.

One innovative form of music therapy, Guided Imagery and Music (GIM), has evolved from research at the Maryland Psychiatric Research Center in Baltimore, Maryland. Music, observed to be a most effective guide and structure for mind-expanding drug experience, was demonstrated to greatly enhance and deepen nondrug experiential spaces evoked through concentration—relaxation exercises used in stimulating internal imagery. GIM evolved as a process which involves listening to music in a relaxed state for the purpose of allowing imagery, symbols, and deep feelings to arise from the inner self. The materials so evoked may then be used for therapeutic intervention or self-understanding. The GIM process allows individuals to get in touch with their own unique creative flow. A particularly wholistic* approach for the viewing of the psyche, GIM helps those who experience it to get in touch not only with psychodynamics, but also with the transpersonal aspects of the self.

## Groups and Associations

(985) **NATIONAL ASSOCIATION FOR MUSIC THERAPY, INC.**
Box 610
Lawrence, KS 66044

(913) 842-1909

Registration for music therapists on college level complying with specified standards established by the NAMT.

(986) **AMERICAN ASSOCIATION FOR MUSIC THERAPY**
Department of Music and Music Education
777 Education Building
Washington Square
New York, NY 10003

(212) 598-3491

Offers certification in music therapy based on academic background and experience in the field.

## Schools, Centers, and Clinics

(987) **WELL-SPRINGS**
11667 Alba Road
Ben Lomond, CA 95005

(408) 336-8594

*Kay Ortmans, Director*

A teaching and therapy center with programs designed for the professional therapist. These include therapy and training in "Alignment-through-Music" and movement to release blocked energies. Additional programs are also available in chalk and clay creative writing. Week long training sessions are given throughout the year.

**INSTITUTE FOR CREATIVE AGING** (wholistic workshops)/Malibu, CA **(see 94)**

(988) **SPECTRUM RESEARCH INSTITUTE**
231 Emerson Street
Palo Alto, CA 94301

(415) 328-0264

*Steven Halpern, MA, Director*

Conducts research into the physiological and psychological effects of "meditative music." Distributes information on the subject of music and consciousness, and has available a recording (LP or cassette) entitled *Spectrum Suite: A Meditative Environment*, which has successfully been used in a variety of clinical and experimental settings. (The latter was formerly released as *Christening for Listening*.)

**LONE MOUNTAIN COLLEGE** (graduate programs in dance and music therapies)/San Francisco, CA **(see 909)**

(989) **INSTITUTE FOR CONSCIOUSNESS AND MUSIC TRAINING SEMINARS**
417 East Belvedere
Baltimore, MD 21212

(301) 433-1472

*Helen Bonny, RMT, PhD, Director*

Promotes workshops, lectures, and intensive training seminars in guided imagery with music (G.I.M.) in the Baltimore area and at other central points across the United States. Once-a-month weekend workshops and five-day intensive workshops followed by five-week seminars are held three times a year starting in the months of February, July, and October. For those persons who want full endorsement and training in G.I.M., a year's internship is also provided for the professional practitioner.

*Spelled holistic in original text.*

(990) **INNER SOUND INSTITUTE**
1572 Beacon Street, #3
Brookline, MA 02146

(617) 734-1428

*Steven Schatz, Director*

Offers a 12-week, individually-oriented training program in alternative music therapy. The method uses deep relaxation to induce altered states of consciousness. The methods and models of psychosynthesis encourage the integration of the unconscious material evoked. Techniques used in the training include toning, chanting, guided imagery, fantasy work, affirmations, and grounding with mandalas, writing, and drawing. The Institute also offers individual sessions "for those who choose to open and unfold from center, through working with the heart, the body, and the mind." Founded 1975."

**INTERFACE** (wholistic center)/Newton, MA **(see 131)**

**ESSEX COUNTY HOSPITAL CENTER** (clinical training)/Cedar Grove, NJ **(see 940)**

(991) **TURTLE BAY MUSIC SCHOOL**
Arts in Therapy Program
244 East 52nd Street
New York, NY 10022

(212) 753-8811

*Jean Mass, Director*

Offers one-year certification training program, including six-months clinical internship in music therapy. Also has available training workshops for drama, dance, and art therapy. Advanced intertherapy workshops are given for graduates of the music therapy program.

**HAHNEMANN MEDICAL COLLEGE** (clinical training)/Philadelphia, PA **(see 974)**

**HERTFORDSHIRE COLLEGE OF ART & DESIGN** (programs in music therapy)/Hertfordshire, England **(see 979)**

**MIDDELOO TRAINING SCHOOL FOR CREATIVE ACTIVITIES AND GROUP WORK** (music therapy program)/Amersfoort, The Netherlands **(see 951)**

**ITA-WEGMAN-KLINIK** (anthroposophical clinic)/Arlesheim, Switzerland **(see 813)**

**SANATORIUM SONNENECK** (anthroposophical clinic) Badenweiler, Switzerland **(see 815)**

**FRIEDRICH HUSEMANN-KLINIK** (anthroposophical clinic)/West Germany **(see 817)**

**LUKAS KLINIK** (anthroposophical clinic)/West Germany **(see 814)**

**SANATORIUM FÜR DYNAMISCHE THERAPIE STUDENHOF** (anthroposophical clinic)/West Germany **(see 823)**

# Schools (Universities)

*Since November 1975 the following colleges and universities have been recognized by the National Association for Music Therapy, Inc.* **(985)** *as being either in the process of securing or as having already secured approval of the National Association of Schools of Music for their degree programs in music therapy. Each of them awards the Bachelor's degree, and those which are indicated award the Master's degree. Master's degree programs have more variation than the undergraduate programs, and those interested in graduate study should get curriculum information directly from the accredited institution of their choice.*

(992) **ARIZONA STATE UNIVERSITY**
Tempe, AZ 85281

(602) 565-3371

*Betty Isern Howery, Department of Music*

Undergraduate program in music therapy.

(993) **CALIFORNIA STATE UNIVERSITY**
Long Beach, CA 90840

(213) 498-4111

*Kay Roskam, RMT, Department of Music*

Undergraduate program in music therapy.

(994) **UNIVERSITY OF THE PACIFIC**
Stockton, CA 95204

(209) 946-2011

*Suzanne B. Hanser, RMT, Department of Music Therapy*

Undergraduate program in music therapy.

(995) **COLORADO STATE UNIVERSITY**
Fort Collins, CO 80523

(303) 491-1101

*Frederick Tims, RMT, Department of Music Education*

Undergraduate program in music therapy.

(996) **CATHOLIC UNIVERSITY OF AMERICA**
Washington, DC 20064

(202) 635-5000

*Helen L. Bonny, RMT, PhD, Department of Music Therapy*

Probationally approved department of music therapy.

(997) **UNIVERSITY OF MIAMI**
Coral Gables, FL 33124

(305) 284-2211

*Constance Willeford, RMT*

Offers Master of Arts degree in music therapy.

(998) **FLORIDA STATE UNIVERSITY**
Tallahassee, FL 32306

(904) 644-2525

*Diane Greenfield, RMT, Director of Music Therapy*

Offers Master of Arts degree in music therapy.

**(999) UNIVERSITY OF GEORGIA**
Athens, GA 30601

(404) 542-3738

*Richard M. Graham, RMT, Department of Music*

Offers doctorate program in music therapy.

**(1000) DePAUL UNIVERSITY**
25 East Jackson Boulevard
Chicago, IL 60604

(312) 321-8000

*James Harris, RMT, Director of Music Therapy*

Undergraduate program in music therapy.

**(1001) ILLINOIS STATE UNIVERSITY**
Normal, IL 61761

(309) 436-7631

*Daniel Stephens, RMT, Music Department*

Undergraduate program in music therapy.

**(1002) INDIANA UNIVERSITY—FORT WAYNE**
Fort Wayne, IN 46803

(219) 482-5746

*Carol I. Collins, RMT, Department of Music*

Undergraduate program in music therapy.

**(1003) UNIVERSITY OF KANSAS**
Lawrence, KS 66045

(913) 864-2700

*William W. Sears, RMT, Department of Music Education–Music Therapy*

Offers doctorate program in music therapy.

**(1004) LOYOLA UNIVERSITY**
New Orleans, LA 70118

(504) 863-2011

*Charles Braswell, RMT, Chairman of Music Therapy*

Offers Master of Arts in music therapy.

**(1005) MICHIGAN STATE UNIVERSITY**
East Lansing, MI 48823

(517) 355-1855

*Robert F. Unkefer, RMT, Department of Music*

Offers Master of Arts in music therapy.

**(1006) WESTERN MICHIGAN UNIVERSITY**
Kalamazoo, MI 49001

(616) 383-1600

*Brian Wilson, RMT, Department of Music*

Undergraduate program in music therapy.

**(1007) UNIVERSITY OF MINNESOTA**
Minneapolis, MN 55455

(612) 373-2851

*Judith Jellison, RMT, Department of Music Education*

Undergraduate program in music therapy.

**(1008) COLLEGE OF SAINT TERESA**
Winona, MN 55987

(507) 454-2930

*Mary Nichols, RMT, Department of Music*

Offers degree programs in music, art, and dance therapies.

**(1009) WILLIAM CAREY COLLEGE**
Hattiesburg, MS 39401

(601) 582-5050

*Carylee Hammons, RMT, School of Music*

Offers degree program in music therapy.

**(1010) LINCOLN UNIVERSITY**
Jefferson City, MO 65101

(814) 751-2325

*Carolyn Hancock, RMT, Department of Music*

Undergraduate program in music therapy.

**(1011) UNIVERSITY OF MISSOURI—KANSAS CITY**
Kansas City, MO 64111

(816) 276-2731

*Wanda Lathom, RMT, Conservatory of Music*

Undergraduate program in music therapy.

**(1012) MARYVILLE COLLEGE**
13550 Conway Road
St. Louis, MO 63141

(314) 434-4100

*Sister Ruth M. Sheehan, RMT, Department of Music*

Undergraduate program in music therapy.

**(1013) MONTCLAIR STATE COLLEGE**
Upper Montclair, NJ 07043

(201) 893-4443

*Barbara Wheeler, RMT, Department of Music*

Undergraduate program in music therapy.

**(1014) EASTERN NEW MEXICO UNIVERSITY**
Portales, NM 88130

(505) 562-2731

*Joseph Moreno, RMT, Department of Music*

Undergraduate program in music therapy.

**(1015) EAST CAROLINA UNIVERSITY**
Greenville, NC 27834

(919) 757-6851

*Ruth Boxberger, RMT, School of Music*

Undergraduate program in music therapy.

**(1016) OHIO UNIVERSITY**
Athens, OH 45701

(614) 594-5511

*Michael Kellogg, RMT, School of Music*

Undergraduate program in music therapy.

(1017) **UNIVERSITY OF DAYTON**
Dayton, OH 45469

(513) 229-0123

*Marilyn Sandness, RMT, Music Division of Performing and Visual Arts Department*

Undergraduate program in music therapy.

(1018) **COLLEGE OF MT. ST. JOSEPH ON THE OHIO**
Mt. St. Joseph, OH 45051

*Sister Miriam Elizabeth Dunn, RMT, Department of Music*

Undergraduate program in music therapy.

(1019) **PHILLIPS UNIVERSITY**
Enid, OK 73701

(405) 237-4433

*Betty Shirm, RMT, School of Music*

Undergraduate program in music therapy.

(1020) **WILLAMETTE UNIVERSITY**
Salem, OR 97301

(503) 370-6300

*Maurice W. Brennen, RMT, Music Therapy Department*

Undergraduate program in music therapy.

(1021) **COMBS COLLEGE OF MUSIC**
Philadelphia, PA 19119

(215) 818-7500

*Helen Braun, RMT, Music Therapy Department*

Undergraduate program in music therapy.

(1022) **DUQUESNE UNIVERSITY**
Pittsburgh, PA 15219

(412) 434-6080

*Richard Gray, RMT, Department of Music*

Undergraduate program in music therapy.

(1023) **BAPTIST COLLEGE**
Music Therapy Department
Charleston, SC 29411

(803) 797-4011

Undergraduate program in music therapy.

(1024) **WEST TEXAS STATE UNIVERSITY**
Canyon, TX 79016

(806) 656-0111

*Martha Estes, RMT, Department of Music*

Undergraduate program in music therapy.

(1025) **SOUTHERN METHODIST UNIVERSITY**
Dallas, TX 75275

(214) 692-2000

*Charles Eagle, RMT, Coordinator of Music Therapy*

Offers Master of Arts in music therapy.

(1026) **TEXAS WOMAN'S UNIVERSITY**
Denton, TX 76204

(817) 382-3913

*Donald Michel, RMT, Department of Music*

Offers Master of Arts in music therapy.

(1027) **SHENANDOAH CONSERVATORY OF MUSIC**
Winchester, VA 22601

(703) 667-8714

*Marian Sung, RMT*

Undergraduate program in music therapy.

(1028) **UNIVERSITY OF WISCONSIN—EAU CLAIRE**
Eau Claire, WI 54701

(715) 836-2284

*Dale Taylor, RMT, Department of Music*

Undergraduate program in music therapy.

(1029) **ALVERNO COLLEGE**
Milwaukee, WI 53215

(414) 671-5400

*Sister M. Josepha Schorsch, RMT, Department of Music*

Undergraduate program in music therapy.

(1030) **UNIVERSITY OF WISCONSIN—MILWAUKEE**
Milwaukee, WI 53201

(414) 963-5584

*Leo Muskatevc, RMT, Department of Music*

Undergraduate program in music therapy.

(1031) **UNIVERSITY OF WISCONSIN—OSHKOSH**
Oshkosh, WI 54901

(414) 424-4224

*Nancy Hinant, RMT, Department of Music*

Undergraduate program in music therapy.

## Journals and Publications

(1032) **JOURNAL OF MUSIC THERAPY**
N.A.M.T.
Box 610
Lawrence, KS 66044

Professional publication of the N.A.M.T. containing research and other papers in the field of music therapy. Quarterly issues from 1964 to the present are available.

(1033) **NEWSLETTER OF THE AMERICAN ASSOCIATION OF MUSIC THERAPY**
Department of Music and Music Education
777 Education Building
Washington Square
New York, NY 10003

(212) 598-3491

Papers and research relating to the field of music therapy.

## Products and Services

(1034) **UNITY RECORDS**
Box 12
Corte Madera, CA 94925

(415) 924-7667

Independent record company specializing in "consciousness music" . . . music intended to raise the consciousness, heal, and instill a more gentle, transcendental approach to living. A free catalog of records and cassettes is available.

(1035) **INSTITUTE FOR CONSCIOUSNESS AND MUSIC**
31 Allegheny Avenue
Towson, MD 21204

(301) 377-2640

*Helen Bonny, RMT, PhD, Director*

Nonprofit organization which provides services to professionals interested in the field of guided imagery with music (G.I.M.). A book, *Music and Your Mind*, and a 16-mm film of the same title provide basic information. Additional materials in the form of music, tapes, records, and informational brochures are available.

(1036) **FOLKWAYS RECORD CO.**
43 West 61st Street
New York, NY 10023

(212) 586-7260

Has one of the most extensive selections of multicultural ethnic recordings, most of them recorded during actual ritual and ceremonial gatherings.

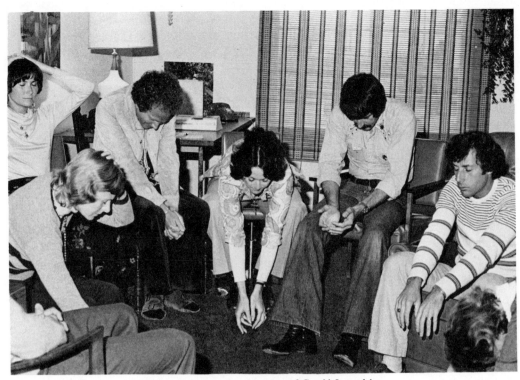

Taking the brain out and washing out old tears, photo courtesy of Gerald Jampolsky.

# Hypnosis/Active Imagination
*Gerald G. Jampolsky, MD*

Hypnotic, trancelike states have been known from very early times, especially among the Oriental peoples, and these states have frequently been associated with mystical and religious practices. An increase in the interest in hypnotic phenomena occured in 1779, when Franz Mesmer published his theory of animal magnetism. In the United States Clark Hull wrote his classic, *Hypnosis and Suggestibility,* in 1933, and Milton H. Erickson later became known as the "father of modern-day hypnosis."

During World War II there was a resurgence of interest in hypnosis for the treatment of what was then diagnosed as "shell shock," "battle fatigue," or "hysterical paralysis." Slowly, in the 1940s and 1950s, hypnosis began to gain a reputation as a psychotherapeutic tool in the fields of medicine, psychology, and dentistry. Though the American Medical Association approved hypnosis as an acceptable mode of treatment in 1958, acceptance among the medical community has been slow, and some medical schools have only recently begun to include hypnosis in their curricula.

Despite the general acceptance of hypnosis as a therapeutic tool and extensive research in the field, the scientific nature of the suggestive state of hypnosis is still considered controversial. Much has been learned about the psychophysiological response of a patient in a hypnotic state, but "What is a trance?" and "What constitutes the various states of hypnosis?" are still under debate. No agreement has been reached on what constitutes a hypnotic state.

In the United States hypnotherapy has generally been conducted with the patient in only a light hypnotic state. Originally limited to phobic and hysterical states, it has since been used in conjunction with virtually every medical specialty. With increased enlightenment regarding the role that the mind plays in all illnesses, whether functional or organic, it became clear that hypnosis could assist in the treatment of all illnesses. In the past decade, it has been particularly useful in helping cancer patients to deal with pain and assisting dying patients to harmonize their mind, body, and psychological and spiritual forces.

With children hypnosis has been used to successfully treat a number of conditions, including bed-wetting, poison oak, dermatitis, asthma, stuttering, learning blocks, and even cancer. With adults it has been used to assist patients to stop smoking and to lose weight. It is also used in anesthesiology and to treat psychosomatic conditions. Increasingly, age regression is being used to bring about emotional detachment from traumatic events in the past that have been short-circuiting present functioning. Such time distortion has proved helpful not only in eliminating pain but also in helping the patient to live more in the time frame of "now."

The growing trend toward using hypnosis is explained by the fact that it can serve as a shortcut to other, more standard psychotherapeutic techniques. Moreover, by teaching autohypnosis, professionals have been able to assist patients to play a more active role in their own healing process, while gaining a more wholistic viewpoint of the relationship of mind, body, and psychological and spiritual self-concepts. Through hypnotherapy patients can participate in creating a positive health profile.

"Active imagination," a term coined by Carl Jung, has recently come into popular use; it denotes a process in which the mind makes use of mental pictures to modify misperceptions of one's inner and outer spaces. Today a number of psychotherapeutic techniques make use of such imagery, including psychosynthesis, gestalt therapy, meditation, primal scream, psychodrama, hypnotic, autogenic, and suggestive therapies, biofeedback, and Jacobson relaxation techniques.

The first step in active imagination is quieting the mind. In essence, subjects must learn to stop thinking. A variety of different techniques exists to accomplish this goal: for example, concentrating on a mantra (as in many types of meditation), Herbert Benson's method of counting one's breathing, or developing a mental picture of where one would like to be (such as relaxed on a beach).

The second step is to create in one's mind a positive, active motion picture of what one would like to experience. In a sense, subjects create a precognitive picture of what they would like to experience, fuse with that picture, and then allow that active imagination picture to come into the present as a current reality. Thus, this method bypasses cognitive thinking. By enabling one to dissolve the emotional attachment to previous experiences, active imagination helps do away with fears related to the past-future paradigm. It allows the unconscious and conscious mind to fuse in a positive pleasurable picture.

In addition, suggestions are made to help the subject stop using words such as *impossible, can't, difficult, try, but, however, should,* and *ought.* These words take energy away from experiencing the nowness of the moment and tend to make the past superimpose itself on the present. For the same reason, subjects are also encouraged to make fewer comparisons and spend less time evaluating concepts.

In essence, subjects are encouraged to diminish their left brain functioning, which makes use of logical, rational, sequential thought processes and linear time. As a result, subjects may experience a sense of cohesion and oneness with the environment, which permits an experience of love both within and without. The active imagination method allows subjects to take responsibility for, and to actively participate in, their own healing process.

## Groups and Associations

(1037) **THE AMERICAN SOCIETY OF CLINICAL HYPNOSIS**
2400 East Devon Avenue, Suite 218
Des Plaines, IL 60018

(312) 297-3317

National society devoted to the scientific study of hypnosis and its therapeutic applications. Brings together professionals in medicine, dentistry, and psychology to establish standards for training, to share information, and to stimulate research and its publication. Publishes the *Journal of Clinical Hypnosis* (editor: Sheldon B. Cohn, MD). Member organization of the World Federation of Mental Health and affiliate of the American Association for the Advancement of Science. Holds workshops which have been approved by AMA for Category 1 of Continuing Education Credit. Membership open to MDs, DOs, DDSs, DMDs, and PhDs in psychology and certain allied fields. Founded 1957.

**NATIONAL INSTITUTE FOR PSYCHOTHERA-PIES**/New York, NY (see 1045)

## Schools, Centers, and Clinics

**HEALTH AWARENESS INSTITUTE** (holistic)/Phoenix, AZ (see 74)

**HUMAN PROCESS INSTITUTE** (psychotherapy)/Encino, CA (see 1052)

**WHOLISTIC MEDICINE AND PERSONAL GROWTH CENTER**/Hawthorne, CA (see 84)

**PSYCHOTHERAPY CENTER**/Los Angeles, CA (see 1054)

**AUTOGENIC HEALTH CENTER**/Oakland, CA (see 98)

**SAN ANDREAS HEALTH CENTER** (holistic therapy and workshops)/Palo Alto, CA (see 101)

**CHILD PSYCHOLOGY INSTITUTE OF SAN DIEGO** (humanistic)/San Diego, CA (see 1058)

**BIOFEEDBACK INSTITUTE OF SAN FRANCISCO** (psychotherapy)/San Francisco, CA (see 1059)

**FAMILY PRACTICE CENTER** (growth center)/Santa Rosa, CA (see 116)

**PSYCHOPHYSICS FOUNDATION** (bodymind workshops)/Miami, FL (see 594)

**KENTUCKY CENTER OF PSYCHOSYNTHESIS**/Lexington, KY (see 1138)

**BIOFEEDBACK INSTITUTE**/Brookline, MA (see 739)

**INSTITUTE FOR PSYCHOENERGETICS** (psychophysical workshops)/Brookline, MA (see 128)

**(1038) PSYCHE RESEARCH INSTITUTE**
10701 Lomas Northeast, Suite 210
Albuquerque, NM 87112

(505) 292-0370

An extension of the Center for Hypnosis Training and Consultation, the Institute is involved in the investigation of hypnosis, meditation, biofeedback, sensory isolation and related techniques as a means of studying consciousness. The Institute teaches courses for both professionals and the general public, and lectures by invitation throughout the United States. Instructional cassette tape recordings are available in hypnosis, meditation and altered states of consciousness.

**(1039) THE SOCIETY FOR CLINICAL AND EXPERIMENTAL HYPNOSIS**
129A Kings Park Drive
Liverpool, NY 13088

(315) 652-7299

*Marian Kenn, Administrative Director*

Offers 3 ½-day workshops in hypnosis in medicine, psychotherapy, and dentistry. The workshops aim to provide participants with the opportunity to learn hypnotic techniques and therapeutic applications for use in their own professional activities. Membership open to psychologists, physicians, and dentists at doctoral level who use therapeutic hypnosis.

**BEHAVIOR THERAPY CENTER OF NEW YORK**/New York, NY (see 1115)

**CENTER FOR HIGHER CONSCIOUSNESS** (hypnosis)/Cleveland Heights, OH (see 146)

**YORK UNIVERSITY** (transpersonal)/Downsview, Ontario, Canada (see 68)

## Journals and Publications

**BRAIN/MIND BULLETIN** (multidisciplinary)/Los Angeles, CA (see 184)

**THE JOURNAL OF CLINICAL HYPNOSIS**/Des Plaines, IL (see 1037)

**(1040) INTERNATIONAL JOURNAL OF CLINICAL AND EXPERIMENTAL HYPNOSIS**
111 North 49th Street
Philadelphia, PA 19139

Official publication of the Society for Clinical and Experimental Hypnosis (1039). Publishes original contributions dealing with hypnosis in psychology, psychiatry, the medical and dental specialties, and allied areas of science. Founded 1952.

## Products and Services

**HEALTH RESEARCH** (books)/Mokelumne Hill, CA (see 209)

**BUTTERFLY MEDIA DIMENSIONS** (cassette tapes)/N. Hollywood, CA (see 210)

**CENTER FOR HEALTH EDUCATION** (cassette tapes)/Palo Verdes, CA (see 211)

**COGNETICS** (cassette tapes)/Saratoga, CA (see 214)

**HARTLEY FILM PRODUCTIONS** (audiovisual)/Cos Cob, CT (see 219)

**(1041) PSYCHOLOGICAL SERVICES**
936 Courthouse Road, Suite 3
Gulfport, MI 39501

Offers cassette tape-recorded programs in self-hypnosis, assertiveness training, and other techniques of psychological self-improvement. Hypnosis tapes aim to assist in such areas as stopping smoking, developing psychic powers, improvement of golf or tennis, weight control, and development of breast size in women.

**PSYCHE RESEARCH INSTITUTE** (cassette tapes)/Albuquerque, NM (see 1038)

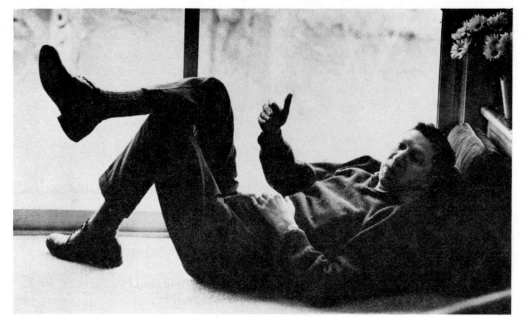

Abraham Maslow, pioneer in Humanistic Psychology, photo courtesy of
Bertha Maslow and the Association for Humanistic Psychology.

# Humanistic Psychology

*Thomas C. Greening, PhD*

*"He gave me his impressions of the white man, and said that they were always upset, always
looking for something, and that as a consequence, their faces were lined with wrinkles, which he
took to be a sign of eternal restlessness. Ochwiay Biano also thought that whites were crazy since
they maintained that they thought with their heads, whereas it was well-known that only crazy
people did that. This assertion by the chief of the Pueblos so surprised me that I asked him how he
thought. He answered that he naturally thought with his heart."*

*C.G. Jung*

Among the origins of humanistic psychology is the work of Kurt Goldstein, MD, with brain-injured
patients. It was Dr. Goldstein who originated the concept of self-actualization; he observed that his
patients demonstrated a drive toward growth in spite of their injuries, a drive that enabled them to achieve
progress beyond what would be predicted from the medical prognosis alone. This expanded view of
human potentialities has become a cornerstone of humanistic psychology.

Abraham Maslow wrote of "high-level wellness" and urged us to look beyond our usual standards of
"adjustment" and absence of gross pathology to see the human capacity and desire for continued
development. This view has enriched the fields of psychotherapy, group thereapy, research psychology,
and education. Recent developments in healing meditation, biofeedback, self-control of autonomic
functioning, and self-care programs have dramatically demonstrated how the self-actualization drive can
manifest itself in areas where passive reliance on expert medical intervention previously predominated.
We are rediscovering what Kurt Goldstein demonstrated years ago—that the power of mind over matter is
a great medical resource too often neglected in modern scientific medicine.

Humanistic psychology provides a theoretical context, a loose but widespread confederation of
explorers, and a forum for the sharing and integrating of findings. Conferences conducted by the
Association for Humanistic Psychology increasingly include sessions on health enhancement, healing
processes, and alternatives to mechanical and depersonalized medical strategies. A central tenet of
humanistic psychology is that we are whole persons who can best be understood and helped by approaches
that respect the complex interaction of our entire way of being. Thus, artificial separation into part

functions is regarded as a pathogenic oversimplification unlikely to enlist the health-seeking forces latent within us. Maslow liked the concept of "synergy," which so well expresses the interdependency and mutual supportiveness of the various subsystems that join together in our simplest as well as our most complex endeavors.

Good nutrition, for example, requires a combination of such factors as cognitive knowledge; the motivation to live well; collaboration to produce, procure, and prepare good food; stress-free digestion; and efficient metabolism. People need to be aware of the many component parts in the process of obtaining good nutrition, and they need to have the motivation and the faith that they can make a difference in running that aspect of their lives. Maslow's theory of the hierarchy of needs postulates that as lower-level needs are met, people do not settle for homeostatic quiescence but instead keep searching for ways to fulfill the next level of need. Thus, even within the rather basic level of the need for food, we see that people want this to be an experience that is fulfilling in as many ways as possible—e.g., nutritionally, aesthetically, and socially.

Another example is childbirth. Developments such as natural drug-free childbirth, husband-coaching, early mother-child bonding, and nonviolent birth all originated outside of humanistic psychology but have been picked up, integrated and elaborated, and publicly shared by humanistic psychologists through lay and professional meetings, journal articles and books, and practiced in a variety of settings. Childbirth has too long been an area in which concern for medical safety crowded out the dignity and conscious, shared experience of the key participants. Humanistic psychology, with its valuing of experiencing and its belief in people's capacity to become more responsible for their own well-being, provides an integrating organizational and theoretical focus for people seeking to improve childbirth, just as it does for other workers attempting to apply psychology to the actualization of our full human potential.

Cancer is a dread disease usually treated surgically and chemically. It takes quite a leap of faith to regard it as an opportunity for fundamental life review, stimulation of spiritual growth, and movement into more fulfilling ways of being. But here also humanistic psychology has provided theories, forums, and opportunities for cross-fertilization for workers seeking to activate cancer patients to participate as energetic self-healers rather than as resigned victims. A dramatic shift in attitudes is possible in patients who grasp that self-concepts, the will to live, primary relationships, and emotional states can powerfully influence rate of tumor growth and response to radiation. We do not yet know much about the actual means by which our ideas about our bodies and cancer, our emotions, and our physiological processes are connected so as to affect recovery. But evidence is accumulating rapidly that we are well advised to treat the whole person, not just the cancer.

Sidney Jourard was an active humanistic psychologist and president of the Association for Humanistic Psychology. He studied the phenomenon of "inspiriting" and "dispiriting" experiences and their relationship to physical illness. His extensive research demonstrated that we have a basic need to disclose ourselves to others, to establish deep and open human contact by making ourselves known. People who fall ill are often emotionally isolated from others either as the result of characterological withholding or loss of a relationship. Jourard believed that we cannot really know ourselves unless we discover ourselves in the act of sharing openly.

## Groups and Associations

(1042) **THE INSTITUTE FOR THE STUDY OF HUMAN KNOWLEDGE**
Box 176
Los Altos, CA 94022

(415) 948-9428

*Robert Ornstein, PhD, President*

Sponsors workshops and symposia with authorities from the fields of neurology, psychiatry, mythology, and Eastern thought. Aims at bringing to public awareness new possibilities, such as a complete psychology of consciousness and human development, a medicine which considers the whole person, and an education of the full range of human capacities.

(1043) **ASSOCIATION FOR HUMANISTIC PSYCHOLOGY**
325 Ninth Street
San Francisco, CA 94103

(415) 626-2375

*Eleanor Criswell, EdD, Current President*

International institute for the advancement of humanistic psychology. Maintains a PhD-level graduate program in humanistic psychology, a monthly *Newsletter*, a quarterly *Journal of Humanistic Psychology*, an annual meeting featuring both the theory and the practice of humanistic psychology, regional meetings throughout the United States, international meetings in Latin America and Europe, and local chapters and groups throughout the world. Networks exist for members who wish to be in communication with others who share their special interest. The Association also publishes a yearly roster of AHP members, reprints selected materials at low cost, and maintains lists of colleges with humanistically oriented programs, growth centers, and books in the field. Founded 1961.

### (1044) AMERICAN GROUP PSYCHOTHERAPY ASSOCIATION
1995 Broadway
New York, NY 10023

(212) 787-2618

Nonprofit, multidisciplinary competency organization. Offers a journal, *The International Journal of Group Psychotherapy*, an annual training institute and conference, a referral service, newsletter, and various publications. Founded 1942.

### (1045) NATIONAL INSTITUTE FOR PSYCHOTHERAPIES
330 West 58th Street, Suite 200
New York, NY 10019

(212) 582-1566

*Henry Grayson, PhD, Executive Director*

Devoted to heightening the communication and sharing of knowledge among the major schools of psychotherapy. Combines a postgraduate training program in psychotherapy with clinical and research services. The training program includes study, supervision and practice in bioenergetics, gestalt, hypnosis, and psychoanalysis. Workshops and symposia are held in such areas as parapsychology and healing. Membership is open to psychiatrists, psychologists, pastoral counselors, and psychiatric nurses who hold degrees from recognized universities, are members of their representative professional organizations, and have had 100 hours supervision in psychotherapy.

## Schools, Centers, and Clinics

**HEALTH AWARENESS INSTITUTE** (treatment and educational center)/Phoenix, AZ **(see 74)**

### (1046) RIGGS AND ASSOCIATES
Psychological Services Center
710 South Brookhurst, Suite 1
Anaheim, CA 92804

(714) 635-2350

*M. David Riggs, Executive Director*

3700 Ingraham
San Diego, CA 93109

(714) 272-3335

A multidisciplinary service organization specializing in the application of psychological, physiological, and spiritual principles for the furtherance of individual and interpersonal

growth. Techniques used include individual and group psychotherapy, hypnosis, guided imagery, relaxation techniques, meditation, biofeedback, and healing-touch.

**BERKELEY WOMEN'S HEALTH COLLECTIVE** (psychotherapy)/Berkeley, CA **(see 77)**

### (1047) CENTER FOR BEING
1521 San Pablo Avenue
Berkeley, CA 94702

(415) 525-3685

*John Lonsbury, MA, Director*

Devoted to emotional education through reexperience. Uses a phenomenological model of therapy which is neither medical nor cathartic. Creative and purposive expression is cultivated while passing through recurring emotion cycles. The self is treated as an organic process.

### (1048) METAMORPHOSIS
1812 Short Street
Berkeley, CA 94702

(213) 841-6500

*Marie Jorgensen Brewer, Director*

Dedicated to self-discovery and integration of the whole person through workshops, groups, and individual counseling. Reichian bodywork, T.A., gestalt, family therapy, movement, massage, dream work, and guided fantasy are the techniques used.

**PSYCHOSOMATIC MEDICINE CLINIC** (holistic clinic)/Berkeley, CA **(see 78)**

### (1049) SENIOR ACTUALIZATION AND GROWTH EXPLORATIONS
Claremont Office Park
41 Tunnel Road
Berkeley, CA 94705

(415) 841-9858

*Elizabeth F. Bexton, Administrator*

A program to alter negative cultural attitudes about aging, and assist people over 60 in realizing old age as a period of rich, creative culmination and growth. Toward this end, SAGE offers group therapy and fantasy exercises, counseling, dance, music, and art; and instruction in breathing, meditation, autogenic training, biofeedback, massage, and special exercises. SAGE holds regular workshops across the country on topics related to gerontology, self-development, and changing attitudes toward aging. Three video tapes on the SAGE program are available for rent or purchase. Founded 1974.

### (1050) ARCANA WORKSHOPS
407 North Maple Drive
Suite 214
Beverly Hills, CA 90210

(213) 273-5949

*Marguerite L. Rompage, Director of Training Programs*

Teaches and practices a system of integrative therapy designed to integrate the component parts of the human being and to integrate the individual into his/her total environment. Uses group techniques, meditation, and the principle that many seeming aberrations are actually symptoms of growth. Founded 1955.

## (1051) THE ESALEN INSTITUTE
Big Sur, CA 93920

(408) 667-2335

*Janet Lederman, Co-Director of Education*

1793 Union Street
San Francisco, CA 94123

(415) 771-1710

*Dulce Murphy, Director*

A multidimensional educational laboratory, a way of life. Teachers of virtually all New Age and wholistic persuasions may be present in formal workshops or in the communal baths. Workshops in all areas of human potential, mythology, massage, movement, psychology, and art are offered in both short-term and long-term formats. A catalog fully describing the course offerings is available by subscription. Activities are offered both in San Francisco and Big Sur, where groups may stay as long as a month.

## (1052) HUMAN PROCESS INSTITUTE
16200 Ventura Boulevard, #416
Encino, CA 91436

(213) 784-9406

*Valerie G. Cummings, MA, Director*

Provides individual, group, and family counseling/psychotherapy using a "process-interactional" approach focusing on the integration of the body, mind, and emotions of the whole person. Techniques include gestalt, bioenergetics, hypnotherapy, communication theory, and training assertiveness and psychopharmacology. Also offers crisis counseling and a 24-hour crisis line: (213) 784-9406. Founded 1974.

## WHOLISTIC MEDICINE AND PERSONAL GROWTH CENTER/Hawthorne, CA (see 84)

## BARAKA (holistic clinic)/Los Angeles, CA (see 87)

## HOLISTIC HEALTH CENTER (workshops)/Los Angeles, CA (see 90)

## (1053) PSYCHOLOGICAL SERVICE ASSOCIATES
1314 Westwood Boulevard
Los Angeles, CA 90024

(213) 474-6545

A group of psychologists using a variety of methods, including neo-Reichian therapy and guided meditation, to assist patients in healing themselves of illnesses with a psychogenic component. Members of the group also conduct training and education programs for professionals and the lay public. Founded 1953.

## (1054) THE PSYCHOTHERAPY CENTER, INC.
1620 Westwood Boulevard
Los Angeles, CA 90024

(213) 474-5111

*Donald D. Lathrop, MD, Director*

Uses Jungian and gestalt approaches to psychotherapy in individual, family, and group contexts. Techniques emphasized are hypno-relaxation, dream work, and communi-

cations facilitation. Specialized programs include sexual reeducation, child and adolescent counseling, parenting, leisure/lifestyle, surgical counseling, speech and hearing, substance abuse, and death, dying, and terminal illness. The staff are actively exploring nutrition, meditation, yoga, and psychic development. Founded 1975.

## (1055) WOMEN'S INSTITUTE & HEALTH CENTER, INC.
7151 West Manchester Avenue, Suite One
Los Angeles, CA 90045

(213) 641-2911

*Marilynn J. Pratt, MD, Founder and Director*

Provides preventive medical care and Jungian-oriented psychotherapy for women. Classes for women also offered in yoga and self-defense. Also directs research projects related to women's health.

## INSTITUTE FOR CREATIVE AGING (geriatric therapy)/Malibu, CA (see 94)

## (1056) HEART HAUS CENTER
968 Greenhill Road
Mill Valley, CA 94941

(415) 383-4859

The Center has programs available in gestalt therapy, Reichian and Alexander techniques. A biofeedback, transcendental meditation and psychosynthesis program is also available.

## (1057) GROWTH SEMINAR TRAINING
5461 Lawton Avenue
Oakland, CA 94618

(415) 841-6500 ext. 456

*Jim Spillane*

Offers a workshop which is an overview of growth opportunities in the Bay Area. There are guest speakers from the leading programs in gestalt, hypnosis, bodywork, self-realization, movement, and related areas. The workshop concludes with a Disco dance lesson.

## SAN ANDREAS HEALTH CENTER (holistic clinic and school)/Palo Alto, CA (see 101)

## HUMAN POTENTIAL CAMP (both adults and children)/ Point Arena, CA (see 169)

## JOHNSTON COLLEGE (degree programs in transpersonal)/Redlands, CA (see 1154)

## LIFE AND HEALTH MEDICAL GROUP (clinic)/Redlands, CA (see 102)

## (1058) CHILD PSYCHOLOGY INSTITUTE OF SAN DIEGO
2616 Front Street
San Diego, CA 92103

(714) 235-4001

*Clifford S. Marks, PhD, Director*

Offers individual, family, and group therapy for children and adults. Method is an eclectic integration of T.A., gestalt, bioenergetics, psychodrama, techniques from *est*, hypnosis, rational-emotive, and biocentric therapy. Children over two years old are accompanied with play therapy. Other techniques used by professionals at the center include biofeedback, Rolfing, massage, iridology, prayer, polarity, yoga, kinesiology, energy balancing, dream interpretation, nutritional counseling, sexual therapy, and parapsychological techniques. Founded 1972.

## (1059) BIOFEEDBACK INSTITUTE OF SAN FRANCISCO
3428 Sacramento Street
San Francisco, CA 94118

(415) 921-5455

*George D. Fuller, PhD, Clinical Director*

A multidisciplinary clinic using EEG, EMG, GSR, temperature, blood pressure, and heart rate biofeedback training, with adjunctive autogenic training, hypnosis, guided imagery, and psychotherapy. Researches clinical applications of biofeedback, provides continuing education for professionals, and develops programs for agencies, businesses, and organizations.

## (1060) THE FAMILY GROUP INSTITUTE
527 Irving Street
San Francisco, CA 94122

(415) 731-1095

*Ruth Berlin, MSW, Co-Director*

Works with individuals, groups, couples, and families in group contexts. The interpersonal arena is a resource for enabling intrapersonal growth as well as that of the family. In addition to the more usual forms of individual and group therapy, the Institute also makes use of family group therapy, consisting of male and female cotherapists and three to four families. A broad spectrum of techniques are used including gestalt work, psychosynthesis, guided imagery, meditation, and bodywork.

## (1061) FORT HELP
169 Eleventh Street
San Francisco, CA 94103

(415) 864-HELP

*Joel Fort, MD, Founder*

Offers therapy to individuals, couples, and families as well as group therapy for overeating, sexual enrichment, body awareness, encounter, gay awareness, people over 60, and feminism. Founded 1970.

## (1062) LIFE COUNSELING INSTITUTE OF AMERICA
2101 Pacific Avenue
San Francisco, CA 94115

(415) 563-1779

*David C. Gordon, Director*

Individual therapy and some group work in the framework of life counseling, "a wholistic approach to life and to the total human being." Aims to actualize feelings of oneness with people, nature, and cosmos in a "unification experience."

## (1063) QUADRINITY CENTER, INC.
1005 Sansome Street
San Francisco, CA 94111

(415) 397-0466

*Bob Hoffman, Director*

990 East Arques
Sunnyvale, CA 94086

(408) 732-6572

*Atten: Miriam and Julius Brandstatter*

Teachers of the Fischer-Hoffman Process, a method of altering the effects of parental conditioning that center around poor self-esteem and the inability to establish and maintain loving personal relationships. The approach was developed through the collaboration of Dr. Siegfried Fischer, a deceased psychiatrist, with a psychic, Bob Hoffman. The Quadrinity concept holds that the spiritual, diamond-like self becomes obscured by the negative love programming of mother and father. The Process removes this "encrusted dirt" so that the four aspects of humanity: physical body, and nonphysical spiritual, intellectual, and emotional mind, exist in loving, integrated harmony. The thirteen-week process is described in detail in *Getting Divorced from Mother and Dad*, E.P. Dutton, 1976. Founded 1967.

## (1064) THETA SEMINARS
301 Lyon Street
San Francisco, CA 94117

(415) 929-1743

*Leonard Orr, President*

A professional association of individuals offering seminars in rebirthing. The rebirthing process, developed by the organization, claims to "transform the subconscious impression of birth from one of primal pain to pleasure. The effects on life are immediate; as negative energy patterns held in the mind start to dissolve, 'Youthing' replaces aging and life becomes more fun." Theta Seminars are offered in several major U.S. cities.

*AFFILIATE CENTERS*

**FULL CIRCLE ASSOCIATES**
645 Las Lomas Avenue
Pacific Palisades, CA 90272

(213) 299-0639

**THETA GROWTH CENTER OF THE HIGH SIERRA**
P.O. Box 2342
Truckee, CA 95734

(916) 587-4487

**THETA BOULDER**
P.O. Box 1693
Boulder, CO 80306

(303) 443-4028

**THETA TAMPA**
2011 First
Indian Rocks Beach, FL 33535

(813) 823-6986

**THETA MIAMI**
1430 Northwest 197th Street
Miami, FL 33169

(305) 653-3578

**THETA HAWAII**
966 Prospect Street
Honolulu, HI 96822

(808) 533-4681

**THETA BOSTON**
75 Jason Street
Arlington, MA 02146

(617) 646-6758

(1065) **COUNSELORS AND CONSULTANTS**
3082 Driftwood Drive
San Jose, CA 95128

(408) 736-6806

*Edward G. Momrow, PhD, Director*

An eclectic group practice using psychodynamic, transactional, transpersonal, and humanistic approaches. Psychodynamic assessments, group therapy, individual therapy, conjoint marital therapy, and marathons are techniques used. Referrals are accepted from physicians, lawyers, and clergy.

(1066) **PSYCHOTHERAPY AND GROWTH CENTER**
1745 Saratoga Avenue
San Jose, CA 95129

(408) 246-6033

*Walter E. Jessen, PhD, Director*

Works with psychosomatic, somatic, behavioral, and life problems by developing a specialized technology for each patient to participate in his own healing. Technologies involve behavioral prescription, hypnosis, meditation, biofeedback, directed sensory awareness, and fantasy work to alter neurophysiological and psychological function.

(1067) **THE CENTER WITHIN**
1715 Lincoln Avenue
San Rafael, CA 94901

(415) 456-4588

Offers a primal feeling process designed to "gradually unfold the layers of the personality to reveal the feeling child within, and integrate this new awareness into a real life."

**ASSOCIATED PSYCHOLOGISTS OF SANTA CLARA**/Santa Clara, CA **(see 114)**

**UNIVERSITY OF CALIFORNIA EXTENSION** (holistic workshops)/Santa Cruz, CA **(see 172)**

**FAMILY PRACTICE CENTER** (holistic clinic)/Santa Rosa, CA **(see 116)**

(1068) **SYNERGY SEMINARS**
P.O. Box 855
Sausalito, CA 94965

(415) 332-5410

*Hardy Jones, Director*

Uses a technique of directed meditation, called Consulting, to enable patients to connect with the roots of psychosomatic disturbances. Psychotherapy aimed at confronting one's total situation is offered. Synergy also offers workshops on themes related to healing and consciousness. Founded 1976.

(1069) **ELYSIUM INSTITUTE**
814 Robinson Road
Topanga, CA 90290

(213) 455-9026

*Nancy Andrews, Registrar*

Provides practical and experiential opportunities for human growth, in nontherapeutic group contexts. Interpersonal group activity is guided and occurs in a supportive setting. It is emphasized that the experience is not intended as a substitute for therapy. Facilities include four acres of tree-shaded lawn, swimming pool, hydro pool, sauna, tennis courts, and other recreational activities. Clothing is optional. A quarterly journal, *Elysium: Journal of the Senses*, is published by the Institute. Founded 1968.

(1070) **TOPANGA CENTER FOR HUMAN DEVELOPMENT**
2247 North Topanga Canyon Boulevard
Topanga, CA 90290

(213) 455-1342

*Mary E. Miller, Executive Director*

Offers workshops in gestalt, bioenergetic, neo-Reichian, transpersonal, encounter, and transactional approaches to psychotherapy; also yoga, nutrition, paraprofessional group leaders training, Kirlian photography, American Indian healing, and spirituality. On going personal growth groups and weekend drop-in encounter groups are offered as well.

(1071) **WILBUR HOT SPRINGS**
Wilbur Springs, CA 95987

(916) 473-2306

*Richard Louis Miller, PhD, Director*

The benefits of natural hot mineral baths are supplemented with journal writing, gestalt and Rogerian psychotherapy, meditation, polarity balancing, massage, nutrition, Sufi dancing, and skills in country living. Special Koshare-Residential experiences in contemporary psychology are available.

(1072) **ASPEN CENTER FOR HUMAN GROWTH**
P.O. Box 361
Aspen, CO 81611

(303) 925-4399

*Louis K. Lowenstein, PhD, Director*

Operates only in the summer, offers week-long groups in encounter, gestalt and psychosynthesis. Sessions are experiential and geared toward self-awareness. Founded 1972.

(1073) **BOULDER WORKSHOP: Experiences in Personal Growth**
2889 Valmont Road
Boulder, CO 80301

(303) 449-5230

Offers workshops in techniques designed to promote personal growth. These include marathon encounter, gestalt therapy, Aikido, sensory awareness, bioenergetics, biofeedback, meditation, decision making, the I Ching, assertiveness training, and psychosynthesis.

## (1074) ASSERTIVENESS TRAINING INSTITUTE OF DENVER
1011 Adams Street
Denver, CO 80206

(303) 322-9385

*Pat Palmer, Founder*

Offers assertiveness training from a humanistic and transpersonal framework. Includes right brain training, progressive relaxation, modeling, covert rehearsal, and how to deal with anger verbally or in gestalt process. Founded 1975.

## (1075) THE CENTER FOR NEW BEGINNINGS
200 South Sherman Street
Denver, CO 80209

(303) 777-8004

*Clyde Reid, Director*

Provides individual and group psychotherapy from a Jungian perspective. Courses in Jungian psychology are offered with credit extended through the University of Northern Colorado (graduate level). Founded 1974.

## (1076) SHORELINE TRAINING AND EMPLOYMENT SERVICES
Apple Doll House Farm
12 Durham Road
Guilford, CT 06437

(203) 453-4888

*Eleanor Pascalides*

Maintains a program of horticultural therapy for retarded and handicapped persons. Patients become involved in greenhouse management, wood splitting, lawn maintenance and organic gardening. New techniques and the effects of environment on behavior are being researched. Founded 1975.

## (1077) NEW HAVEN CENTER FOR HUMAN RELATIONS
400 Prospect Street
New Haven, CT 06511

(203) 776-1333

Offers workshops and classes in psychodrama, gestalt, T.A., massage, and bioenergetics.

**INTEGRAL HEALTH SERVICES** (holistic clinic and workshops)/Putnam, CT **(see 120)**

## (1078) ENCOUNTERS
5225 Connecticut Avenue, Suite 209
Washington, DC 20015

(202) 363-3033

*Lawrence Tirnauer, PhD, Director*

Presents workshops on dreams, bioenergetics, gestalt groups, nondirective groups, encounter, and couples groups. Founded 1968.

## (1079) SISYPHUS HUMANISTIC INSTITUTE OF FLORIDA
1720 Canal Court
Merrit Island, FL 32952

(305) 783-3913

*Howard R. Bernstein, PhD, Director*

Offers individual, couples, and group work in gestalt therapy. Also offered in gestalt are weekend and residential workshops and professional training programs. Other techniques used include massage, movement, music, and meditation. Founded 1973.

## (1080) TRANSPERIENCE CENTER
3041 Grand Avenue
Coconut Grove
Miami, FL 33133

(305) 444-4412

*Alan M. Rockway, PhD, Clinical Director*

Provides individual and group counseling and growth experiences, with emphasis on nonsexist love relationships, bisexuality, gay consciousness, and love alternatives. Direct Love Transperience is accomplished with three people, meditating and experiencing male and female energy simultaneously. Training is offered for professionals and paraprofessionals wishing to work with clients in alternative lovestyles. Founded 1976.

## (1081) HUMANISTIC GROWTH INSTITUTE
P.O. Box 5345
Tallahassee, FL 32301

(904) 576-9017

*Lloyd Goodwin, PhD, Director*

Offers a five-step program in individual therapy, drawing from gestalt, T.A., Living Love, yoga, dream work, nutrition, and meditation. Marriage/relationship and divorce counseling are also offered. Periodic seminars are offered in creative divorce, meditation, dreams, relaxation techniques, and death and dying.

## (1082) COUNSELING AND SEXUAL ENRICHMENT CENTER OF ATLANTA
5675 Peachtree-Dunwoody Road, C-522
Atlanta, GA 30342

(404) 355-7439

*Lawrence D. Baker, MD, and Frances Nagata, RN, MS, Co-Directors*

Offers individual and group therapy focusing on sexual enrichment. There are special groups for women unable to reach orgasm, and for women who do not have partners participating in the program. Schools of thought used in the program are systems theory, behavioral therapy, T.A., psychodynamic theory, and gestalt. Audio-visual materials for sex education are available.

## (1083) NORTHSIDE COUNSELING CENTER
204 Northside Medical Center
Atlanta, GA 30328

(404) 252-7552

*James E. Kilgore, ReLD, Director*

Specializes in marriage and family counseling, child evaluation, and the training of marriage and family counselors. Also provides personal growth groups, marriage enrichment programs, and "Systematic Training for Effective Parenting." Founded 1972.

(1084) **OASIS CENTER FOR HUMAN POTENTIAL**
12 East Grand Avenue
Chicago, IL 60611

(312) 266-0033

*DeLacy Brubaker, Executive Director*

Offers seminars and lectures in meditation, gestalt, bodywork, T'ai Chi, bioenergetics, encounter yoga, Eastern religion, organizational development, psychodrama, astrology, and whole person health. Also offers a twelve-month Facilitator Training Program. Founded 1967.

(1085) **CONTEMPORARY ADLERIAN LEARNING CENTER**
Fountain Square Building
1601 Sherman
Evanston, IL 60201

(312) 869-4624

*Jane E. Meyers, MA, CSW, Director*

Uses Primary Relationship Therapy, based on Adlerian theory. In a therapeutic relationship with a therapist/parent, honesty, openness, and caring are cultivated. As the patient assumes the role of child, the sessions consist largely of cuddling and fantasy. With the adolescent period, emphasis is on issues: friendships, sexual relationships, career, and personal values. The result is a healing of the client's self-perception. Acceptance and self-respect are developed and the client feels in control of and totally responsible for his/her life.

(1086) **THE WHOLISTIC HEALTH CENTER**
137 South Garfield
Hinsdale, IL 60521

(312) 986-5252

*Donald A. Tubesing, PhD, Executive Vice-President*

Associated with the Department of Preventive Medicine and Community Health of the University of Illinois, the Center provides counseling and medical care for problems related to the stresses of life, especially major life changes. It attempts to treat the whole person, on both the physical and spiritual levels. Detailed reports developed by the Center on the philosophy of wholistic health care, as well as on the background and development of the Wholistic Health Center, are available from the above address.

(1087) **THE SELF ACTUALIZATION INSTITUTE**
7835 Maple Street
New Orleans, LA 70118

(504) 866-4915

*Barbara Braunstein, Director*

A developing educational center dedicated to helping individuals realize their pure center of love. Plans programs, workshops, and services in Rolfing, gestalt, bioenergetics, meditation, yoga, T'ai Chi, massage, polarity, shiatsu, acupuncture, nutrition, herbs, homeopathy, anatomy and physiology. Founded 1976.

(1088) **SARGASSO: CENTER FOR GROWTH AND DEVELOPMENT**
1105-D Spring Street
Silver Spring, MD 20910

*Doris J. Waldbaum, PhD, Director*

Encourages the development of personal resources for self, institution, and community. Offers participatory workshops in meditation, sensory awareness, gestalt, psychodrama, dance, art, music, couples, sexual conflict, and women in transition. Founded 1975.

(1089) **NEW ENGLAND CENTER FOR PERSONAL AND ORGANIZATIONAL DEVELOPMENT**
Box 575E
Amherst, MA 01002

Offers summer workshops in gestalt, massage, yoga, women's consciousness raising, and psychosynthesis.

(1090) **EXPANSION INC.**
41 North Road
Bedford, MA 01730

(617) 275-2320

*E.M. Conney, MS, Co-Director*

". . . a self-supporting mental health organization committed to the growth of people." Individualized, growth-oriented therapy is conducted in individual, couple, family, and group contexts. Specialized programs exist for children, sexual counseling, adolescent problems, terminal illness, and over-60 groups. Techniques include art therapy, acupuncture, and movement therapy. Founded 1973.

(1091) **BOSTON PSYCHOLOGICAL CENTER FOR WOMEN**
376 Boylston
Suite 603
Boston, MA 02116

(617) 266-0136

*Nona S. Ferdon, PhD, Director*

Counseling and psychotherapy center for women. Approaches include gestalt, bioenergetics, T.A., and nutritional analysis, all conducted in both individual and group settings. Founded 1975.

(1092) **CROSSROADS COUNSELING CENTER**
665 Beacon Street
Boston, MA 02215

(617) 266-7805

A group of humanistic therapists offering support for persons wanting to go through barriers to growth and enhanced well-being. Staff draws from gestalt, existential, basic encounter, bioenergetics, meditation, sex therapy, and *est*. Services include individual, couples, family, and group psychotherapy; workshops in human sexuality, women's issues, and relationships skills; and counseling groups for men, women, middle-aged, men/women growth, and couples.

(1093) **PSYCHOMOTOR INSTITUTE**
25 Huntington Avenue, Suite 415
Boston, MA 02116

(617) 261-2622

*Louisa P. Howe, PhD, Registrar*

Teaches and practices a method of therapy and emotional reeducation called "psychomotor" or "Pesso System of Psychomotor" (PSP). "It is a method that invites the expression of emotion through motor as well as vocal action by offering appropriate and satisfying motor and vocal responses *(accommodation)* to feelings as they become manifest . . . During a psychomotor structure *accommodators* (and often their stand-ins or extensions in the form of cushions or beanbag chairs) assume the roles of persons significant to the enactor of the structure within the personal-historic context in which the enactor feels impelled to work. Usually this context goes back to childhood, with the significant interactive roles being those of the parents . . . The task of the leader or therapist is mainly that of making sure that the arena for symbolic action and interaction is safely controlled, that fully satisfying expressions of the enactor's feelings occur, and that these expressions are given appropriately matching responses by accommodators." Founded 1970.

### (1094) BROOKLINE MEDICAL ASSOCIATES
7 Harvard Square
Brookline, MA 02146

(617) 738-4501

Emphasis on direct-feeling work, primal, and other expressive therapies. Emotional working occurs by: moving from pain and its dynamic corollaries (fear, impotence, etc.) toward affective self-affirmation (territorial anger, potency, worth, joyous participation), and toward developing an "action logic" through experiencing the organic continuity between mind, body, and emotions.

### (1095) CENTER FOR EXPRESSIVE THERAPY AND COUNSELING
67 Thatcher Street
Brookline, MA 02146

(617) 734-7715

172 Main Street
Brockton, MA 02401

(617) 583-2411

Offers individual, marital, family, and group counseling, as well as expressive therapy, an affective approach developed from gestalt and primal theory.

### (1096) COMMUNITY SEX INFORMATION
10 Sewall Avenue
Brookline, MA 02146

(617) 267-3300

Offers counseling and psychotherapy for individuals, couples, families, and groups. Aims to ". . . cultivate a responsible attitude toward human sexuality and all other aspects of personal and societal living."

### (1097) COMPREHENSIVE THERAPIES, P.C.
1018 Beacon Street
Brookline, MA 02146

(617) 566-6699

Provides individual, couple, family, group, and sexual therapy in a humanistic, open context. Also offered are business and industrial consultation, residential treatment, death and dying counseling, marathon encounter, parenthood training, school consultations, and consciousness raising groups. Nutritional counseling, gestalt, yoga, and massage are incorporated into the total approach.

### (1098) EIKOS
Therapeutic Environments
7 Harvard Square
Brookline, MA 02146

(617) 738-4500

A non-profit residential care facility devoted to the rehabilitation of persons in need of a supportive and/or therapeutic community. People with short or long term needs are welcome. ". . . frequently functions as a creative and economical alternative to hospitalization," or for "weaning people from excessive dependence on psychiatric hospitalization or unhealthy family situations."

### (1099) PEQUOD (CAMBRIDGE) INC.
1145 Massachusetts Avenue
Cambridge, MA 02138

(617) 354-6259

A collectively operated community mental health center, private and nonprofit, offering individual, couple, family, and group counseling, training, and consulting. Founded 1970.

### (1100) STORY STREET ASSOCIATES
14 Story Street
Cambridge, MA 02138

(617) 661-7776

Offers individual, family, couple and group therapies, psychodiagnostic evaluation and testing, consultation, and referral services with a humanistic orientation. Also sponsors the *Story Street Lyceum*, an educational workshop series in the healing arts.

### (1101) ASSOCIATES FOR HUMAN RESOURCES, INC.
191 Sudbury Road
Box 727
Concord, MA 01742

(617) 259-9624

*Marie Maeks, Executive Director*

A guild of professionals in humanistic behavior offering therapy to individuals, couples, and families. Contemporary therapies used include gestalt, bioenergetics, transactional analysis, Alexander technique, meditation, psychosynthesis, assertiveness training, couples groups, and body-mind workshops and practicums. A year-long training program and internships are offered in humanistic psychology. Founded 1968.

### (1102) CAPE COUNSELING CENTER
54 Main Street
Hyannis, MA 02601

(617) 775-1728

*Arthur F. Thurber, PhD, Director*

Counseling center and outpatient alcoholic clinic, drawing from humanistic, behavioral, and gestalt schools of psychology.

## (1103) WALNUT HOUSE ASSOCIATES
Weston Road, Box 291A
Lincoln, MA 01773

(617) 259-8180

*Leie Lindmann Carmoddy and Sean Carmoddy, Co-Founders*

Offers individual, couple, and family therapy; minigroups, organization facilitation, and counselor/leadership training. Techniques from a variety of disciplines are used including gestalt, T.A., fantasy, sexuality, mystical teachings, psychodrama, meditation, bioenergetics, dreamwork, and healing. Special programs offered are the "Intrinsic Process," a twelve-week healing process integrating tne Fischer-Hoffman process with Buddhist concepts; "Eclectic Training," a theoretical/experiential program for the training of counselors and group leaders covering the techniques listed above; "Fantasy Reading," a training workshop for professional consultants; and "Life Reading Interpretation," based on a theory of reincarnation in which each individual has a particular lesson to learn in this life.

## (1104) GOULD FARM
Monterey, MA 01245

(413) 528-1804

*Kent D. Smith, Director*

A nonsectarian recuperation and rehabilitation center for individuals experiencing anxiety, depression, fatigue, or mental illness. Offers a caring atmosphere, individual and group therapy, and an environment conducive to work, rest, and growth. Patients with brain damage, who have suffered from severe psychosis, or who are assaultive or suicidal are not accepted. Founded 1913.

## ACUPUNCTURE CENTER OF MASSACHUSETTS
(psychotherapy)/Newton, MA **(see 130)**

## (1105) ASSOCIATES FOR CREATIVE THERAPY
P.O. Box 161
Newtonville, MA 02160

(617) 965-2315

Collective of therapists with humanistic orientation. Techniques include gestalt, T.A., bioenergetics, fantasy, and art. Services include supportive counseling, psychotherapy, and professional training. Researching possibilities of using humanistic mode in residential treatment, establishing a center for separated and divorced people, work in family dynamics applying T.A. theory, and developing "feminist" and "masculinist" therapies. Fees are on a sliding scale.

## (1106) WOMEN'S MENTAL HEALTH COLLECTIVE, INC.
326 Somerville Avenue
Somerville, MA 02143

(617) 625-2729

Offers free and low-cost feminist psychotherapy to women living in the Somerville area.

## (1107) EXPERIENTIAL WEEKENDS
2005 Penncraft Court
Ann Arbor, MI 48103

(313) 769-0046

*Bob and Margaret Blood, Directors*

Offers weekend workshops in couples enrichment, dreams, sexual enrichment, and personal decision-making. Founded 1973.

## (1108) THE MEDITATION CENTER
631 University Avenue, N.E.
Minneapolis, MN 55413

(612) 338-8838

*Usharbudh Arya, MA, DLitt, Director*

A teaching center for dissemination of knowledge about meditation, yoga, and psychotherapy from a yogic perspective. A research program currently under way is exploring the efficacy of meditation in the treatment of alcoholism and drug addiction. Teachers are trained at the Center and then sent to various hospitals and detoxification centers. Training is also offered to counselors and therapists in biofeedback and in the therapeutic uses of meditation and yoga. The Center also maintains an extensive audiovisual library on these subjects.

## (1109) SAGARIS—THE WOMEN'S THERAPY COLLECTIVE
2619 Garfield Avenue South
Minneapolis, MN 55408

(612) 825-7338

A feminist therapy collective for women offering individual and group psychotherapy, and special focus groups in sexuality, anger, massage, and self-healing. Therapeutic techniques used include gestalt and bodywork. A nine-month training program in feminist therapy is available. Founded 1974.

## (1110) WOMANKIND
5001 Olson Memorial Highway
Minneapolis, MN 55422

(612) 546-5001

Womankind is a growth center for the development of positive feelings of self-identification within woman. To attain this, educational and counseling services are available by a sensitive and professionally trained staff. Modalities used include gestalt therapy, meditation, body awareness and movement, art therapy and bioenergetics.

## (1111) GREATER KANSAS CITY COUNSELING CENTER
501 East Armour Boulevard
Kansas City, MO 64109

(816) 931-6374

*John W. Johnston*

The laboratory/clinic for The International University's programs in psychology, guidance, and counseling. Directed research, seminars, and directed practicum sessions are designed for the use of the university community. Counseling services of a humanistic orientation are available to the university and surrounding community. Founded 1972.

## (1112) CENTRAL BERGEN COMMUNITY MENTAL HEALTH CENTER
26 Park Place
Paramus, NJ 07652

(201) 265-8200

*Aristide H. Esser, MD, Director*

A community-oriented mental health treatment center, emphasizing deinstitutionalization and placement in the general community. Biofeedback, acupuncture, and self-help techniques are sometimes used. Founded 1971.

(1113) **PLAINFIELD CONSULTATION CENTER**
831 Madison Avenue
Plainfield, NJ 07060

(201) 757-4921

*Lawrence Kesner, PhD, Director*

Employs gestalt theory in individual, family, marital, child, adolescent, and group psychotherapy.

**DESERT LIGHT FOUNDATION** (holistic clinic and school)/Albuquerque, NM **(see 134)**

(1114) **ENTAYANT INSTITUTE**
Box 120
Centerport, NY 11721

(212) 767-2780

*Don Busch, Director*

Sponsors workshops held in the Adirondacks, often lasting several days each. Topics are growth oriented. Some have included guided fantasy, dream interpretation, interspecies communication, gestalt therapy, color heaing, and T'ai Chi Ch'uan. About 40% of the workshops are for professionals in the helping professions. Also sponsors ongoing gestalt groups and Friday and Saturday evening socials with Entayant leaders.

(1115) **BEHAVIOR THERAPY CENTER OF NEW YORK, P.C.**
111 East 85th Street
New York, NY 10028

(212) 722-2300

*Leonard A. Bachelis, PhD, Center Director*

A group of professional psychologists specializing in behavior therapy, biofeedback, relaxation training, and hypnosis.

(1116) **CENTER FOR EXPRESSIVE PSYCHO-THERAPY**
104 East 40th Street, Suite 407
New York, NY 10016

(212) 490-2363

*Arthur Robbins, EdD, Director*

A professional cooperative incorporating art, music, and movement with verbal communication in "expressive psychotherapy." Specific services include individual and group therapy, family and marriage therapy, childhood therapy, old age counseling, crisis intervention, community consultation, and addiction problems.

**CREATIVITY LABORATORIES** (psychosexual training)/New York, NY **(see 597)**

(1117) **DIALOGUE HOUSE LIBRARY**
80 East Eleventh Street
New York, NY 10003

(800) 221-5844

*Ira Progoff, PhD, Director*

Offers weekend workshops in the Intensive Journal, a tool for self-awareness and realization. Books and cassette tapes on the Intensive Journal and Jungian psychology are available by mail order.

(1118) **THE DI MELE CENTER FOR RECONNEC-TIVE PSYCHOTHERAPY**
15 East 40th Street
New York, NY 10021

(212) 889-5555

*Armand F. Di Mele, CSW, CRC, Director*

A multimodal wholistic treatment approach focusing on reclaiming the client's natural feeling self and his/her personal wisdom. Therapy is done both in groups and individually. Techniques used include psychoanalysis, gestalt, primal, and bioenergetics. The Center coordinates the treatment plan in a team approach.

(1119) **HUMANISTIC PSYCHOLOGY CENTER OF NEW YORK**
285 Central Park West
New York, NY 10024

(212) 873-3668

*Carmi Harari, EdD, Director*

Provides individual, group, couple, and family therapy. Training programs are offered for group leaders, using encounter, sensitivity, and group dynamic approaches. The Center's orientation is humanistic/Existential/phenomenological. Founded 1956.

(1120) **INSTITUTE FOR RATIONAL LIVING**
45 East 65th Street
New York, NY 10021

(212) 535-0822

2435 Ocean Avenue
San Francisco, CA 94127

(415) 334-3450

330 Dartmouth Street
Boston, MA 02116

(617) 536-1756

Maintains a counseling center and research and community education program. Some of the areas covered include weight control, dealing with feelings, stopping habits such as smoking or drinking, marriage reassessment and/or restructuring, rational child rearing, and rational self-actualization.

(1121) **THE NEW YORK INSTITUTE FOR THE DYNAMIC-AFFECTIVE PSYCHOTHERAPIES**
15 East 40th Street
New York, NY 10016

(212) 889-5555

*Armand F. Di Mele, CSW, CRC, President*

Provides a center for affect-oriented psychotherapists to exchange information and grow mutually through experiential workshops, seminars, lectures, and research. Stresses the integration of contributions from the dynamic psychologies and the affective therapies. Members of the Institute have training in such areas as primal therapy, hypnosis, and the Alexander technique.

### (1122) WAINWRIGHT HOUSE
Center for the Development of Human Resources
260 Stuyvesant Avenue
Rye, NY 10580

(914) 967-6080

An established educational center for Jungian psychology, religion, and inner growth. Special programs include: Receptive Listening, a twenty-year-old course geared to self-understanding, enrichment of relationships, and mind/body/spirit integration; S.C.O.P.E., an educational program for people desiring to enrich the second half of life, with courses in foreign languages, yoga, psychodrama, and the arts; and healing workshops, studying the source and reality of spiritual healing. Contemporary approaches to psychology which have been recently integrated into the program include psychosynthesis, gestalt, T.A., and psychodrama. Founded 1941.

### (1123) MANDALA CENTER, INC.
3637 Old Vineyard Road
Winston Salem, NC 27104

(919) 768-7710

*Richard V. Woodard, Administrator*

A center with outpatient and inpatient facilities for interdisciplinary, psychiatric care. Mandala offers direct helping services to the acutely ill, the mildly disturbed, or the normal individual wishing to expand his/her potential. Services offered are individual, couple, child, family, and group psychotherapy, pastoral counseling, vocational guidance and rehabilitation, psychological testing, chemotherapy, electrotherapy, and other somatic therapy services. Founded 1973.

**MERETA GROUP** (counseling and psychotherapy)/Columbus, OH **(see 147)**

### (1124) CENTER FOR THE WHOLE PERSON
122 South Sixteenth Street
Philadelphia, PA 19102

(215) 546-1687

Route 1, Box 84
Mays Landing, NJ 08330

(609) 625-1611

304 West 104th Street
New York, NY 10025

(212) 222-9445

801 College Street
Toronto, Ontario, Canada

Offers experiential educational programs in Primal Integration, an eclectic approach drawing from bioenergetic, Rogerian, Transactional Analysis, primal, gestalt, rational emotive therapy, and encounter sources. Services include individual and group sessions, one-day and weekend

marathons, five- and seven-day intensive communities, one-year professional training programs, and extended professional workshops. Founded 1962.

### (1125) FRIENDS HOSPITAL
Roosevelt Boulevard and Adams Avenue
Philadelphia, PA 19124

(215) 289-5151

Maintains a program for the use of horticulture as a psychiatric therapy.

### (1126) HUMANISTIC PSYCHOTHERAPY STUDIES CENTER
2127 Pine Street
Philadelphia, PA 19103

(215) 732-8887

*David Morgenstern, PhD, Founder and Director*

Offers individual and group psychotherapy, training programs for student therapists, marathons, consultations and presentations for community groups, and a series of courses for practicing psychotherapists, psychologists, and other interested persons. The Center does not stress any particular techniques, but aims to help the whole person change to a more positive self-enhancing view of self and others. Founded 1974.

### (1127) WOMEN ASSOCIATES
402 West Mt. Airy Avenue
Philadelphia, PA 19119

(215) 248-4916

Collective of women professionals in psychology, education, and organizational development. Uses an eclectic approach in individual and group counseling, and human relations training and consultation. Workshops are offered in such areas as assertiveness training, sex role awareness, interpersonal communications, and women's life patterns. Founded 1975.

### (1128) CENTER FOR HUMAN DEVELOPMENT
221 Shady Avenue
Pittsburgh, PA 15206

(412) 361-1400

*Marjorie Gatz, Director*

Humanistic growth center with ongoing groups geared to realization of personal awareness. Special groups are offered in meditation, male sexuality, psychodrama, bioenergetics, yoga, and organizational development. Professional training programs in gestalt therapy are available. Founded 1967.

### (1129) CAMBRIDGE HOUSE
1900 North Cambridge Avenue
Milwaukee, WI 53202

(414) 273-6333

Self-awareness and professional training programs in gestalt, bioenergetics, body movement and dance, sensory awareness, creativity and communication groups, T.A., encounter, meditation, and yoga. Founded 1956.

### (1130) COLD MOUNTAIN INSTITUTE
Granville Island
Vancouver, BC, Canada V6H 3M5

(604) 684-5355

Box 2, Masons Landing
Cortes Island, BC, Canada VOP IKO

*James Sellner, Director*

Holds workshops and seminars in acupuncture, encounter, nutrition, fantasy, art therapy and gestalt. BA and MA degree programs are available in cooperation with Antioch College. Founded 1968.

**(1131) THE CANADIAN ACADEMY OF PSYCHO-TRONICS**
43 Eglinton Avenue East, Suite 803
Toronto, Ontario, Canada M4P 1A2

(416) 481-6419

*Terry Burrows, BSc, MD, General Secretary*

A professional medical association of Family Practice physicians exploring the use of psychotronics, "the interdisciplinary science of the study of the mutual interactions of consciousness, energy and matter," in medicine. Courses in biofeedback, humanistic psychology, and psychosomatics in family practice are offered, as well as an "Eidetic Biofeedback Training Program," approved by the college of Family Physicians of Canada for continuing medical education study credit. Individuals who have contributed to psychotronics are invited to join the Academy as fellows; this is the only membership classification. Publications available through the Academy are announced in the bibliographic section of a periodic Bulletin. Founded 1973.

## Journals and Publications

**BRAIN/MIND BULLETIN** (psychotherapy)/Los Angeles, CA **(see 184)**

**(1132) AHP NEWSLETTER**
Association for Humanistic Psychology
325 Ninth Street
San Francisco, CA 94103

(415) 626-2375

*Carol Guion and Christina Kelly*

Monthly newsletter containing AHP news, calendar of national activities in humanistic psychology and many related fields, book reviews, and letters from AHP members.

**COMMON GROUND** (multidisciplinary source listings Bay area)PSan Francisco, CA **(see 187)**

**(1133) JOURNAL OF HUMANISTIC PSYCHOLOGY**
325 Ninth Street
San Francisco, CA 94103

(415) 626-2375

*Thomas C. Greening, PhD, Editor*

The journal of the Association for Humanistic Psychology. "Publishes experiential reports, theoreetical papers, personal essays, research studies, applications of humanistic psychology, humanistic analyses of contemporary culture,

and occasional poems. Topics of special interest are authenticity, encounter, self-actualization, self-transcendence, search for meaning, creativity, personal growth, psychological health, being-motivation, values, identity, and love." Founded 1961.

**(1134) MADNESS NETWORK NEWS**
2150 Market Street
San Francisco, CA 94114

A politically oriented newspaper written by former psychiatric patients, emphasizing breaking through institutionalized psychiatry.

**NEW AGE JOURNAL** (multidisciplinary)/Brookline, MA **(see 196)**

**INTERNATIONAL JOURNAL OF GROUP PSYCHOTHERAPY**/New York, NY **(see 1044)**

**SEEKER** (New York area multidisciplinary source listing)/**(see 202)**

**HUMAN DIMENSIONS** (multidisciplinary journal)/**(see 203)**

## Products and Services

**CELESTIAL ARTS** (book publishers)/Millbrae, CA **(see 208)**

**BUTTERFLY MEDIA DIMENSIONS** (cassette tapes of live recordings)/**(see 210)**

**OPEN EDUCATION EXCHANGE** (holistic directory)/Oakland, CA **(see 100)**

**CENTER FOR HEALTH EDUCATION** (cassette tapes)/Palos Verde, CA **(see 211)**

**NEW DIMENSIONS FOUNDATION** (cassette tapes)/San Francisco, CA **(see 212)**

**COGNETICS** (multidisciplinary cassette tapes)/Saratoga, CA **(see 214)**

**(1135) BIG SUR RECORDINGS**
2015 Bridgeway
Sausalito, CA 94965

(415) 332-5960

Records lectures and conferences for a number of wholistic groups, including the Association of Humanistic Psychology, Esalen Institute, C.G. Jung Institute, and the Menninger Foundation. A tape library of over 450 titles, on topics including biofeedback, acupuncture, altered states of consciousness, American Indians, mythology, contemporary psychologies, world religions, meditation, and healing, is available as a whole or as single tapes. A catalog will be sent on request.

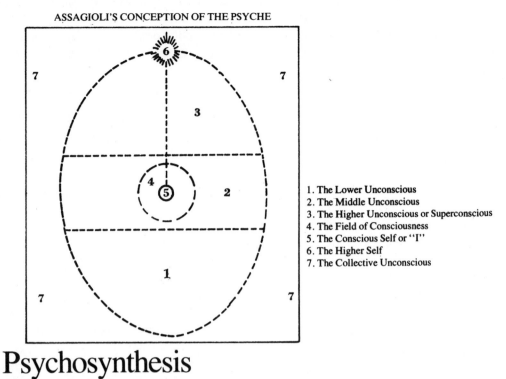

ASSAGIOLI'S CONCEPTION OF THE PSYCHE

1. The Lower Unconscious
2. The Middle Unconscious
3. The Higher Unconscious or Superconscious
4. The Field of Consciousness
5. The Conscious Self or "I"
6. The Higher Self
7. The Collective Unconscious

# Psychosynthesis

## *Martha Crampton, MA*

*"Our civilization represses not only "the instincts" not only sexuality, but any form of transcendence. Among one-dimensional men, it is not surprising that someone with an insistent experience of other dimensions that he cannot entirely deny or forget, will run the risk either of being destroyed by the others, or of betraying what he knows."*

*R. D. Laing*

Psychosynthesis is an approach to human development that is inclusive and wholistic in its orientation. Its central aim is the discovery and expression in daily living of the Self—the principle of unification and purpose at the core of human identity. The Self is seen as the integrating principle through which conflicts and polarities are reconciled; it enables us to find unity, harmony, and fulfillment within ourselves as well as meaningful relatedness to society and to the universe.

Psychosynthesis was founed by an Italian psychiatrist, Roberto Assagioli (1888-1974), who was a colleague of Freud and Jung and a pioneer of psychoanalysis in Italy. Through his studies of the philosophical and spiritual traditions of East and West, and through his own experience of what is today called the "transpersonal" realm, he concluded that a truly comprehensive approach to the study of man must include the higher dimensions of human consciousness and must take account of our specifically human ability to cooperate consciously with the process of our own evolution.

Psychosynthesis has achieved increasing recognition over the past ten years. Its practitioners have developed and utilized a wide variety of techniques, according to the needs of the situation. The open-ended framework has integrated methods from other therapies and growth disciplines such as gestalt, abreaction therapy, creative expression modalities, behavior modification, and meditative approaches. The techniques used may include guided imagery, body awareness and body movement, role playing, art media, and dreamwork, to mention but a few. The particular methods chosen are less significant than the consciousness of the person using them.

In psychosynthesis emphasis is placed on establishing contact with the integrating center of the personality, as first the "I," or personal self, and later the transpersonal Self. As this occurs, our will is liberated so that it becomes possible for us to make and carry out choices that are clear and constructive. It is through this integrating center that we can take our own evolution in hand. From this vantage point we recognize the essential wholeness of our being and conflicts that previously seemed insoluble fall into place. Polarities that once appeared antagonistic (e.g., open/closed; rigid/flowing) we soon see as complementary. We can examine the various aspects of the personality "from center" in light of our emerging sense of direction, so that we can make wise decisions about work on particular elements that may need further development or integration, such as the body, the emotions, the intellect, the imagination, the intuition, or the will.

To be able to contact the Self, or integrating principle of our personality, we must learn to extricate our true center of identity from the various other aspects of ourselves with which we are habitually identified. Often we are so caught up in, and controlled by, some partial aspect of our personality—such as our emotions, our thoughts, the roles we play, or our "subpersonalities" (structured complexes)—that we are unaware of our deeper and more inclusive center of identity. Our vision and our will may be severely restricted by this condition of identification with some partial reality. Only when we have learned to "disidentify" from all the aspects of our personality can we experience the "I" as something distinct from the many parts and free from their control; and only then can the "I" fulfill its function of bringing the various parts into harmony with one another.

When the person has achieved a certain level of personality integration, and sometimes earlier, a natural evolutionary process will draw his attention to the transpersonal dimension. Resisting this process of unfoldment can create severe problems, as it means resisting the force of nature. Just as we can suffer from repression of our more primitive impulses, so we can be harmed equally by repression of the sublime. There is a fundamental tendency within human nature to fulfill itself, which, in the more advanced stages of personality integration, necessitates the owning and expression of our "higher" and more truly human impulses. Assagioli spoke of the locus of these higher impulses as the "superconscious" and considered the exploration of this realm to be of great importance. The superconscious is the source of such activities and impulses as altruistic love and will, humanitarian action, artistic and scientific inspiration, spiritual insight, and the drive for purpose and meaning in life.

After we have dealt with the unresolved elements from the past, and after we have harmonized and developed the conflicting and undeveloped aspects of the personality, the psychosynthetic process then culminates in the release of transpersonal energies that enable us to contribute creatively to society and to express in daily living the higher qualities of our being.

## Schools, Centers, and Clinics

**HOLISTIC HEALTH CENTER** (workshops and clinic)/Los Angeles, CA **(see 90)**

**HEART HAUS CENTER** (holistic center)/Mill Valley, CA **(see 1056)**

**WELLNESS RESOURCE CENTER** (preventive)/Mill Valley, CA **(see 96)**

**SAN ANDREAS HEALTH CENTER** (holistic clinic and school)/Palo Alto, CA **(see 101)**

(1136) **HIGH POINT FOUNDATION**
647 North Madison Avenue
Pasadena, CA 91101

(213) 796-8355

*Edith Stauffer, Executive Director*

5337 North Millbrook
Fresno, CA 93710

(209) 222-2034

1085 Longridge Road
Oakland, CA 94610

615 Main Street
Edmonds, WA 98020

Nonprofit educational corporation founded "on the belief that all persons have an innate capacity for unfoldment." Offers classes and workshops based on the psychological concepts of psychosynthesis, which teaches the existence of a unifying center, a point of synthesis above the conflicting forces that constantly operate within. This center brings balance and harmony and uses them in creative expression in the outer life. Techniques used in psychosynthesis include psychodrama, gestalt learning, body movement and awareness, meditation, creative use of art and music, and personal systematic study.

**JOHNSTON COLLEGE** (degree courses in transpersonal)/Redlands, CA **(see 1154)**

**FAMILY GROUP INSTITUTE** (workshops in psychosynthesis)/San Francisco, CA **(see 1060)**

(1137) **PSYCHOSYNTHESIS INSTITUTE**
3352 Sacramento Street
San Francisco, CA 94118

(415) 922-9182

*Jim and Susan Vargiu, Founders*

Nonprofit organization dedicated to making psychosynthesis available to the public. Services provided include individual psychosynthesis for those interested in pursuing in-depth work on their own growth; single evening presentations for those wishing an evening's exploration of specific life issues; thematic programs for the person seeking a deep and focused look at specialized personal and professional themes; and fundamentals of psychosynthesis, an experiential and theoretical course designed for people interested in a breadth-and-depth investigation of psychosynthesis. In addition, professional training programs in psychosynthesis are offered to helping professionals. Publications in the field of psychosynthesis and related areas are available through the Institute. The Institute publishes a periodic news calendar of its activities. Founded 1969.

**ASPEN CENTER FOR HUMAN GROWTH** (workshops and growth center)/Aspen, CO **(see 1072)**

**BOULDER WORKSHOP** (growth center)/Boulder, CO **(see 1073)**

(1138) **KENTUCKY CENTER OF PSYCHOSYN-THESIS**
1226 Lakewood Drive
Lexington, KY 40502

(606) 269-6588

*John H. Parks, MD, Director*

Offers individual psychosynthesis, hypnosis, homeopathy, and orthomolecular psychiatry. Founded 1974.

**INSTITUTE FOR HUMANISTIC AND TRANSPER-SONAL EDUCATION**/Amherst, MA **(see 1147)**

**ASSOCIATES FOR HUMAN RESOURCES** (workshops in psychosynthesis)/Concord, MA **(see 1101)**

**WAINWRIGHT HOUSE** (growth center)/Rye, NY **(see 1122)**

(1139) **CANADIAN INSTITUTE OF PSYCHOSYN-THESIS, INC.**
3496 Marlowe Avenue
Montreal, Quebec
Canada H4A 3L7

(514) 488-4494

*Martha Crampton, MA, Director*

Offers both personal growth and professional training programs. The personal growth activities include interpersonal and personal growth groups as well as individual sessions. The professional training programs are offered to qualified individuals seeking a certificate of competence as a psychosynthesist, and to professionals and students in medicine, psychology, management, and religion who wish to use psychosynthesis principles in their work. The training includes personal and interpersonal psychosynthesis, conceptual study, observation of experienced practitioners, study of videotaped sessions, guiding skills training, and supervision of individual and group work. The program of training for psychosynthesists normally requires three full years of study for local persons and is designed so that regular employment can be maintained. The training format for out-of-town students is flexible to accommodate individual situations. Members of the Institute staff are available to give lectures or workshops on psychosynthesis and related topics.

(1140) **THE INSTITUTE OF PSYCHOSYNTHESIS**
Highwood Park
Nan Clark's Lane
Mill Hill
London, England

Offers both personal growth and professional training programs.

(1141) **CENTRE FRANÇAIS DE PSYCHOSYNTHÈSE**
61, rue de la Verrerie
75004 Paris, France

Offers both personal growth and professional training programs.

(1142) **INSTITUTO DI PSICOSINTESI**
16 Via San Domenico
50133 Florence, Italy

Offers both personal growth and professional training programs.

## Journals and Publications

(1143) **SYNTHESIS, THE REALIZATION OF THE SELF**
830 Woodside Road
Redwood City, CA 94061

(415) 365-2698

*James Vargiu, Editor*

Biannual journal of articles on psychosynthesis and related areas. Contributing authors have included Robert Assagioli, Viktor Frankl, Lama Govinda, and Elizabeth Kubler-Ross. Included in each workbook is an article outlining the principle of a particular aspect of personal growth, specific exercises for its application, illustrated examples, questions and answers, and suggested reading. Originated in 1974.

**JOURNAL OF HUMANISTIC PSYCHOLOGY**/San Francisco, CA **(see 1043)**

**HUMAN DIMENSIONS** (multidisciplinary journal)/Williamsville, NY **(see 203)**

## Products and Services

**CELESTIAL ARTS** (book publishers)/Millbrae, CA **(see 208)**

**BUTTERFLY MEDIA DIMENSIONS** (cassette tapes)/N. Hollywood, CA **(see 210)**

**CENTER FOR HEALTH EDUCATION** (cassette tapes)/Palos Verde, CA **(see 211)**

**NEW DIMENSIONS FOUNDATION** (cassette tapes)/San Francisco, CA 94111 **(see 212)**

**COGNETICS** (cassette tapes)/Saratoga, CA **(see 214)**

**BIG SUR RECORDINGS** (audiovisual and cassette tapes)/Sausalito, CA **(see 1135)**

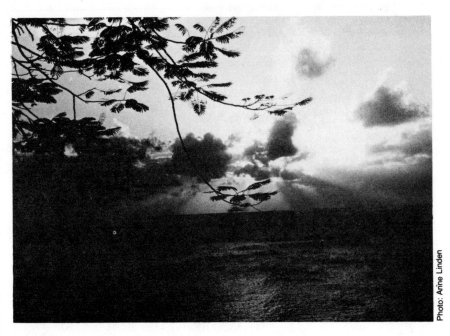

Photo: Anne Linden

# Transpersonal Psychology

## Frances Vaughan Clark, PhD

*"The cardinal discovery of transpersonal psychology is that the collective psyche, the deepest layer of the unconscious, is the living ground current from which is derived everything to do with a particularized ego possessing consciousness: Upon this it is based, by this it is nourished, and without this it cannot exist."*

Eric Neumann, The Origins and History of Consciousness

In recent years transpersonal psychology has emerged as the fourth force in psychology, the other three being psychoanalysis, behaviorism, and humanistic psychology. Transpersonal psychology expands the field to include the study of consciousness, particularly those states associated with the optimum development of human potential. Transpersonal psychology integrates physical, emotional, mental, and spiritual dimensions of growth and affirms the validity of the spiritual quest as an intrinsic part of self-realization. The scope of inquiry includes the teachings of Eastern spiritual disciplines, which have, over thousands of years, developed powerful methods for expanding consciousness and controlling internal states. In the West the scientific investigation of consciousness and the technology of biofeedback (which brings under conscious control many physiological functions that used to be considered involuntary) are a recent development. Transpersonal psychology aims at synthesizing Eastern wisdom and Western science, and is exploring new ways of transforming consciousness of both self and society.

Current research in transpersonal psychology includes the empirical investigation of transpersonal experiences, meditation, biofeedback, psychic phenomena, states of consciousness, maps of consciousness, wholistic healing, energy transformation, body disciplines, applications to education and psychotherapy, and many other related subjects.

Transpersonal experience is defined as that which transcends ego boundaries and the ordinary limitations of time and space. Transpersonal experiences include mystical, religious, and psychic experiences, as well as other altered states of expanded consciousness that frequently are attained through the practice of mental or physical disciplines, or both, and sometimes occur spontaneously. Transpersonal psychology is concerned with the empirical investigation of such experiences and with their integration into an expanded vision of health and wholeness. Transpersonal experience is validated rather than discounted, although it is not sought as an end in itself. Its significance is related to its effects and the quality of life that ensues.

Transpersonal psychology does not espouse any particular belief system but considers beliefs to be frameworks for ordering experience, important in shaping reality. Each individual, becoming conscious, can freely choose his/her own path and beliefs. Transpersonal psychology affirms the human capacity for transcending conditioning and beliefs that limit growth and awareness, and sees the individual as capable of taking full responsibility for his/her own life. Beyond self-actualization is the possibility of self-transcendence, with an emphasis on the value of service in the world. The transpersonal orientation offers a wholistic view of the individual and the environment as integral parts of a unified whole in which inner and outer experience reflect each other. The inner work on consciousness is therefore accorded equal importance with outer work in the world.

In the field of education transpersonal psychology seeks to balance awareness of inner and outer experience and integrate the development of body, mind, emotions, and spirit. Education of the whole person includes educating both the rational, intellectual faculties associated with the left hemisphere of the brain and the intuitive faculties associated with the right hemisphere. Transpersonal education includes personal, interpersonal, and intrapersonal work and goes beyond the personality to explore the essential experience of being, which affirms the underlying oneness of life and the interrelatedness of all beings.

In the field of psychotherapy transpersonal psychology refers to values and attitudes of the therapist rather than any specific techniques of therapy. Impulses toward spiritual growth are acknowledged as inherent in the healthy person and are nurtured in the therapeutic process, which deals with values, meaning, and purpose as intrinsic aspects of self-awareness. A transpersonal therapist also gives the client the opportunity to experience the transpersonal dimensions of his/her own being. Transpersonal therapy includes work with inner experiences such as dreams, imagery, and altered states of consciousness, but is not limited to any particular method. Attention is given to changing the context rather than the content of experience. Transpersonal psychotherapy seeks a balanced integration of physical, emotional, mental, and spiritual development throughout life.

## Groups and Associations

**(1144) ASSOCIATION FOR TRANSPERSONAL PSYCHOLOGY**
345 California Avenue
Palo Alto, CA 94306

(415) 327-2066

*Miles Vich, Executive Director*

A group of individuals sharing an interest in transpersonal psychology and transpersonal values. Some members are interested in, or are practicing professionally in; education, psychotherapy, research, and spiritual disciplines. Others are philosophers or friends who support the transpersonal orientation. The Association provides a vehicle for those who want to communicate with each other about their transpersonal ideas, experiences, work, and process. Members receive a Newsletter and the *Journal of Transpersonal Psychology*. Founded 1971.

**(1145) COLORADO ASSOCIATION FOR TRANS-PERSONAL PSYCHOLOGY**
P.O. Box 3125
Grand Junction, CO 81501

(303) 245-3880

*Michael Hensley*

Educational network of Coloradoans interested in transpersonal psychology. Coordinates workshops, conferences, and meetings throughout the state.

## Schools, Centers, and Clinics

**BIOLOGY OF THE MIND/BODY** (workshop)/Davis, CA **(see 80)**

**NATIONAL CENTER FOR THE EXPLORATION OF HUMAN POTENTIAL**/San Diego, CA **(see 106)**

**(1146) INTEGRAL COUNSELING CENTER**
California Institute of Asian Studies
3736 Twentieth Street
San Francisco, CA 94110

(415) 648-2644

*Paul E. Herman, PhD, and Bruce Cole, MA, Directors*

Offers crisis and ongoing growth counseling to individuals, couples, and groups. Orientation is transpersonal integration of Eastern disciplines and Western humanistic and behaviorist psychology. Tools include gestalt, psychosynthesis, meditation, yoga, dreamwork, Jungian psychology, guided fantasy, autogenic training, bioenergetics, and behavior modification.

**PSYCHOSYNTHESIS INSTITUTE**/San Francisco, CA **(see 1137)**

**COUNSELORS AND CONSULTANTS**/San Jose, CA **(see 1065)**

**TOPANGA CENTER FOR HUMAN DEVELOPMENT** (personal growth and workshops)/Topanga, CA **(see 1070)**

**ASSERTIVENESS TRAINING INSTITUTE OF DENVER**/Denver, CO **(see 1074)**

**(1147) INSTITUTE FOR HUMANISTIC AND TRANSPERSONAL EDUCATION**
Box 575
Amherst, MA 01002

(413) 367-2385

*Jack Canfield, MEd, Director*

Trains teachers to teach children in wholistic ways, using body, emotions, imagination, intuition, and transpersonal self. Teachers are instructed in nutrition, massage, herbs, fasting, psychosomatic symptomology, reflexology, yoga, guided imagery, gestalt, psychosynthesis, bioenergetics, meditation, Arica exercises, and dream work. Founded 1975.

**(1148) CENTRAL COUNSELING SERVICE**
219 West 81st Street, 9A
New York, NY 10024

(212) 799-9460

*Theodore R. Smith, Jr., DMin, Director*

Practices metapsychiatry, "... an approach to psychotherapy which is basically existential analysis on a spiritual foundation. Although human beings are social and psychological creatures, they are more deeply spiritual beings (conscious beings aware of themselves). Metapsychiatry analyzes the false suppositions humans make, and attempts to shed light on man's being as spiritual, loving, aware, and positive, enabling the seeker to build on this fundamental foundation." Founded 1969.

**INTERNATIONAL INSTITUTE OF INTEGRAL SCIENCES** (psychic)/Montreal, Canada **(see 68)**

**(1149) YORK UNIVERSITY**
The Centre for Continuing Education and Growth Opportunities
4700 Keele Street
Downsview, Ontario, Canada M3J 2R6

(416) 667-3276

*Howard Eisenberg, MD, MSc, Director*

Offers courses and workshops for medical and psychological professionals, as well as the general public, in various approaches of the human potential movement. Particular offerings include biofeedback, bioenergetics, hypnosis, art therapy, parapsychology, primal therapy, yoga, group leadership, T.A., psychodrama, dreams, and encounter.

## Schools (Universities)

**(1150) NYINGMA INSTITUTE**
1815 Highland Place
Berkeley, CA 94709

(415) 843-6812

MA degree in the essentials of Buddhism, a two-year program based on interplay of meditation and intellectual understanding. Also, nondegree study programs.

**(1151) CALIFORNIA INSTITUTE OF TRANSPERSONAL PSYCHOLOGY**
250 Oak Grove Avenue
Menlo Park, CA 94025

(415) 326-1960

*Robert Frager, PhD, Director*

Offers a PhD program in transpersonal psychology which integrates experiential and theoretical training in the physical, emotional, intellectual, and spiritual aspects of the person. Bodywork includes Aikido, Alexander technique, dance and movement therapy, bioenergetics, Reichian therapy, yoga, T'ai Chi, sexual therapy, and massage. Group work involves gestalt, T.A., psychodrama, Rogerian, and collective decision making; Jungian analysis and psychosynthesis are offered as individual approaches. Spiritual work is supported within the contexts of the Jewish, Christian, Buddhist, and Hindu traditions. Special nondegree workshops in transpersonal psychology are offered throughout the year. Founded 1975.

**(1152) JOHN F. KENNEDY UNIVERSITY**
12 Altarinda Road
Orinda, CA 94563

(415) 254-0200

*Dr. Pascal Kaplan*

BA degree in psychology and MA degree in counseling psychology with subject field specialization in transpersonal counseling, mysticism, and parapsychology.

**(1153) PACIFIC GRADUATE SCHOOL**
645 University Avenue
Palo Alto, CA 94301

(415) 321-1895

*Robert Kantor, President*

PhD program in clinical psychology includes transpersonal orientation. Course approved by California Department of Education.

**(1154) JOHNSTON COLLEGE**
University of Redlands
Redlands, CA 92373

(714) 793-2121

*Hugh Redmond, PhD, Director*

Provides fully accredited external MA program in transpersonal and humanistic psychology, in addition to an undergraduate program in psychology and education. Students may design their education around the theme of wholistic health. Facilities include a biofeedback laboratory and meditation room. Courses are offered in healing, transpersonal psychology, psychosynthesis, and mysticism.

**(1155) ANTIOCH COLLEGE WEST**
1161 Mission Street
San Francisco, CA 94103
ATTN: Graduate Program in Psychology

(415) 864-2575

Master's degree program in psychology for certificate in family and child counseling may include transpersonal psychology. A fully accredited college.

### (1156) CALIFORNIA INSTITUTE FOR ASIAN STUDIES
3494 21st Street
San Francisco, CA 94110

(415) 648-1489

Degree in integral counseling. MA program and PhD program in East-West psychology and others.

### (1157) HUMANISTIC PSYCHOLOGY INSTITUTE
325 Ninth Street
San Francisco, CA 94103

(415) 626-4494

External degree programs leading to PhD.

### (1158) NAROPA INSTITUTE
1441 Broadway
Boulder, CO 80302

(303) 444-0202

Last two years of BA degree in Buddhist studies and BFA degree in expressive arts and visual arts.

### (1159) WESTERN COLORADO UNIVERSITY
P.O. Box 2102
Grand Junction, CO 81501

(303) 245-3880

*Michael L. Hensley, Advisor in Psychology and Education*

Studies in transpersonal psychology acceptable toward BA and MA in general psychology.

### (1160) ILLINOIS CENTER FOR PSYCHOLOGICAL RESEARCH
324 Tuohy
Park Ridge, IL 60068

(312) 825-4277

BA and MA degrees in transpersonal and humanistic psychology.

### (1161) THOMAS JEFFERSON COLLEGE
Allendale, MI 49401

(616) 895-6611

Four-year curriculum in transpersonal psychology leading to a Bachelor of Philosophy degree (BPh).

### (1162) FRIENDS WORLD COLLEGE
Lloyd Harbor
Huntington, NY 11743

(516) 549-1102

*Arthur Meyer, Director of Admissions*

BA degree can include study of psychology in Switzerland, social work in London, living in a Buddhist monastery in Bangkok, working on an archeological dig in Mexico, and similar alternatives. Individual field study and work with scholars, professionals, and others seeking global perspectives and answers to world problems. In lieu of exams and lectures, students keep journals of their growth.

### (1163) NOOGENESIS PROGRAM
c/o Vermont College of Community Involvement
90 Main Street
Burlington, VT 05401

(802) 862-5620

*Judith Orloff, Director*

Offers a BA program in transpersonal psychology. Students become familiar with bioenergetics, movement, yoga, meditation, massage, Jungian and Reichian psychology, androgyny, mysticism, psychic healing through classes, workshops and internships. AA program also available. Founded 1975.

## Journals and Publications

**BRAIN/MIND BULLETIN**/Los Angeles, CA **(see 184)**

**COMMON GROUND** (multidisciplinary source listings Bay area)/San Francisco, CA **(see 187)**

**JOURNAL OF HUMANISTIC PSYCHOLOGY**/San Francisco, CA **(see 1043)**

### (1164) THE JOURNAL OF TRANSPERSONAL PSYCHOLOGY
P.O. Box 4437
Stanford, CA 94305

(415) 327-2066

*Miles A. Vich, Editor*

Biannual journal concerned with "transpersonal values and states, unitive consciousness, metaneeds, peak experiences, ecstasy, mystical experience, being, self-actualization, transcendence of self, spirit, sacralization of everyday life, oneness, cosmic awareness, individual and specieswide synergy, the theories and practices of meditation, spiritual paths, compassion, and related concepts, experiences and activities." Features include original articles, book reviews, and bibliographies. Founded 1969.

**SEEKER** (multidisciplinary newsletter directory NY area)/New York, NY **(see 202)**

## Products and Services

**CELESTIAL ARTS** (book publishers)/Millbrae, CA **(see 208)**

**BUTTERFLY MEDIA DIMENSIONS** (multidiscpplinary recordings)/N. Hollywood, CA **(see 210)**

**CENTER FOR HEALTH EDUCATION** (cassette tapes)/Palos Verde, CA **(see 211)**

**NEW DIMENSIONS FOUNDATION** (cassette tapes)/San Francisco, CA **(see 212)**

**COGNETICS** (cassette tapes)/Saratoga, CA **(see 214)**

**BIG SUR RECORDINGS** (multidisciplinary audio-visuals)/Sausalito, CA **(see 1135)**

**HARTLEY FILM PRODUCTIONS** (multidisciplinary audiovisuals)/Cos Cob, CT **(see 219)**

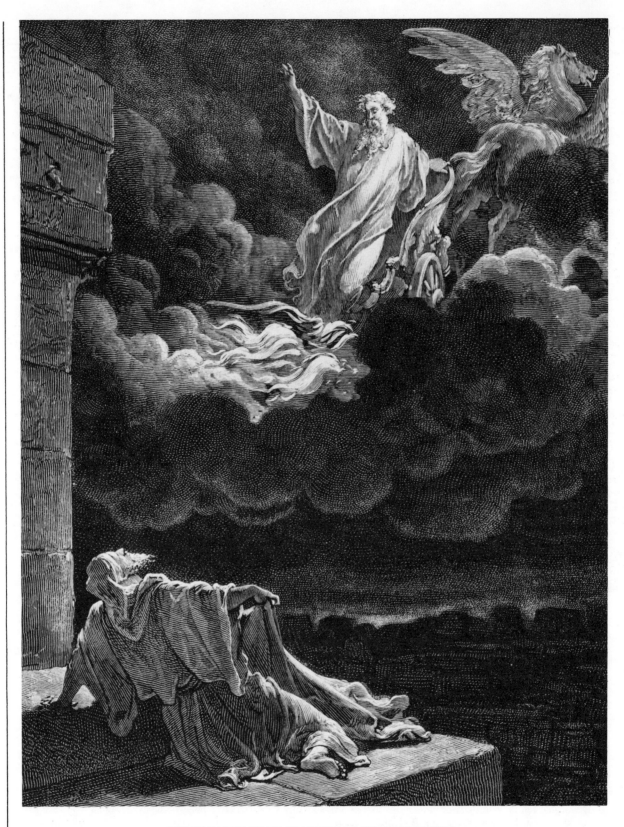

**ELIJAH TAKEN UP TO HEAVEN IN A CHARIOT OF FIRE**
Behold, there appeared a chariot of fire, and horses of fire, and parted them both
asunder; and Elijah went up by a whirlwind into heaven. (II Kings 2: 11, 12);
courtesy Dover Publications, from *The Dore Bible Illustrations*. New York:
Dover Publications, 1974.

# Life After Life

*Raymond A. Moody, Jr., PhD, MD*

*"Death does not mean the end of life; the grave is not the goal of men, no more than the Earth the goal of seeds. Life is the consequence of death: the seed may seem to die, but from its grave the tree arises into life."*

*155:16 Aquarian Gospel of Jesus the Christ*

In recent months, much attention has been drawn to the occurrence of what may be called "near-death experiences." Such experiences are reported to take place in at least three kinds of situations:

1. When a person has a close brush with death in life-threatening danger, such as accidents, severe injury, or illness;
2. When a person is believed, adjudged, or in some cases pronounced clinically dead or undergoes cardiac and/or respiratory arrest but is resuscitated; and
3. When a person actually does die and is not resuscitated but—while dying—describes unusual phenomena, which are later reported by others present at the deathbed.

Investigators of near-death experiences have been impressed by the great number of experiences of this type and by their similarities. In the hundreds of instances of such experiences that I have gathered, there seem to be fifteen features that recur in many reports. By combining these features one can construct a kind of composite picture of near-death experiences:

*A man is dying and, as he reaches the point of greatest physical stress, he hears himself pronounced dead by his doctor. He begins to hear an uncomfortable noise, a loud ringing or buzzing, and at the same time feels himself moving very rapidly through a long dark tunnel. After this, he suddenly finds himself outside of his own physical body, but still in the immediate physical environment, and he sees his own body from a distance, as though he is a spectator. He watches the resuscitation attempt from this unusual vantage point and is in a state of emotional upheaval.*

*After a while, he collects himself and becomes more accustomed to his odd condition. He notices that he still has a "body," but one of a very different nature and with very different powers from the physical body he has left behind. Soon other things begin to happen. Others come to meet and to help him. He glimpses the spirits of relatives and friends who have already died, and a loving, warm spirit of a kind he has never encountered before—a being of light—appears before him. This being asks him a question, nonverbally, to make him evaluate his life and helps him along by showing him a panoramic, instantaneous playback of the major events of his life. At some point he finds himself approaching some sort of barrier or border, apparently representing the limit between earthly life and the next life. Still he finds that he must go back to Earth, that the time for his death has not yet come. At this point he resists, for by now he is taken up with his experiences in the afterlife and does not want to return. He is overwhelmed by intense feelings of joy, love, and peace. Despite his attitude, though, he somehow reunites with his physical body and lives.*

*Later he tries to tell others, but he has trouble doing so. In the first place, he can find no human words adequate to describe these unearthly episodes. He also finds that others scoff, so he stops telling other people. Still, the experience affects his life profoundly, especially his views about death and its relationship to life.\**

What, though, would be the purpose of investigating them? First, persons whose near-death experiences embody the more transcendental features of this composite come back convinced that life after death is a reality. Thus, it is remotely possible that these experiences, upon examination, might yield clues toward the solution of the age-old riddle of the survival of bodily death.

Regardless of whether they can be used to substantiate the existence of life after death, such experiences in themselves are of importance for those of us in the healing arts and professions. Recent

---

\*From *Life After Life*. Courtesy Mockingbird Press, Covington, Georgia, 1975.

years have seen the development of a medical technology that enables us to bring people back from a state that 100 years ago would have been called "death," and many people thus "brought back" talk of unusual spiritual experiences that seemed to take place in the interim. In a sense, then, near-death experiences can be seen as an occasional "side effect" of a medical procedure—namely, cardiopulmonary resuscitation—now coming into widespread use.

The question then arises, How ought the practitioner respond when a patient undergoing this procedure reports a spiritual experience? Many patients have related that when they tried to tell their physicians, nurses, or others about what had happened, they were told that "It was just a dream," or "You had a hallucination," and the matter was dropped. Their own feelings, however, were that what they had experienced was very real and had a great influence on their subsequent views of reality and life. After being rebuffed in their initial attempts to explain their experiences to others, many have concluded that they were alone, that no one else had ever had an experience of this type. Reassuring such patients that they are not alone—that, though no scientific explanation of such happenings has been established, they are rather common—could well have been a beneficial effect.

Another possible point of clinical significance for the study of near-death experiences has been mentioned by several physicians. Numerous people who have been believed dead by attending personnel have later quoted, word for word, what was said during the resuscitation procedure. Thus, we should remain sensitive to what is being said in the presence of a supposedly unconscious patient, even one who appears, by some criteria, to be dead.

Near-death experiences illustrate the way in which medical and spiritual concerns overlap and perhaps are even indistinguishable. For even in our encounters with the most advanced and sophisticated devices of technological medicine, we as human beings may find ourselves confronted with those awesome possibilities which constitute our most ancient spiritual heritage.

*. . . a diseased organism contains the same forces and impulses as a healthy one, but these are no longer able to say in balance. They have come to a crisis which might, for instance, be a crisis of development. Development, a process inseparable from human nature, represents the transition from one state of balance to a new one that has to be achieved. An old equilibrium is given up so that a higher one may be attained. However this may be, in whatever form the crisis may present itself: through the disruption of the balance some parts of the whole are given an advantage, others put at a disadvantage. Some wilt, others flourish and develop in excess. Harmony, the very expression of wholeness, is deeply disturbed, and the whole is "hurt," it is ill. Not only is it at war with itself; in one way or other, depending on the nature of the disturbance in equilibrium, it also loses its healthy relation to the forces of the world outside. This will either come in too strongly, or it will not be properly mastered. And so damage from outside is added to disruption within. The internal imbalance establishes the disposition to disease, and the outside world gives rise to secondary effects, e.g. the development of bacterial infection and the like.*

*. . . Disease—as a brilliant aphorism by Novalis—becomes a musical problem, a dissonance that must not be allowed to fall back into the harmony which preceded it but must be resolved into a better harmony that is to follow. An illness properly gone through will lead to better health. The idea of disease and its justification, indeed its necessity, in a world of beings who are developing further, is becoming apparent, and from this one can then work towards an idea of healing.*

*Wilhelm Pelikan*

From *Heilpflanzenkunde*, Vol. I: Philosophisch—Anthroposophischer Verlag am Goetheanum, Dornach, Switzerland. Translation reprinted from *The British Homeopathic Journal*.

# Biography of Contributors

**Wyrth Post Baker, MD**
Chairman, Board of Trustees, American Institute of Homeopathy, Falls Church, Virginia; Founder, International Academy of Metabology, Pasadena, California; President, American Foundation for Homoeopathy, Falls Church, Virginia; President, Board of Examiners in Medicine and Osteopathy. Commission on Licensure for the District of Columbia, Washington, D.C.

**Helen L. Bonny, PhD, RMT**
Founder, Institute for Consciousness and Music, Baltimore, Maryland.

**Joseph A. Boucher, ND**
Chairman, Board of Directors, National College of Naturopathic Medicine, Portland, Oregon; President, Canadian Naturopathic Association, Vancouver, British Columbia; Secretary, Naturopathic Physicians Association of British Columbia, Vancouver, British Columbia.

**Robert A. Bradley, MD**
Pioneer in the field of natural childbirth; developer of the Bradley Method of Husband-Coached Childbirth.

**Richard O. Brennan, DO**
Founder and Chairman, Board of Trustees, International Academy of Preventive Medicine, Houston, Texas; Medical Director, Bellevue Metabolic Clinic, Houston, Texas; author of *Nutrigenetics* (New York City: M. Evans, 1975)

**David E. Bresler, PhD**
Director, Pain Control Unit, and Assistant Adjunct Professor, Departments of Anesthesiology, Gnathology and Psychology, University of California Schools of Medicine and Dentistry and College of Letters and Sciences; Los Angeles, California; Director, Center for Integral Medicine, Pacific Palisades, California.

**Charles V.W. Brooks**
Author of *Sensory Awareness* (Big Sur, California: Esalen Institute, 1974).

**Rick J. Carlson, JD**
Assistant Adjunct Professor of Medicine, Boston University School of Medicine, Boston, Massachusetts; Senior Research Associate, The Institute of Medicine, National Academy of Sciences, Washington, D.C.; author of *The End of Medicine* (New York City: Wiley, 1975), *The Dilemmas of Corrections* (Lexington, Massachusetts: Lexington Press, 1976), and *A New Medicine: Holistic Approaches to Health* (Cambridge, Massachusetts: Ballinger, in press).

**J. Dudley Chapman, DO, DSc**
Editor-in-chief, *Osteopathic Physician* (O.P. Journal), New York City; former President, American College of Osteopathic Obstetrics and Gynecology, University of Ohio, College of Osteopathic Medicine, Athens, Ohio.

**Frances Vaughan Clark, PhD**
President, Association for Transpersonal Psychology, Palo Alto, California.

**Harris L. Coulter, PhD**
Medical historian and author of *Homeopathic Medicine* (St. Louis: Formur, 1972) and *Divided Legacy: A History of the Schism in Medical Thought* (3 volumes; Washington, D.C.: Weehawken, 1973-1977).

**Richard Courtney**
President, Canadian Conference on the Arts, Toronto, Canada, and Professor of Arts and Education, Ontario Institute for Studies in Education, Toronto, Canada.

**Major B. DeJarnette, DC, DO**
Pioneer in the field of cranial technique; developer of Sacro Occipital Technic; founder of the Sacro Occipital Research Society International, Nebraska City, Nebraska.

**Martha Crampton, MA**
Director, Canadian Institute of Psychosynthesis, Montreal, Quebec, Canada.

**Marjorie de la Warr**
Co-founder, Delawarr Laboratories, Oxford, England; author, teacher, practitioner, and pioneer in the field of radionics.

**Julius Dintenfass, DC**
Former Chairman, New York State Board of Chiropractic Examiners, Albany, New York; former Director of Chiropractic, New York City Department of Health; author of *Chiropractic: A Modern Way to Health* (New York: Pyramid, 1966).

**William W. Eidson, PhD**
Professor and Chairman, Department of Physics and Atmospheric Science, Drexel University, Philadelphia, Pennsylvania; former Chairman, Department of Physics, University of Missouri—St. Louis, St. Louis, Missouri; visiting scientist at Kansas State University, Manhattan, Kansas; University of Washington, Seattle, Washington; Argonne National Laboratories, Chicago, Illinois, and Oak Ridge National Laboratories, Oak Ridge, Tennessee.

**Norman R. Farnsworth, PhD**
Professor and Head, Department of Pharmacognosy and Pharmacology, College of Pharmacy, University of Illinois, at the Medical Center, Chicago, Illinois; author of numerous papers and books in the field of pharmacognosy and pharmacology.

**David L. Faust**
Writer and lecturer; former Research Associate with Logical Technical Services, New York City (formerly under contract with Advanced Research Projects Agency, U.S. Department of Defense, Washington, D.C., engaged in the study and examination of Kirlian photography); member, Biophysics Research Staff, Drexel University, Philadelphia, Pennsylvania.

**Josef Garai, PhD**
Former Professor and Chairman, Art Therapy Department, Pratt Institute, Brooklyn, New York.

**Robert M. Giller, MD**
Author and lecturer; Former instructor, (course entitled: New Light on Therapeutic Energies), New School for Social Research, New York City; private practice, New York City.

**Bernard Gittleson**
Founder, Time Pattern Research Institute, West Caldwell, New Jersey; President, Biorhythm Computers, Inc., New York City; author of *Biorhythm: A Personal Science* and *Biorhythm Sportsforecasting* (New York: Arco, 1975 and 1977).

**George J. Goodheart, DC**
Pioneer in and developer of Kinesiology; founder and Director of Research, International College of Applied Kinesiology, Detroit, Michigan; lecturer and author of numerous works in the field of Kinesiology.

**Raymond L. Gottlieb, OD**
Researcher and lecturer; consultant to the California Department

of Rehabilitation, Santa Rosa, California; private practice, Santa Rosa, California, specializing in developmental vision therapy.

**Elmer Green, PhD**
Researcher; Director, Voluntary Controls Program, Menninger Foundation, Topeka, Kansas.

**Jerry Green, JD**
Attorney, private practice in Mill Valley, California, specializing in holistic medicine; faculty member, Holistic Life Foundation, San Francisco, California.

**Thomas C. Greening, PhD**
Editor, *Journal of the Association of Humanistic Psychology*, San Francisco, California.

**Doris B. Haire**
President, American Foundation for Maternal and Child Health, Inc., New York City; former President, International Childbirth Association, Milwaukee, Wisconsin; member, U.S. Food and Drug Administration Consumer Advisory Committee and Forum on Patient Prescription Drug Labeling, Washington, D.C.; member, Committee on the Prevention of Fetal and Perinatal Disease, National Institute of Health, Bethesda, Maryland; and a contributing author of *Prevention of Embryonic Fetal and Perinatal Disease* (Bethesda, Maryland: Fogarty International Center, at the National Institute of Health, 1976).

**Gerald G. Jampolsky, MD**
Consultant to The Center for Attitudinal Healing, Tiburon, California; former Chairman of the School of Health Committee of the California Medical Association, San Francisco, California; in private practice, Tiburon, California.

**Joseph Janse, DC**
President, National College of Chiropractic, Lombard, Illinois.

**Bernard Jensen, DC, ND**
Pioneer and a developer in the science of Iridology; Director, Hidden Valley Health Ranch, Escondido, California.

**Mario Jones, MD**
Author, researcher and lecturer in the field of medical astrology.

**Leslie J. Kaslof**
Founder, International Institute for Biological and Botanical Research, and The National Council on Wholistic Therapeutics and Medicine, Brooklyn, New York. President United Communications Research Publications, Woodmere, New York; author of the *Herb And Ailment Cross-Reference Chart;* active member of the Society for Economic Botany and the New York Academy of Sciences.

**Sheila Kitzinger, BLitt**
Researcher and educator; developer of the Kitzinger Psychosexual Approach to Childbirth.

**Dolores Krieger, RN, PhD**
Professor of Nursing, New York University, School of Education, Health, Nursing and the Art Professions, Division of Nursing, New York City; developed the first university based course (at NYU) at the Masters level on healing by human field interaction; contributing editor, *The Persistent Reality* (Wheaton, Illinois: Quest Books, in press); member, Sigma Pheta Tau (national honor society for nursing); has appeared on NBC, Not For Women Only, as well as many other talk shows on national and local TV; and is New York Regional and National consultant on Spinal Cord Injuries to the Veterans Administration, Washington, DC.

**Richard J. Kroening, MD**
Medical Director, Pain Control Unit; and Assistant Adjunct Professor of Anesthesiology, School of Medicine, and Joint Direc-

tor, TMJ clinic, School of Dentistry, University of California, Los Angeles, California.

**Michio Kushi**
Lecturer and teacher of macrobiotics; author of numerous articles on macrobiotics.

**Philip Lansky**
Author, researcher and lecturer.

**Robert Masters, PhD**
Author, lecturer, and Director of Research, Foundation for Mind Research, Pomona, New York.

**Shizuto Masunaga**
Author of *Zen Shiatsu* (Elmsford, New York: Japan Publications, 1977), and noted authority in the field of shiatsu.

**Willie B. May, BS, DDS**
Founding and charter member, American Equilibration Society, Edwardsville, Illinois; charter member, American Academy of Craniomandibular Orthopedics, Wantagh, New York; in private practice, Albuquerque, New Mexico.

**William A. McGarey, MD**
Co-founder with Gladys McGarey, M.D., and Clinical Director, A.R.E. Clinic, Phoenix, Arizona; Director, Medical Research Division, Edgar Cayce Foundation, Virginia Beach, Virginia; author of *Edgar Cayce on Healing* (New York City: Paperback Library, 1972), *Acupuncture and Body Energies* (Phoenix, Arizona: Gabriel, 1973), and *There Will Your Heart Be* (New York City: Prentice-Hall, 1976).

**Raymond A. Moody, Jr., PhD, MD**
Author of *Life after Life* (Covington, Georgia: Mockingbird Press, 1975, and New York City: Bantam, 1975); former Assistant Professor of Philosophy, East Carolina University, Greenville, North Carolina.

**John N. Ott, ScD (Hon.)**
Chairman and former Executive Director, Environmental Health and Light Research Institute, Sarasota, Florida; President, Ott Laboratories, Inc., Chicago, Illinois; and author of *Health and Light* (Old Greenwich, Connecticut: Devin Adair, 1973).

**Pierre Pannetier**
Successor to Dr. Randolph Stone, developer of polarity therapy; Director, Polarity Center, Orange, California.

**Laura Perls, DSc**
Co-developer with Fritz Perls of Gestalt therapy; and President of the New York Institute for Gestalt Therapy, New York City.

**Harold T. Perry, DDS, PhD**
Professor and Chairman, Department of Orthodontics, Northwestern University, Chicago, Illinois.

**Ida P. Rolf, PhD**
Developer of Rolfing; founder, Rolf Institute, Boulder, Colorado.

**Illana Rubenfeld**
Teacher and practitioner of Alexander Technique; developer of Gestalt Synergy; Adjunct Assistant Professor of Humanistic Psychology, New York University School of Continuing Education, New York City; and lecturer, New York University, School of Social Work, New York City; founder and Director, The Ilana Rubenfeld Center for Gestalt Synergy, New York City.

**Edward W. Russell, MA**
Author of *Design for Destiny* (London: Neville Spearman, 1971) and *Report on Radionics* (London: Neville Spearman, 1973).

**Claire Schmais, MA, DTR**
Coordinator, Dance Therapy Masters Program, Hunter College, New York City; Adjunct Assistant Professor, Cornell University Medical College, Payne Whitney Clinic, New York City, and State University of New York, Purchase, New York; founding member, American Dance Therapy Association, Columbia, Maryland; Chairperson, Dance Therapy Committee, American Association of Health, Physical Education and Recreation, Washington, D.C.

**Walter H. Schmitt, Jr., DC**
Treasurer and Education Committee Chairman, International College of Applied Kinesiology, Detroit, Michigan.

**Katsusuke Serizawa, MD**
Professor and head of Physiotherapeutic hospital, Tokyo University of Education, Tokyo, Japan; author of *Massage: The Oriental Method* (Elmsford, New York: Japan Publications, 1972) and *Tsubo* (Elmsford, New York: Japan Publications, 1976).

**C. Norman Shealy, MD**
Director, Pain Rehabilitation Center, LaCrosse, Wisconsin; Assistant Clinical Professor, Department of Psychology, University of Wisconsin, Madison, Wisconsin; author of *The Pain Game* (Millbrae, California: Celestial Arts, 1976), *Occult Medicine Can Save Your Life* (New York City: Dial Press, 1975), and *90 Days to Self-Health* (New York City: Dial Press, 1977).

**Felix Gad Sulman, MD, DMD**
Head, Bioclimatology Unit, Department of Applied Pharmacology, Hebrew University-Hadassah Medical Center, Jerusalem, Israel.

**William A. Tiller, PhD**
Professor and Chairman, Department of Material Science and Engineering, Stanford University, Palo Alto, California.

**Michael P. Volen, MD**
Clinical Medical Director, Pain Control Unit; Associate Physician Department of Anesthesiology, School of Medicine, University of California, Los Angeles, California.

**Aubrey Westlake, MB, BChir, MRCS**
Vice-President, Psionic Medicine Society, and pioneer in the field of wholistic medicine; author, *The Pattern of Health* (Berkeley, California: Shambhala, 1973) and *Life Threatened: Menace and Way Out* (London: Stuart Watkins, 1967).

**Ruth T. Wilf, CNM, PhD**
Nurse-midwife and childbirth educator, Booth Maternity Center, Philadelphia, Pennsylvania; Community Outreach Chairman, International Childbirth Education Association; Chairman, Board of Directors, Family Support Center, Yeadon, Pennsylvania; Board of Consultants, National Association of Parents and Professionals for Safe Alternatives in Childbirth; Member, editorial board, Birth and the Family Journal, Berkeley, California.

**Otto Wolff, MD**
Author, pioneer and lecturer in the field of Anthroposophical medicine; Director, Ita Wegman Clinic, Arlesheim, Switzerland.

**Olga N. Worrall, PhD, DHL**
Author, pioneer and healer; Director, New Life Clinic, Mt. Washington Methodist Church, Baltimore, Maryland.

**Leonard A. Worthington, LLB**
Attorney; member, Executive Committee, Board of Directors, Hastings College of Law, San Francisco, California; former member, State Bar Committee for Administration of Justice, Northern Sector, San Francisco, California.

# Suggested Reading List

## CHILDBIRTH

### Pregnancy and Childbirth

Anderson, Cheryl. *Free Delivery*. P.O. Box 34263, Station D, Vancouver, British Columbia, 1975.

Arms, Suzanne. *Immaculate Deception: A New Look at Women and Childbirth in America*. Boston: Houghton Mifflin Co., 1975.

Bing, Elizabeth. *Six Practical Lessons for an Easier Childbirth*. New York: Bantam, 1967.

Boston Women's Health Book Collective. *Our Bodies, Ourselves*. New York: Simon and Schuster, 1973. Revised, 1976.

Bradley, Robert A. *Husband-Coached Childbirth*. New York: Harper & Row, 1965, 1974.

Brewer, Gail and Tom. *What Every Pregnant Woman Should Know: About Diet and Drugs in Pregnancy*. New York: Random House, 1977.

Brook, Danae. *Naturebirth, You, Your Body, and Your Baby*. New York: Pantheon, 1976.

Dick-Read, Grantley. *The Practice of Natural Childbirth*. First published under the title of *Childbirth Without Fear* in 1944. Republished in New York: Harper and Row, 1976.

Ehrenreich, Barbara and English, Deirdre. *Witches, Midwives and Nurses*. New York: Feminist Press, 1973.

Eloesser, Leo, Galt, Edith J., and Hemingway, Isabel. *Pregnancy, Childbirth and the Newborn: A Manual for Rural Midwives*. Mexico City: Instituto Indigenista Inter-americano, 1959.

Ewy, Donna and Roger. *Preparation for Childbirth: A Lamaze Guide*. Boulder, Colorado: Pruett Publishing Co., 1970.

Fitzgerald, Herman, Long, Schildroth, and Ventre. *Home Oriented Maternity Experience*, H.O.M.E., Inc., Home Oriented Maternity Experience, 511 New York Ave., Takoma Park, Washington, D.C. 20012. 1976.

Hazell, Lester Dessez. *Commonsense Childbirth*. New York: Berkeley Publishing Corp., 1976.

Howells, John G., ed. *Modern Perspectives in Psycho-Obstetrics*. New York: Brunner/Mazel, 1972.

Kitzinger, Sheila. *The Experience of Childbirth*. New York: Taplinger Publishing Co., 1972.

———. *Giving Birth: The Parents' Emotions in Childbirth*. New York: Taplinger, Publishing Co., 1971.

Klaus, Marshall and Kennell, John. *Maternal-Infant Bonding, The Impact of Early Separation or Loss on Family Development*. St. Louis, Missouri: The C.V. Mosby Co., 1976.

Lamaze, Fernand. *Painless Childbirth*. First English translation published in Great Britain from the French *Qu'est-ce Quel l'accouchement sans douleur?* New York: Pocket Books. Reprinted in 1972.

Lang, Raven. *Birth Book*. Ben Lomond, California: Genesis Press, 1972.

Leboyer, Frederick. *Birth Without Violence*. New York: Alfred A. Knopf, 1975.

Medvin, Jeannine O'Brien. *Prenatal Yoga*. Albion, California: Freestone Publishing Co., 1974.

Milinaire, Caterine. *Birth*. New York: Harmony Books, 1974.

Myles, Margaret F. *A Textbook for Midwives*. London: Churchill Livingstone, 1972.

Nilsson, Ingelman-Sundberg and Wirsen. *A Child Is Born*. New York: Dell Publishing Co., 1969.

Noble, Elizabeth. *Essential Exercises for the Childbearing Year*. Boston: Houghton Mifflin, 1976.

Shaw, Nancy Stoller. *Forced Labor: Maternity Care in the United States*. Elmsford, New York: Pergamon Press, 1974.

Sousa, Marion. *Childbirth at Home*. Englewood Cliffs, New Jersey: Prentice-Hall, 1976.

Stewart, David and Lee, eds. *Safe Alternatives in Childbirth*. Chapel Hill, North Carolina: National Association of Parents and Professionals for Safe Alternatives in Childbirth, 1976.

Tanzer, Deborah. *Why Natural Childbirth*. New York: Doubleday, 1972.

Ward, Charlotte and Fred. *The Home Birth Book*. Washington, D.C.: INSCAPE Publishers, 1976.

Wessel, Helen. *Natural Childbirth and the Family*. New York: Harper & Row, 1973.

White, Gregory J. *Emergency Childbirth*. Franklin Park, Illinois: Police Training Foundation, 1968.

## BREASTFEEDING

Applebaum, Richard. *A breast of the Time*. 7914 S.W. 104th Street, Miami, Florida 33156. Privately published by author, 1969.

Eiger, Marvin and Olds, Karen. *The Complete Book of Breast-feeding*. New York: Workman, 1972.

Jelliffe, D.B. and E.F.P., guest eds. *The Uniqueness of Human Milk*. The American Journal of Clinical Nutrition, 1971.

Kippley, Sheila. *Breastfeeding and Natural Child-Spacing: The Ecology of Mothering*. New York: Harper & Row, 1974.

La Leche League International. *The Womanly Art of Breast-feeding*. Franklin Park, Illinois: La Leche League International, 1963.

Pryor, Karen. *Nursing Your Baby*, New York: Pocket Books, 1973.

Raphael, Dana. *The Tender Gift: Breastfeeding*. Englewood Cliffs, New Jersey: Prentice-Hall, 1973.

### Child Care and Development

Bowlby, John. *Attachment and Loss*. Vol. I. New York: Basic Books, 1969

———. *Child Care and the Growth of Love*. Baltimore, Maryland: Penguin Books, 1965.

Bricklin, Alice G. *Mother Love: The Book of Natural Child Rearing*. Philadelphia: Running Press, 1975.

Fraiberg, Selma H. *The Magic Years: Understanding and Handling the Problems of Early Childhood*. New York: Charles Scribners' Sons, 1959.

LeShan Eda J. *The Conspiracy Against Childhood*. New York: Atheneum, 1971.

———. *Natural Parenthood: Raising Your Child Without a Script*. A Signet Book from New American Library, 1970.

Montagu, Ashley. *Touching: The Human Significance of the Skin*. New York: Harper & Row, 1971.

Newton, Niles. *The Family Book of Child Care*. New York: Harper & Row, 1957.

Salk, Lee, and Kramer, Rita. *How to Raise a Human Being: A Parents' Guide to Emotional Health from Infancy to Adolesence*. New York: Random House, 1969.

Salk, Lee. *What Every Child Would Like His Parents to Know*. New York: Warner Books, 1972.

Thevenin, Tine. *The Family Bed: An Age-Old Concept in Child Rearing*. Box 16004, Minneapolis, Minnesota: Privately published by author, 1976.

Von Heydebrand, Caroline. *Childhood: A Study of the Growing Soul*. New York: Anthroposophic Press, 1970.

### Nutrition

Citizen's Committee on Infant Nutrition (Center for Science in the Public Interest). "White Paper on Infant Feeding Practices": Washington, D.C., 1974.

Davis, Adelle. *Let's Have Healthy Children*. New York: New American Library, 1972.

Lappe, Frances Moore. *Diet for a Small Planet*. New York: A Friends of the Earth/Ballantine Book, 1971.

Williams, Phyllis S. *Nourishing Your Unborn Child*. New York: Avon Books, 1975.

## INTEGRATIVE MEDICAL SYSTEMS

### Homeopathy

Allen, H.C. *Keynotes and Characteristics of the Materia Medica with Nosodes*. New York: Johnson Reprint Co., 1975.

Blackie, Margery G. *The Patient, Not the Cure. The Challenge of Homeopathy*. London: Macdonald and Jane's, 1976.

Boericke, William. *Materia Medica with Repertory*. New York: Johnson Reprint Co., 1927.

Boger, C.M. *A Synoptic Key of the Materia Medica*. Calcutta: Salzer and Co.

Clarke, J.H. *The Prescriber*. England: Health Science Press, 1968.

Coulter, Harris L. *Divided Legacy: A History of the Schism in Medical Thought. Volume I. The Patterns Emerge: Hippocrates to Paracelsus. Volume II. Progress and Regress: J.B. Van Helmont to Claude Bernard*. Washington, D.C.: Wehawken, 1973.

———. *Homeopathic Medicine*. St. Louis, Missouri: Formur, 1973.

Gibson, D.M. *First Aid Homeopathy in Accidents and Ailments*. England: British Homeopathic Association, 1975.

Hahnemann, Samuel. *Organon of Medicine*. Translated in 1921 from the German by William Boericke. Reprinted New Delhi: Jain Publishing Co.

———. *The Chronic Diseases*. Translated from the German edition of 1835 by Louis H. Tafel. Reprinted New Delhi: Jain Publishing Co., 1972.

Kent, James. *Repertory of the Homeopathic Materia Medica*. New York: Johnson Reprint Co., 1974.

Mitchell, George Ruthven. *Homeopathy: The First Authoritative Study of its Place in Medicine Today*. London: Allen, 1975.

Roberts, Herbert. *Art of Cure by Homeopathy*. New York: Johnson Reprint Co., 1942.

Sharma, C.H. *A Manual of Homeopathy and Natural Medicine*. London: Turnstone Books, 1975.

Shepherd, Dorothy. *Magic of Minimum Dose*. England: Health Science Press, 1964.

———. *More Magic of Minimum Dose*. England, Health Science Press, 1974.

———. *A Physician's Posy*. England: Health Science Press, 1969.

Stephenson, James H. *A Doctor's Guide to Helping Yourself with Homeopathic Remedies*. West Nyack, New York: Parker Publishing Co., 1976.

Vithoulkas, George. *Homeopathy, Medicine of the New Man. A Complete Introduction to the Natural System of Medicine*. New York: Avon Books, 1972.

### Osteopathy

Chaitow, Leon. *Osteopathy*. England: Thorsons, 1974.

Still, Andrew T. *Autobiography of A.T. Still*. Kirksville, Missouri: Privately published by author, 1897.

———. *Osteopathy, Research & Practice*. Kirksville, Missouri: Press of the Journal Printing Co., 1910.

———. *Philosophy of Osteopathy*. Kirksville, Missouri: Privately published by author, 1899.

Truhlar, Robert E. *Doctor A.T. Still in the Living*. Cleveland, Ohio: Privately published by Robert E. Truhlar, DO, 1950.

Webster, George V. *Sage Sayings of Still*. Los Angeles: Wetzel, 1935.

### Chiropractic

*Annals of the Swiss Chiropractors Association*, Vol. IV, V, VI, Geneva, Switzerland: Imprimeries, Populaires, 1969.

*Basic Chiropractic Procedure Manual*, R. C. Schafer, ed., 2nd edition. Des Moines, Iowa: American Chiropractic Association, 1977.

Dintenfass, Julius. *Chiropractic A Modern Way to Health*. New York: Pyramid Publications, 1970.

Harper, W. D. *Anything Can Cause Anything*. San Antonio, Texas: W. D. Harper, 1964.

Higley, Henry G. *The Intervertebral Disk Syndrome*. Des Moines, Iowa: American Chiropractic Association, 1965.

Illi, F. W. *The Vertebral Column*. Lombard, Illinois: National College of Chiropractic, 1951.

Inglis, Brian. *The Case for Unorthodox Medicine*. New York: G. P. Putnam Sons, 1965.

Janse, J., Houser, R.H., and Wells, B.F. *Chiropractic Principles and Technique*. Lombard, Illinois: National College of Chiropractic, 1947.

Levine, Mortimer. *The Structural Approach to Chiropractic*. New York: Comet Press, 1964.

### Applied Kinesiology

Goodheart, George J. *Applied Kinesiology—1977 Workshop Procedure Manual*. Detroit: Privately published, 1977. also available—Dr. Goodheart's Workshop Procedure Manuals from 1964, 1971, and 1973-76.

Walther, David S. *Applied Kinesiology–The Advanced Approach In Chiropractic*. Pueblo, Colorado: Privately published, 1976.

Stoner, Fred. *The Eclectic Approach to Chiropractic*. 2nd edition. Las Vegas: Privately published, 1976.

Thie, John F., with Marks, Mary. *Touch For Health*. Santa Monica, California: DeVorss, 1973.

Kendall, Henry O., and Florence P., and Wadsworth, Gladys E. *Muscles, Testing and Function*. 2nd ed. Baltimore: Williams and Wilkins, 1971.

Additional "Collected Papers" available through the International College of Applied Kinesiology, 542 Michigan Bldg., Detroit, MI 48226.

### Naturopathic Medicine

Abbot, A.E., ed. *The Art of Healing*. London: Emerson Press, 1963.

Airola, Paavo. *How To Get Well*. Phoenix, Arizona: Health Plus Publishers, 1974.

———. *Are You Confused?* Phoenix, Arizona: Health Plus Publishers, 1971.

Benjamin, Harry. *Everybodys Guide To Nature Cure*. Northamptonshire, England: Thorsons, 1961.
Bragg, Paul. *How To Keep Your Heart Healthy and Fit*. Desert Hot Springs, California: Health Science Publishers, 1975.
Bricklin, Mark. The *Practical Encyclopedia of Natural Healing*. Emmaus, Pennsylvania: Rodale Press, 1976.
Clark, Linda. *Handbook of Natural Remedies For Common Ailments*. Old Greenwich, Connecticut: Devin-Adair, 1976.
Clements, G.R. *The Law of Life and Human Health*. Boston: Christopher Publishing House, 1926. Reprinted Mokelumne Hill, California: Health Research, 1972.
Clymer, R. Swinburne. *Making Health Certain*. Quakertown, Pennsylvania: The Humanitarian Society, 1921.
————. *The Natura Physician*. Quakertown, Pennsylvania: Philosophical Publishing Co., 1933.
Densmore, Emmet. *How Nature Cures*. Mokelumne Hill, California: Health Research, reprinted, 1976.
Dickey, Lawrence. *Clinical Ecology*. Springfield, Illinois: Charles C. Thomas Publishers, 1976.
Donnsbach, Kurt. *Passport to Good Health*. Santa Anna, California: Rayline Publishing Co., 1972.
————. *Preventive Organic Medicine*. New Canaan, Connecticut: Keats Publishing Co., 1972.
Gallert, Mark L. *Constructive Treatment For Health*. Privately published by author, 1965.
Hotema, Hilton. *The Empyreal Sea*. Mokelumne Hill, California: Health Resarch, 1964.
————. *The Magic Temple*. Mokelumne Hill, California: Health Research, 1968.
————. *Secret of Regeneration*. Mokelumne Hill, California: Health Research, 1963.
————. *Son of Perfection*. Vols. I and II. Mokelumne Hill, California: Health Research.
Jensen, Bernard. *You Can Master Disease*. Solana Beach, California: Bernard Jensen Publishing Co., 1952.
Just, Adolf. *Return to Nature*. Mokelumne Hill, California: Health Research, reprinted, 1970.
Kulvinskas, Viktoras. *Survival into the 21st Century*. Wethersfield, Connecticut: Omangod Press, 1975.
Kuts-Chereaux, A. *Naturae Medicina and Naturopathic Dispensatory*. American Naturopathic Physicians and Surgeons Association. Yellow Springs, Ohio: Antioch Press. 1975.
Mausert, Otto. *Herbs for Health*. ed. and reprinted under the title of *Herbs*. By Elaine M. Muhr. Eugene, Oregon: Privately published, 1974.
Mellor, Constance. *Natural Remedies for Common Ailments*. London: C. W. Daniels and Co., 1973.
Roberts, Herbert. *The Principles and Art of Cure by Homeopathy*. England: Health Science Press, 1942.
Roe, Dapane. *Drug Induced Nutritional Deficiencies*. Westport, Connecticut: Avi Publishing Co., 1976.
Schroeder, Henry. *The Trace Elements and Man*. Old Greenwich, Connecticut: Devin-Adair, 1973.
Sharma, C.H. *A Manual of Homeopathy and Natural Medicine*. London: Turnstone Books, 1975.
Shelton, Herbert. *Getting Well*. Reprinted Mokelumne Hill, California: Health Research.
————. *The Hygienic System*. 7 vol's. Mokelumne Hill, California: Health Research, 1952.
Shelton, Herbert, and Clements, G.R. *Orthopathy*. San Antonio, Texas: The International School of Orthopathy, reprinted Mokelumne Hill, California: Health Research, 1963.
Tilden, J.H. *Diseases of Woman and Easy Childbirth*. Reprinted Mokelumne Hill, California: Health Research, reprinted, 1962.
————. *Impaired Health*. Vol's I and II. Mokelumne Hill, California: Health Research, reprinted, 1960 and 1959, respectively.
Trall, R.T. *The True Healing Art*. Reprinted Mokelumne Hill, California: Health Research.
Wendel, Paul. *Handbook of Diagnosis, Herbal Chemistry, and Their Curative Powers*. Wentzville, Missouri: W.B. Bazan.

As Naturopathy encompasses most natural techniques, additional references may generally be found in any of the source books in this section. (Integrative Medical Systems.)

### Cranial Technique

De Jarnette, M. *Cranial Technic*. Nebraska City, Nebraska: De Jarnette. 70, 72, 73, 74, 75, 76, 77.
Lippincott, R. and Lippincott, H. *A Manual of Cranial Technic*. Meridian, Idaho: Academy of Applied Osteopathy, 1943.
Magoun, H. *Commentaries of Dr. Sutherland's Recordings*. Denver, Colorado: Sutherland Teaching Foundation, 1961.
————. *Osteopathy In The Cranial Field*. Meridian, Idaho: Osteopathic Cranial Academy, 1966.
Journal of The Osteopathic Cranial Association. Meridian Idaho: Osteopathic Cranial Association, 1948 and 1953.
Sutherland, W. *The Cranial Bowl*. Mankato, Minnesota: Sutherland, 1939.

Other authors include Goodheart, King, Alberts, Lavitan, and researchers from the University of Michigan State College of Human Medicine as published in the Journal of the American Osteopathic Association.

### Temporomandibular Joint Technique

Freese, A.S., and Scheman, P. *Management of Temporomandibular Joint Problems*. St. Louis: C.V. Mosby, 1962.
Garliner, D. *Myofunctional Therapy in Dental Practice*. Philadelphia: W.B. Saunders, 1976.
Gelb, H., and contributors. *Clinical Management of Head, Neck and Jaw Dysfunction*. Philadelphia: W.B. Saunders, 1977.
Grieder, A., and Cinotti, W.R. *Periodontal Prosthesis, Volume I*. St. Louis: C.V. Mosby, 1968.
Griffin, C.J., and Harris, R. "The Temporomandibular Joint Syndrome." *Monographs in Oral Science*, Volume 4. Basel, Switzerland: Karger, 1975.
Kraus, H. *Clinical Treatment of Back and Neck Pain*. New York: McGraw-Hill, 1970.
Morgan, Douglas, and contributors. *Diseases of the Temporomandibular Apparatus: A Multidisciplinary Approach*. St. Louis: C.V. Mosby, 1977.
Posselt, Ulf. *The Physiology of Occlusion and Rehabilitation*. Philadelphia: F.A. Davis, 1962.
Sarnat, B.G. *The Temporomandibular Joint*. Springfield, Illinois: Charles C. Thomas, 1951.
Schwartz, L.L. *Disorders of the Temporomandibular Joint*. Philadelphia: W.B. Saunders, 1959.
Schweitzer, J.M. *Oral Rehabilitation*. St. Louis: C.V. Mosby, 1951.
Selye, H. *The Stress of Life*. New York: McGraw-Hill, 1956.
Shore, N.A. *Occlusal Equilibration and Temporomandibular Joint Dysfunction*. Philadelphia: J.B. Lippincott, 1959.
Wolff, H.G. *Headache and Other Head Pain*. New York: Oxford University Press, 1948.

### Developmental Vision Therapy

Ames, L.D., Gillespie, C., and Stress, J.W., *Stop School Failure*. New York: Harper and Row, 1969.
Cohn, N. and Shapiro, J., *Out of Sight into Vision*. New York: Simon and Schuster, 1977.
Corbett, M.D., *Quick Guide to Better Vision*. Englewood Cliffs, New Jersey: Prentice-Hall, 1957.
Furth, M.G. and Wachs, H., *Thinking Goes to School*. New York: Oxford University Press, 1974.
Greenstein, T., *Vision and Learning Disability*. St. Louis: American Optometric Association, 1976.
Jackson, J., *Seeing Yourself See*. New York: E.P. Dutton, 1975.
Kraskin, R.A., *How to Improve your Vision*. North Hollywood, California: Wilshire Books, 1968.
Lee, W.C., *Each of Us an Island*. New York: Vantage, 1976.
Nugent, L.J., "I was Nearly a Drop-out", *Family Circle Magazine*. March, 1971.
Orem, R.C., *Learning to See and Seeing to Learn*. Johnstown, Pennsylvania: Mafex Associates, 1971.
Orem, R.C., *Developmental Vision for Lifelong Learning*. Johnstown, Pennsylvania: Mafex Associates, 1977.
Rosner, J. *Helping Children Overcome Learning Difficulties*. New York: Walker and Co., 1975.
Suchoff, I.B., *Visual Spatial Development in the Child*. New York: State College of Optometry, S.U.N.Y., 1975.
Weiner, H., *Eyes OK I'm OK*. San Rafael, California: Academic Therapy, 1977.
Wold, R.M., *Visual and Perceptual Aspects for the Achieving and Underachieving Child*. Seattle, Washington: Special Child Publications, 1969.

## NUTRITION AND HERBS

### Nutrition

Abrahamson, E.M. *Body, Mind and Sugar*. New York: Pyramid Books, 1971.
Adams, R. and Murray F. *Body, Mind and the B Vitamins*. New York: Larchmont Books, 1972.
——. *Megavitamin Therapy*. New York: Larchmont Books, 1973.
Blaine, T.R. *Mentol Health Through Nutrition*. Secaucus, New Jersey: Citadel Press, 1969.
Brennan, R.O. *Nutrigenetics*. New York: M. Evans & Co., 1975.
Bruch, H. *Eating Disorders*. New York: Basic Books, 1973.
Cheraskin E., Ringsdorf, W.M., Jr., and Clark, J.W. *Diet and Disease*. Emmaus, Pennsylvania: Rodale Books, 1968.
Cheraskin, E., Ringsdorf, W.M., Jr. *New Hope for Incurable Diseases*. Jericho, New York: Exposition Press, 1971.
——. *Predictive Medicine: A Study in Strategy*. Mountain View, California: Pacific Press Publishing Association, 1973.
Coca, A.F. *The Pulse Test*. New York: Arco Books, 1956.
Crawford, Michael and Sheilagh. *What We Eat Today*. London: Neville Spearman, 1972.
Cureton, T.K. *The Physiological Effects of Wheat Germ Oil on Humans in Exercise*. Springfield, Illinois: Charles C. Thomas, 1972.
Currier, W.D. *Dizziness Related to Hypoglycemia: The Role of Adrenal Steroids and Nutrition*. Reprinted from the *Journal of Applied Nutrition* #1 and 2, 1969.
Davis, Adelle. *Let's Get Well*. New York: Harcourt Brace Jovanovich, 1965. Paperback, Signet, 1972.
Frederick, Carlton. *Eating Right for You*. New York: Grosset & Dunlap, 1972.
——. *Food Facts and Fallacies*. New York: Galahad Books, 1965.
Galdston, I. *Beyond the Germ Theory: The Role of Deprivation and Stress in Health and Disease*. New York: Health Education Council, 1954.
Gorman, ClK. "Hypoglycemia: A Brief Review." *Medical Clinics of North America* **49: #4**, 947-959, July 1965.
Hawkins, D.R., and Pauling, L.C. *Orthomolecular Psychiatry: Treatment of Schizophrenia*. San Francisco: W.H. Freeman and Co., 1973.
Hunter, Beatrice Trum. *Consumer Beware! Your Food and What's Been Done to It*. New York: Simon & Schuster, 1976.
Hurd, Frank and Rosalie. *Ten Talents Cook Book*. Grand Rapids, Michigan: Life Line Health Center, 1968.
Lasagna, L. *The Doctor's Dilemma*. New York: Harper and Brothers, 1962.
Locke, David M. *Enzymes–The Agents of Life*. New York: Crown Publishers, 1969.
Mackarness, Richard. *Eating Dangerously: The Hazards of Hidden Allergies*. New York: Harcourt Brace Jovanovich, 1976.
Murphy, W.B. "Some Things You Might Not Know About the Foods Served to Children." *Nutrition Today* **7: #5**, 34-35, September-October 1972.
Pauling, L.C. The New Medicine? *Nutrition Today* **7: #5**, 18-23, September-October 1972.
——. Orthomolecular Psychiatry. *Science* **160: #3825**, 265-271, 19 April 1968.
Roberts, S.E. *Exhaustion: Causes and Treatment*. Emmaus, Pennsylvania: Rodale Press, 1967.
Rodale, J.I. *Natural Health, Sugar and the Criminal Mind*. New York: Pyramid Books, 1968.
Rosenberg, Harold and Feldzamen, A.N. *The Doctor's Book of Vitamin Therapy*. New York: G.P. Putnam's Sons, 1974.
Schroeder, Henry A. *The Trace Elements and Man*. Old Greenwich, Connecticut: Devin-Adair, 1973.
Shelton, Herbert. *Food Combining Made Easy*. San Antonio, Texas: Sheltons Publishing Company, 1973.
——. *Superior Nutrition*. San Antonio, Texas: Sheltons Publishing Company, 1972.
Watson, G. *Nutrition and Your Mind*. New York: Harper and Row, 1972.
Williams, R.J. *Nutrition Against Disease: Environmental Protection*. New York: Pitman Publishing Co. 1971.
——. *Biochemical Individuality*. New York: Wiley, 1956.

### Macrobiotics

Dufty, William. *You Are All Sanpaku*. Secaucus, New Jersey: University Books, 1965.
——. *Sugar Blues*. Radnor, Pennsylvania: Chilton Books, 1975.
Carrel, Alexis. *Man the Unknown*. New York: Harper & Row, 1935.
Kushi, Aveline. *How to Cook with Miso*. Tokyo: Japan Publications, 1978.
Kushi, Michio. *The Book of Macrobiotics: The Universal Way of Health and Happiness*. Tokyo: Japan Publications, 1977.
——. *The Book of Do-In*. Tokyo: Japan Publications, 1978.
——. *The Teachings of Michio Kushi, Vol. I*. Boston: East West Foundation, 1972.
——. *The Origin and Destiny of Man: The Teachings of Michio Kushi, Vol. II*. Boston: East West Foundation, 1971.
——. *The Order of the Universe: The Teachings of Michio Kushi, Vol. III*. Boston: East West Foundation, 1977.
——. *Spiritual Practices*. Boston: East West Foundation, 1978.
Kushi, Michio; with Tara, William, ed. *Oriental Diagnosis*. London: Red Moon Press, 1976.
Kushi, Michio; with Esko, Edward and Van Cauwenberghe, Marc, eds. *The Macrobiotic Approach to Major Illnesses*. Boston: East West Foundation, 1978.
Ohsawa, George. *Cancer and the Philosophy of the Far East*. Binghamton, New York: Swan House, 1971.
——. *The Unique Principle: The Philosophy of Macrobiotics*. San Francisco: The Ohsawa Foundation, 1973.
——. *A Practical Guide to Far-Eastern Macrobiotic Medicine*. San Francisco: The Ohsawa Foundation, 1973.
——. *Zen Macrobiotics*. Los Angeles: The Ohsawa Foundation, 1965.
——. *The Book of Judgement*. Los Angeles: The Ohsawa Foundation, 1965.
——. *The Macrobiotic Guidebook for Living*. Los Angeles: The Ohsawa Foundation, 1965.
Ohsawa, Lima. *The Art of Just Cooking*. Tokyo: Autumn Press, 1974.
Manaka, Yoshio. *Laymen's Guide to Acupuncture*. Rutland, Vermont: Weatherhill (a division of Tuttle), 1972.
Muramoto, Noboru. *Healing Ourselves*. New York: Avon Books, 1973.
Veith, Ilze, trans. *The Yellow Emperor's Classic of Internal Medicine (Nei Ching)*. Los Angeles: University of California Press, 1949.

## Herbs

Bach, Edward. *Heal Thyself*. England: C.W. Daniels Company, 1931.

——. *The Twelve Healers and Other Remedies*. England: C.W. Daniels Company, 1933.

Bianchini, Francesco, and Corbetta, Francesco. *Health Plants of the World: Atlas of Medicinal Plants*. New York: Newsweek, 1977.

*British Herbal Pharmacopoeia*. London: British Herbal Medicine Association, 1971.

Christopher, John R. *School of Natural Healing*. Provo, Utah: BiWorld, 1976.

Clymer, R. Swinburne. *Nature's Healing Agents*. Philadelphia: Dorrance, 1963.

Committee on Scholarly Communication with the People's Republic of China. *Herbal Pharmacology in the People's Republic of China*. Washington, D.C.: National Academy of Science, 1975.

Culpeper, Nicholas. *Culpeper's English Physician & Complete Herbal Remedies*. North Hollywood, California: Wilshire Book Company, 1972.

Dastur, J.F. *Medicinal Plants of India & Pakistan*. Bombay: D.B. Taraporevala Sons & Co. Private Ltd., 1962.

Densmore, Frances. *How Indians Use Wild Plants for Food Medicine & Crafts*. New York: Dover, 1974.

Gabriel, Ingrid. *Herb Identifier and Handbook*. New York: Sterling Press, 1975.

Geographic Health Studies Program of the John E. Fogarty International Center for Advanced Study in the Health Sciences. *A Barefoot Doctor's Manual*. Washington, D.C.: U.S. Department of Health, Education and Welfare, 1974.

Grieve, Maude. *A Modern Herbal*. Darien, Connecticut: Hafner Publishing Co. Reprinted 1970.

Hand, Wayland D. ed. *American Folk Medicine*. Berkeley, California: University of California Press, 1976.

Harris, Ben Charles. *The Compleat Herbal*. Barre, Massachusetts: Barre Publishing Co., 1972.

Hills, Lawrence D. *Comfrey (Fodder, Food, and Remedy)*. New York: Universe Books, 1976.

Hutchens, Alma R. *Indian Herbalogy of North America*. Kumbakonam, S. India: Homeo House Press, 1969.

Kaslof, Leslie J. *Herb and Ailment Cross Reference Chart*. Brooklyn, New York: United Communications, 1972.

Kervan, Louis C. *Biological Transmutations*. Binghamton, New York: Swan House Publishing Co., 1972.

Kloss, Jethro. *Back to Eden*. Coalmont, Tennessee: Longview Publishing Co., 1939.

Kreig, Margaret B. *Green Medicine: The Search for Plants That Heal*. Chicago: Rand McNally and Co., 1964.

Krochmal, Arnold and Connie. *Guide to Medicinal Plants of the U.S.* New York: Quadrangle, 1973.

Levy, Juliette de Bairacli. *The Complete Herbal Book for the Dog*. New York: Arco, 1973.

Lewis, Walter and Elvin-Lewis, Memory P.F. *Medical Botany: Plants Affecting Man's Health*. New York: Wiley Interscience, 1977.

Messegue, Maurice. *Of Men and Plants*. New York: Macmillan, 1973.

Meyer, Clarence. *American Folk Medicine*. New York: Crowell, 1973.

Millspaugh, Charles F. *American Medicinal Plants*. New York: Dover. Reprinted 1974.

Martinez, Maximino. *Plantas Medicinales De Mexico*. Justo Sierra, Mexico: Ediciones Botas, 1969.

Morton, Julia F. *Folk Remedies of the Low Country*. Miami, Florida: E.A. Seemann Publishing Co., 1974.

Peterson, Roger Tory and McKenny, Margaret. *Field Guide to Wildflowers*. Boston: Houghton Mifflin, 1968.

Rau, Henrietta A. Diers. *Nature's Aid*. New York: Pagent, 1968.

Shih-Chen, Li. Translated and researched by Smith, F. Porter and Stuart, G.A. *Chinese Medicinal Herbs*. San Francisco: Georgetown Press, 1973.

Shook, Edward E. *Advanced Treatise on Herbology*. Mokelumne Hill, California: Reprinted by Health Research.

Shove, Lt.-Col. F. Harper. *Prescriber and Clinical Repertory of Medicinal Herbs*. England: Health Science Press, 1952.

Tompkins, Peter and Bird, Christopher. *The Secret Life of Plants*. New York: Harper and Row, 1972.

Vogel, Virgil J. *American Indian Medicine*. Norman, Oklahoma: University of Oklahoma Press, 1970.

Watt, John Mitchell and Breyer-Brandwijk, Maria Gerdina. *Medicinal and Poisonous Plants of Southern and Eastern Africa*. London: E. & S. Livingston Ltd., 1962.

Weslager, C.A. *Magic Medicines of the Indians*. Wallingford, Pennsylvania; Middle Atlantic Press, 1973.

Wren, R.C. *Potters New Cyclopaedia of Botanical Drugs and Preparations*. England: Health Science Press. Reprinted 1973.

## HEURISTIC DIRECTIONS IN DIAGNOSIS AND TREATMENT

### Subtle Energies

Baxter, C. "Evidence of Primary Perception in Plant Life." *International Journal of Parapsychology* **10**, 1968.

Bentov, Itzhak. *Stalking the Wild Pendulum-on the Mechanics of Consciousness*. New York: E.P. Dutton, 1977.

Blair, Lawrence. *Rhythms of Vision The Changing Patterns of Belief*. New York: Schocken Books, 1975.

Brillouin, L. *Scientific Uncertainty and Information*. New York: Academic Press, 1974.

Brunler, Oscar. *Radiations of the Brain the Body the Earth the Atom*. Privately printed by author, 1948.

Harvalik, Z. V. "Sensitivity Tests on a Dowser Exposed to Artificial D. C. Magnetic Fields." *American Dowser* 13:3, 85 1973, and 14:1, 4 1974.

Kilner, W.J. *The Aura*. New York: Weiser, reprinted, 1973.

Krippner, Stanley, and Rubin, Daniel., eds. *Galaxies of Life*. New York: An Interface Book, Gordon and Breach, 1973.

——. eds. *The Energies of Consciousness*. New York: An Interface Book, Gordon and Breach, 1975.

Merrell-Wolff, Franklin. *Pathways Through Space*. New York: Julian Press, 1973.

Milner, Dennis, and Smart, Edward. *The Loom of Creation*. London and New York: Harper and Row, 1976.

Motoyama, H. "How to Measure and Diagnose the Functions of Meridians." International Association for Religion and Parapsychology 21:2, 1, September 1975.

Nixon, F. *Born to Be Magnetic*, Vols. I and II. P. O. Box 718, Chemainus, British Columbia, Canada: Magnetic Publishers, 1971 and 1973 respectively.

Ostrander, S. and Schroeder, L. *Psychic Discoveries Behind the Iron Curtain*. Englewood Cliffs, New Jersey: Prentice-Hall, 1970.

Regush, Nicholas M., in collaboration with Merta, Jan. *Exploring the Human Aura*. Englewood Cliffs, New Jersey: Prentice Hall, 1975.

Rock, I. *The Nature of Perceptual Adaptation*. New York: Basic Books, 1967.

Tansley, David V *Subtle Body Essence and Shadow*. London: Thames and Hudson, 1977.

Targ, R. and Hurt, D. B. "Learning Clairvoyance and Precognition with an Extra-Sensory Perception Teaching Machine." *IEEE Symposium on Information Theory*, January 1972.

Thie, J. F. *Touch for Health*. Santa Monica, California: De Vorss, 1973.

Tiller, W. A. "Consciousness, Radiation and the Developing Sensory System." Academy of Parapsychology and Medicine Symposium on "Dimensions of Healing," 1972.

——. "Disease as a Biofeedback Mechanism for the Transformation of Man." Phoenix, Arizona: A.R.E. Medical Symposium, January 1973.

——. "Energy Fields and the Human Body, Part II." Phoenix, Arizona: A.R.E. Medical Symposium, January 1972.

——. "Future Medical Therapeutics Based Upon Controlled Energy Fields." Phoenix, Arizona: A.R.E. Medical Symposium, January 1976.

——. "Kirlian Photography, Its Scientific Foundations and Future Potential," *Physiological Physics and Therapies*, ed. D. N. Ghista. New York: Marcel Dekker, 1978.

——. "A Lattice Model of Space and Its Relationship to Multidimensional Physics." Phoenix, Arizona: A.R.E. Medical Symposium, January 1977.

——. "The Positive and Negative Space-Time Frames as Conjugate Systems." Phoenix, Arizona: A.R.E. Medical Symposium, January 1975. *Future Science*, eds. S. Krippner and J. White. New York: Doubleday-Anchor, 1976.

——. "Radionics, Radiesthesia and Physics." Academy of Parapsychology and Medicine Symposium on "The Varieties of Healing Experience," 1971.

——. "Three Relationships of Man." Phoenix, Arizona: A.R.E. Medical Symposium, January 1975. Multidisciplinary Research **4**, Part 1, 143 April 1976.

—— and Cook, Wayne. "Psychoenergetic Field Studies Using a Biomechanical Transducer." Phoenix, Arizona: A.R.E. Medical Symposium, January 1974.

Vasiliev, L.L. *Experiments in Distant Influence*. First published in Russia in 1962, republished New York: E.P. Dutton, 1976.

Young, Arthur M. *The Geometry of Meaning*. New York: Delacorte, 1976.

——. *The Reflexive Universe*. New York: Delacorte, 1976.

### Fields of Life

Detailed information on the experiments of Dr. Burr and his colleagues may be found in his published papers. A partial bibliography from the *Yale Journal of Biology and Medicine* Vol 30 Dec/1957, from 1942 to 1956, is given below.

#### 1942

An electrical study of the human cervix uteri. *Anat. Rec.*, 1942, *82*, 35-36 (with L. Langman).

Electrical correlates of growth in corn roots. *Yale J. Biol. Med.*, 1942, *14*, 581-588.

Electrometric timing of human ovulation. *Amer. J. Obstet Gynec.*, 1942, *44*, 223-230 (with L. Langman).

#### 1943

Neuroid transmission in mimosa. *Anat. Rec.*, 1943, *85*, 12.

Electrical correlates of pure and hybrid strains of corn. *Proc. nat. Acad. Sci.*, 1943, *29*, 163-166.

Electrical polarization of pacemaker neurons. *J. Neurophysiol.*, 1943, *6*, 85-97 (with T.H. Bullock).

An electrometric study of mimosa. *Yale J. Biol. Med.*, 1943, *15*, 823-829.

#### 1944

Moon-madness. *Yale J. Biol. Med.*, 1944, *16*, 249-256.

A biologist considers social security. *Conn. St. med. J.*, 1944, *8*, 165.

Potential gradients in living systems and their measurements. Pp. 1117-1121 in *Medical Physics*. Chicago, The Year Book Publishers, Inc. [c1944].

The meaning of bio-electric potentials. *Yale J. Biol. Med.*, 1944, *16*, 353-360.

Electric correlates of form in Cucurbit fruits. *Amer. J. Botany*, 1944, *31*, 249-253 (with E.W. Sinnott).

Electricity and life: phases of moon correlated with life cycle. *Yale scient. Mag.*, 1944, *18*, 5-6.

#### 1945

Variables in DC measurement. *Yale J. Biol. Med.*, 1945, *17*, 465-478.

Diurnal potentials in the maple tree. *Yale J. Biol. Med.*, 1945, *17*, 727-734.

#### 1946

Electrical correlates of peripheral nerve injury. A preliminary note. *Science*, 1946, *103*, 48-49 (with R.G. Grenell).

Growth correlates of electromotive forces in maize seeds. *Proc. nat. Acad. Sci.*, 1946, *32*, 73-84 (with Oliver Nelson, Jr.).

Surface potentials and peripheral nerve injury: A clinical test. *Yale J. Biol. Med.*, 1946, *18*, 517-525 (with R.G. Grenell).

#### 1947

Tree potentials. *Yale J. Biol. Med.*, 1947, *19*. 311-318.

Electromagnetic studies in women with malignancy of cervix uteri. *Science*, 1947, *105*, 209-210 (with L. Langman).

Field theory in biology. *Sci. Monthly*, 1947, *67*, 217-225.

Surface potentials and peripheral nerve regeneration. *Fed. Proc.*, 1947, *6*, 117 (with R.G. Grenell).

#### 1948

A commentary on full-time teaching. *Conn. St. med. J.*, 1948, *12*, 937-940.

#### 1949

Millivoltmeters. *Yale J. Biol. Med.*, 1949, *21*, 249-253 (with A. Mauro).

A technique to aid in the detection of malignancy of the female genital tract. *Amer. J. Obstet. Gynec.*, 1949, *57*, 274-281.

Electrostatic fields of the sciatic nerve in the frog. *Yale J. Biol. Med.*, 1949, *21*, 455-462 (with A. Mauro).

The Connecticut State Medical Society. *Conn. St. med. J.*, 1949, *13*, 950-955.

#### 1950

Electrometric study of cotton seeds. *J. exp. Zool.*, 1950, *113*, 201-210.

Bioelectricity: potential gradients. Pp. 90-94 in *Medical Physics*. Chicago, The Year Book Publishers, Inc., 1950.

#### 1952

Electrometrics of atypical growth. *Yale J. Biol. Med.*, 1952, *25*, 67-75.

#### 1953

Electrical correlates of ovulation in the rhesus monkey. *Yale J. Biol. Med.*, 1953, *25*, 408-417 (with V.L. Gott).

#### 1954

Confusion or configuration? *The Astronomical League Bulletin*, 1954, *4*, No. 4.

#### 1955

Certain electrical properties of the slime mold. *J. exp. Zool.*, 1955, *129*, 327-342.

Response of the slime mold to electric stimulus. *Science*, 1955, *122*, 1020-1021 (with William Seifriz).

#### 1956

Effect of a severe storm on electric properties of a tree and the earth. *Science*, 1956, *124*, 1204-1205.

Burr, Harold Saxton. *Blueprint for Immortality—The Electric Patterns of Life*. London: Neville Spearman, Ltd., 1972.

## Acupuncture


*Academy of Traditional Chinese Medicine: An Outline of Chinese Acupuncture*. Peking: Foreign Language Press, 1975.

Austin, Mary. Acupuncture Therapy. New York: ASI, 1972.

*A Barefoot Doctor's Manual* (English translation). Washington, D.C.: DHEW Publication No. (NIH) 75-695, 1974 (reproduced in limited quantities).

Chen, James Y.P. *Acupuncture Anesthesia in the People's Republic of China, 1973*. Washington, D.C.: DHEW Publication No. (NIH) 75-769, 1973.

Graystone, Peter, and James, Lynell. *Acupuncture and Pain Therapy—A Comprehensive Bibliography*. Vancouver, B.C.: Biomedical Engineering Services, 1975.

Hwang, Paul T.K.; Wong, Joshua S.L.; and Chan, Pedro C.P. *Acupuncture Made Easy*. Alhambra, California: Chan's Books and Products, 1975.

Kroening, Richard J., and Bresler, David E. *Acupuncture for Management of Facial and Dental Pain (A Work Book)*. Los Angeles: U.C.L.A. Acupuncture Research Project, 1975.

Lavier, J. *Points of Chinese Acupuncture* (trans. by Philip M. Chancellor). Wellingborough, England: Health Science Press, 1974.

Lee, In J., and Lee, Thomas D.H. *Acupuncture Atlas*. Melville, New York: Lycee Trading Corporation, 1975.

Lowe, William C. *Introduction to Acupuncture Anesthesia*. Flushing, New York: Medical Examination Publishing, 1973.

Man, Pang L. *Handbook of Acupuncture Analgesia*. Woodbury, New Jersey: Field Place Press, 1973.

Manaka, Yoshio, and Urquhart, Ian A. *The Layman's Guide to Acupuncture*. New York: Weatherhill, 1972.

Mann, Felix. *Atlas of Acupuncture—Points and Meridians in Relation to Surface Anatomy*. London: William Heinemann, 1972.

Matsumoto, Teruo. *Acupuncture for Physicians*. Springfield, Illinois: Charles C. Thomas, 1974.

Palos, Stephan. *The Chinese Art of Healing*. New York: Bantam 1972.

*The Principles and Practical Use of Acupuncture Anesthesia*. Hong Kong: Medicine and Health Publishing, 1974.

Tan, Leong T.; Tan, Margaret Y.-C.; and Veith, Ilza. *Acupuncture Therapy, Current Chinese Practice*, 2nd edition. Philadelphia: Temple University Press, 1976.

Veith, Ilza. *The Yellow Emperor's Classic of Internal Medicine* Los Angeles: University of California Press, 1972.

Warren, Frank Z. *Handbook of Medical Acupuncture*. New York: Van Nostrand Reinhold, 1976.

Warren, Frank Z., and Huang, Helena L. *Ear Acupuncture*. Emmaus, Pennsylvania: Rodale, 1974.

Wexu, Mario. *A Modern Guide to Ear Acupuncture*. New York:, ASI, 1975.


## Aeriontherapy


Kornblueh, I.H. "Ionization of the Air as a Potential Health Factor," in *10th Convegno della Salute Ferrara*. Modena, Italy: Poligrafico Arioli, 1963.

Krueger, A.P., and Reed, E.J. "Biological Impact of Small Air Ions," *Science* **193**:1209-1213, 1976.

Soyka, Fred. The Ion Effect. New York: E.P. Dutton, 1977.

Sulman, F.G. *Health, Weather, and Climate*. Monograph. Basel, Switzerland: Karger, 1976.


## Light and Health


Feingold, B.F. "Behavioral Disturbances, Learning Disabilities, and Food Additions, *Chemical Technology* **5**:264, 1975.

Hatch, A., et al. "Long-term Isolation Stress in Rats," *Science*, October 1963.

"Light as Antidote to Stress," *New Scientists*, August 20, 1964.

Mayron, Lewis W., et al. "Light, Radiation, and Academic Behavior," *Academic Therapy*, Fall 1974.

Ott, J.N. "Effects of Wavelengths of Light on Physiological Functions of Plants and Animals." *Illuminating Engineering*, April 1965.

———. "Responses of Psychological and Physiological Functions to Environmental Radiation Stress," *Journal of Learning Disabilities*, June 1968.

Sinclair, J.D., and Geller, I. "Ethanol Consumption by Rats under Different Lighting Conditions," *Science* **175**:1143-1144, 1972.


## Kirlian Photography


Boxler, C. and M. Paulson. "Kirlian Photography: A New Tool in Biological Research?" *J. Biol. Phot. Assoc.*, **45**, Number 2, pp. 51-60, April 1977.

Boyers, D.G. and W.A. Tiller. "The Color in Kirlian Photography—Fact or Artifact?" *Functional Photography*, **11**, 3, pp. 20, May 1976.

———. "Corona Discharge Photography," *J. Appl. Phys.*, **44**, pp. 3102-3112, 1973.

Brewer, A.K., *Notes on Kirlian Photography*. Washington, D.C.: Privately published by author, 1975.

Burton, L., W. Joines and B. Stevens. "Kirlian Photography and its Relevance to Parapsychological Research." In *Research in Parapsychology. 1974*. J.D. Morris, W.G. Roll and R.L. Morris, eds., Metuchen, New Jersey: Scarecrow Press, 1975, pp. 107-112.

Burton, L., W. Joines and B. Stevens. "Kirlian Photography in Diagnosis and Early Detection of Disease." Paper presented at the 19th Annual Symposium of the Institute of Electrical and Electronic Engineers. Raleigh, North Carolina, November 1974.

Case, E. and W. Fadner. *Bull. Am. Phys. Soc.* **20,** 427, 1973.

Dakin, H.S. *High Voltage Photography*. San Francisco: H.S. Dakin Co. 1974.

Dombrovsky, B.A., G.A. Sergeyev and B.M. Inyushin, eds. *Bioenergetics Questions (Material of the Scientific Methological Seminar in Alma-Ata)*. Kazakh State University, USSR, 1969. Trans. Southern California Society for Psychical Research, 1972.

Dumitrescu, I. Fl. "Electronography." English translation supplied by author. Bucharest, Romania, 1977.

Dumitrescu, I. Fl. "Electronography—A Scanning Method for the Electromagnetic Exchanges between the Human Body and the Electric Environment." English translation supplied by author. Bucharest, Romania, 1977.

Dumitrescu, I. Fl., N. Golovanov, G. Golovanov and E. Celan. "The Electronography—Method of Exploration of Living Organisms." English translation supplied by author, Bucharest, Romania, 1977.

———. "L'Image Electronographique Des Points D'Acupuncture." French translation supplied by author. Bucharest, Romania, 1977.

Dumitrescu, I. Fl., R. Portocala and R. Herivan. "Microelectrography—A Method of Cell Research," *Revue Roumaine De Biologie—Série De Biologie Animale* **21**, No. 1, pp. 19-22, April-June 1976.

———. "Romanian Contributions to the Developement of Biological Electrography." English translation supplied by author. Bucharest, Romania, 1977.

———. "Rumänischer Beitrag zur Entwiklung der Biologishen Electrographie" *Psychotronik*, **1**, 1, 1977, Innsbruck, Austria, International Association for Psychotronic Research.

Dumitrescu, I. Fl. N. Golovanov, G. Golovanov, and C. Eugen, Letters to the Editor, *Psychoenergetic Systems*, **2**, pp. 308-314, 1977.

———. N. Golovanov, G. Golovanov and E. Celan. "The Electronography—Method of Exploration of Living Organisms." English translation supplied by author, Bucharest, Romania, 1977.

Eidson, W.W. and D.L. Faust. "Corona Discharge Photography: Developing a New Scientific Tool," *Drexel University News* (Alumni Journal) **39**, pp. 7-11, Spring 1977.

———. "Technical Notes on Corona Discharge Photography: Developing a New Scientific Tool," Department of Physics and Atmospheric Science, Drexel University, July 1977.

Faust, D.L. "Instrumentation and Photographic Tekniques Employed in Corona Discharge Photography, Past and Present." Paper presented at 47th Annual Meeting of the Biological Photographic Association, Baltimore, Maryland, August 1977.

Faust, D.L., G.I. Gross, H.J. Kyler and J.O. Pehek. *"Investigations into the Reliability of Electrophotography—Final Technical Report on Phase II*. New York: Logical Technical Services Corp. June 1975.

*"Investigations into the Reliability of Electrophotography—Final Technical Report on Phase III*, AD-A018 806. National Technical Information Service, 295 Port Royal Road, Springfield, Virginia 22151, September 1975.

Hill, Scott. Letter to the Editor on the Kirlian Electrophotography Technique, *Journal Society Psychical Research*, pp. 58-60, London, England, March 1975.

Inyushin, V.M. and P.R. Chekorov. *Biostimulation Through Laser Radiation and Bioplasma* (Kazakh State University, USSR, 1975). Translation by S. Hill and T.D. Ghoshal. Copenhagen, Demark: Danish Society for Psychical Research, 1976.

Kirlian, S.D. and V.K. *Russian Journal Scientific Applied Photography Cinematography*. **6**, 397 (1961). Translations AD299 666 (1963) and Sct-71-3018 (1971) available from National Technical Information Service, 285 Port Royal Road, Springfield, Virginia 22151.

Konikiewicz, L.W. "Kirlian Photography in Theory and Clinical Application," *J. Biol. Photo. Assoc.*, **45**, Number 3, pp. 115-134, July 1977.

Krippner, S., ed. *Energies of Consciousness*. New York: Gordon & Breach, 1975.

Krippner, S. and D. Rubin, eds. *Galaxies of Life: The Human Aura in Acupuncture and Kirlian Photography*. New York: Gordon & Breach, 1973; also published with some changes as *The Kirlian Aura*. New York: Anchor Books, 1974.

Kyler, H.J., J.O. Pehek, D.L. Faust and R.A. Beyer. "Corona Discharge Photography: A Possible Application in Psychophysiology." Paper presented at the 48th Annual Meeting of the Eastern Psychological Association, Boston, Massachusetts, April 1977 (to be submitted for publication).

Lord, D.E. and R.R. Petrini. *High Voltage Photography Applied to Materials Science*. Report UCRL-51702. National Technical Information Service, 285 Port Royal Road, Springfield, Virginia 22151, November 1974.

———. *High Voltage Photography Applied to Materials Testing*. Report UCRL-77388 National Technical Information Service, 385 Port Royal Road, Springfield, Virginia 22151, October 1975.

Milner, D. and E. Smart. *The Loom of Creation*. New York Harper & Row, 1976.

Montandon, H.E. "Psychophysiological Aspects of the Kirlia Phenomenon: A Confirmatory Study," *Journal of the American Society for Psychical Research* **71,** 1, January 1977

Moss, T. and K. Johnson, "Radiation Field Photograph *Psychic Magazine*, July 1972, p. 50.

Omura, Y., "Acupuncture, Intra-Red Thermography and Kirlia Photography," *Acupuncture & Electro-Therapeutic Research International Journal*, **2,** pp. 43-86, 1976.

Ostrander, S. and L. Schroeder. *The ESP Papers: Scientists Spea Out from behind the Iron Curtain*. New York: Bantam, 1976.

———. *Handbook of PSI Discoveries*. New York: Putnam 1974.

———. *Psychic Discoveries Behind the Iron Curtain*. En glewood Cliffs, New Jersey: Prentice-Hall, 1970.

Pehek, J.O., H.J. Kyler and D.L. Faust. "Image Modulation i Corona Discharge Photography," *Science*, Vol. 194, pp 263-270, October 1976.

Pehek, J.O. *Investigations into Electrophotography—Interim Report Phase I*, October 1974. New York: Logical Technica Services Corp., 1974.

———. *Investigations of Electrophotography—Final Technica Report Phase I*. December 1974. New York: Logical Techni cal Services Corp., 1974.

Poock, G.K. "Kirlian Photography: An Engineer's View," *Techni UM* University of Michigan College of Engineering Spring Review (1975), pp. 28-36.

———. "Statistical Analysis of the Electro-bioluminescence o Acupuncture Points," *American Journal of Acupuncture*, **2** No. 4, pp. 257, December 1974.

Prat, S. and J. Schlemmer. "Electrophotography," *J. Biol. Photo Assoc.*, **7,** no. 4, pp. 145-148, June 1939.

Schwartz, Eric. "High Frequency Filter Model for Kirlian Photo graphy," New York: Energy Research Group, 1973.

Targ, R. and J. Cohen. "Kirlian Video Photography," Technica Memorandum SRI Project 3194-3, Menlo Park, California Stanford Research Institute, December 1974.

Tiller, W.A. "Kirlian Photography as an Electro-Therapeutics Re search Tool," *Acupuncture and Electro-Therapeut. Res. Int J.* Vol. 2, pp. 33-42, 1976.

———. "Kirlian Photography, its Scientific Foundations an Future Potential," *Physiological Physics and Therapies* (edited by D.N. Ghista). New York: Marcel Dekker, 1976 Originally available in 1975 as a monograph from Dept. o Materials Science and Engineering, Stanford Univ., Stanford California.

Tiller, W.A. "Are Psychoenergetic Pictures Possible?," *New Scientist*, **62,** 160, 1974.


## Radiesthesia, Psionic Medicine and Radionics


Abrams, Albert. *New Concepts in Diagnosis and Treatment*. Sa Francisco: The Philopolis Press, 1916.

———. *A preliminary Communication concerning the 'Elec tronic Reactions of Abrams'*. London: John Bale, Sons, an Daniellson, Ltd., 1925.

Archdale, F.A. *Elementary Radiesthesia and the Use of the Pen dulum*. Mokelumne Hill, California: Health Research, 1961.

Barr, Sir James, ed. *Abrams Methods of Diagnosis and Treatment* London: W. Heinemann, 1925.

Beasley, Victor R. *Dimensions of Electro-vibratory Phenomena* Boulder Creek, California: University of the Trees Press 1975.

Beasse, Pierre. *A New Rational Treatise of Dowsing*. Printed i 1941 from the French. Reprinted at Mokelumne Hill, Califor nia: Health Research, 1975.

Bhattacharyya, Benoytosh. *Magnet Dowsing*. Calcutta, India: A C. Ghosh Printing House, 1967.

Bird, Christopher. "Dowsing in the USSR" *The America Dowser*. August 1972.

———. "Dowsing in the USA: History, Achievement, an Current Research" *The American Dowser*. August 1973.

Burr, Harold Saxton. *Blueprint for Immortality–The Electric Pat terns of Life*. London: Neville Spearman, Ltd., 1972. U.S edn.: *The Fields of Life*. New York: Ballantine Books, 197

Cave, Francis A. *The Electronic Reactions of Abrams* Mokelumne Hill, California: Reprinted by Health Research

Cookes, H. St. L. *The Brain and Nerve System in Relation to th Earth's Magnetism*. Devon, England: Devon Rustics Ltd 1971.

Crabb, Riley Hansard, ed. *Radionics–The New Age Science Healing*. Vista, California: Borderland Sciences Researc Foundation.

Day, Langston, in collaboration with de la Warr, George. *Ne Worlds Beyond the Atom*. London: Vincent Stuart, 1956.

———. *Matter in the Making*. London: Vincent Stuart, 196

Drown, Ruth Beymer. *The Theory and Technique of the Drown H V. R. and Radio-vision Instruments*. London: Privately pub lished by Hatchard and Co., 1939.

Gallert, Mark L. *New Light on Therapeutic Energies*. Londo James Clark and Co., Ltd., 1966.

———. *Constructive Treatment for Health*. Privately published by author in 1965. Available through the Book Fund, Box 742, Bedford, Virginia 24523.
Hills, Christopher. *Supersensonics*. Boulder Creek, California: University of the Trees Press, 1975.
———. *Radiational Physics–The Ultimate Science and Methods of Radiesthesia*. Boulder Creek, California: University of the Trees Press.
Karagulla, Shafica. *Breakthrough to Creativity–Your Higher Sense Perceptions*. Los Angeles, California: DeVorss, 1967.
Maby, J. Cecil. "The Drown Method of Medical Diagnosis and Therapy", *Psychic Science–Journal of the International Institute of Psychic Investigation*, Vol. XXIII, No. 4, January 1945.
Maclean, Gordon, Sr. *Dowsing, an Introduction to an Ancient Practice*. South Portland, Maine: Privately published by author, 1971.
Mermet, Abbé. *Principles & Practice of Radiesthesia*. London: Watkins. Reprinted 1975.
Reyner, J.H. *Psionic Medicine*. New York: Weisser, 1974.
Richards, W. Guyon. *The Chain of Life*. London: John Bale, Sons, and Daniellson, Ltd., 1934. England: Reprinted by Health Science Press.
Russell, Edward, W. *Design for Destiny*. London: Neville Spearman, Ltd., 1971. New York: Ballantine Books, 1973.
———. *Report on Radionics*. London: Neville Spearman, Ltd., 1973.
Tansley, David V. *Radionics and the Subtle Anatomy of Man*. England: Health Science Press, 1972.
Tomlinson, H. *Divination of Disease*. England: Health Science Press, 1958.
———. *Medical Divination*. England: Health Science Press, 1966.
Tromp, S. W. *Psychical Physics*. London: Elsevier Publishing Co., 1949.
Westlake, Aubrey. *Pattern of Health*. Berkeley, California: Shamballa, 1973.
Wethered, Vernon D. *An Introduction to Medical Radiesthesia & Radionics*. London: C. W. Daniels & Co., 1974.
———. *The Practice of Medical Radiesthesia*. London: L. N. Fowler, 1967.
Wilcox, John. *Radionic Theory and Practice*. London: Herbert Jenkins Ltd., 1960.

### Biorhythms

Anderson, Russell K. "Biorhythm—Man's Timing Mechanism," *American Society of Safety Engineers Journal*, February 1973.
Aschoff, Jurgen, ed. *Circadian Clocks*. Amsterdam: North-Holland Publishing, 1965.
Astrand, Per-Olf and Rodahl, Kaare. *Textbook of Work Physiology*. New York: McGraw-Hill, 1970.
Brown, Frank A.; Hastings, J. Woodland; and Palmer, John D. *The Biological Clock: Two Views*. New York and London: Academic Press, 1970.
Bunning, Erwin. *The Physiological Clock*. New York: Springer-Verlag, 1967.
Colquhoun, W.P., ed. *Biological Rhythms and Human Performance*. London and New York: Academic Press, 1971.
Edholm, O.G., and Bacharach, A.L., eds. *The Physiology of Human Performance*. London and New York: Academic Press, 1965.
Ferguson, George A. *Statistical Analysis in Psychology and Education*. New York: McGraw-Hill, 1971.
Fraisse, Paul. *The Psychology of Time*. New York, Evanston, and London: Harper and Row, 1963.
Gittelson, Bernard. *Biorhythmm: A Personal Science*. New York: Arco, 1975.
Karlins, Marvin, and Andrew, Lewis M. *Biofeedback*. Philadelphia and New York: J.B. Lippincott, 1972.
Luce, Gay Gaer. *Biological Rhythms in Human and Animal Physiology*. New York: Dover, 1971.
———. *Biological Rhythms in Psychiatry and Medicine*. Chevy Chase, Maryland: National Institute of Mental Health, 1970.
———. *Bodytime: Physiological Rhythms and Social Stress*. New York: Pantheon, 1971.
Richter, Paul Curt. *Biological Clocks in Medicine and Psychiatry*. Springfield, Illinois: Charles C. Thomas, 1965.
Thommen, George. *Is This Your Day?* New York: Crown, 1964, 1973.
Ward, Ritchie R. *The Living Clocks*. New York: Alfred A. Knopf, 1971.

### Medical Astrology

Arroyo, Stephen. *Astrology, Psychology and the Four Elements*. Davis, California: CRCS Publications, 1975.
Darling, Harry F., and Oliver, Ruth H. *Astropsychiatry*. Lakemont, Georgia: CSA Press, 1973.
Davidson, William M. *Eight Special Lectures on Medical Astrology*, ed. by Charles A. Jayne. Monroe, New York: Three Brothers Press, 1959.
Ebertin, R. *The Combination of Stellar Influences*, trans. by Alfred B. Roosedale and Linda Kratzsch. Aalen, West Germany: Ebertin-Verlag, 1972.
———. *Applied Cosmobiology*, trans. by Hedi Langman and Jim Ten Hove; ed. by Charles Harvey. Aalen, West Germany: Ebertin-Verlag, 1972.
Tyle, Noel. *The Principles and Practice of Astrology, Vol. IX: Special Horoscope Dimensions*. Minneapolis: Llewellyn Press, 1975.

### Iridology

Collins, F.W. *Disease Diagnosed by Observation of the Eye*. Part I, Vol. I. Newark, New Jersey: Privately published by author, 1908.
Jensen, Bernard. *The Science and Practice of Iridology*. Escondido, California: Jensen Publishing Co., 1952.
Kriege, T. *Fundamental Basis of Irisdiagnosis*. London: L.N. Fowler and Co., 1969.
Lane, Henry Edward. *Diagnosis From the Eye*. Chicago: Kosmos Publishing Co., 1904.
Theil, Peter Johannes. *The Diagnosis of Disease by Observation of the Eye*. Part II, Vol. I. Newark, New Jersey: Published by F.W. Collins.
Weiss, Ralph R. *Irisdiagnosis Notes*. Mokelumne Hill, California: Reprinted by Health Research. Originally published in 1949 by the author.
Wilborn, Robert, and Terrell, James and Marcia. *Handbook of Irisdiagnosis and Rational Therapy*. Mokelumne Hill, California: Health Research, 1961.

## BIOFEEDBACK AND SELF-REGULATION

### Biofeedback

Barber, T.X., et al., eds. *Biofeedback and Self-Control, 1970: An Aldine Annual*. Chicago: Aldine-Atherton, 1971.
———. *Biofeedback and Self-Control: An Aldine Reader*. Chicago: Aldine-Atherton, 1971.
Basmajian, J.V. *Muscles Alive*. Baltimore: Williams and Wilkins, 1967.
Birk, L., ed. *Biofeedback: Behavioral Medicine*. New York: Grune and Stratton, 1973.
Brown, B.B. *New Mind, New Body*. New York: Harper and Row, 1974.
DiCara, L., et al., eds. *Biofeedback and Self-Control, 1974*. Chicago: Aldine, 1975.
Green, Elmer, and Green, Alyce. *Beyond Biofeedback*. New York: Delacorte, 1977.
Haugen, G.B.; Dixon, H.H.; and Dickel, H.A. *A Therapy for Anxiety Tension Reactions*. New York: Macmillan, 1963.
Jacobson, E. *Progressive Relaxation*. Chicago: University of Chicago Press, 1938; paperback, 1974.
Jonas, G. *Visceral Learning: Towards the Science of Self-Control*. New York: Viking, 1973.
Karlins, M., and Andrews, L.M. *Biofeedback: Turning On the Powers of Your Mind*. New York: J.B. Lippincott, 1972.
Luthe, W., ed. *Autogenic Therapy*, volumes 1-6. New York: Grune and Stratton, 1969.
Meares, A. *Relief without Drugs*. Garden City, New York: Doubleday, 1967.
Miller, N.E., et al., eds. *Biofeedback and Self-Control, 1973*. Chicago: Aldine, 1974.
Obrist, P., et al., eds. *Cardiovascular Psychophysiology*. Chicago: Aldine, 1975.
Peper, Erick. *Mind/Body Integration*. New York: Random House, 1977.
Schultz, J.H., and Luthe, W. *Autogenic Training: A Psychophysiologic Approach in Psychotherapy*. New York: Grune and Stratton, 1959.
Shaprio, D., et al., eds. *Biofeedback and Self-Control, 1972*. Chicago: Aldine, 1973.
Stoyva, J.M., et al., eds. *Biofeedback and Self-Control, 1971* Chicago: Aldine-Atherton, 1972.
Tart, C.T., ed. *Altered States of Consciousness*. New York: Wiley, 1969.
Whatmore, George B. *Physiopathology and Treatment of Functional Disorders*. New York: Grune and Stratton, 1974.

### Self Health

Benson, Herbert. *The Relaxation Response*. New York: William Morrow, 1975.
Coué, Emil. *How to Practice Suggestion and Autosuggestion*. New York: American Library Service, 1923.
Luthe, Wolfgang, and Schultz, Johannes. *Autogenic Therapy*, 6 volumes. New York: Grune and Stratton, 1969.
Jacobson, Edmund. *Progressive Relaxation*. Chicago: University of Chicago Press, Midway Reprint, 1974.
Reich, Wilhelm. *The Discovery of the Orgone: The Function of the Orgasm*. New York: Noonday Press, 1971.
Rosa, Karl Robert. *You and AT*. New York: E.P. Dutton, 1973.
Shealy, C. Norman. *90 Days to Self-Health*. New York: Dial Press, 1977.
———. *The Pain Game*. Millbrae, California: Celestial Arts, 1976.

## PSYCHIC AND SPIRITUAL

### Unconventional Healing

Bailey, Alice A. *Esoteric Healing*. London and New York: Lucis Publishing Co., 1953.
Castaneda, Carlos. *A Separate Reality*. New York: Pocket Books, 1973.
———. *Tales of Power*. New York: Simon and Schuster, 1974.
Cooke, Ivan. *Healing: by the Spirit*. Hampshire, England: White Eagle Publishing Trust, 1955.
Cranston, Ruth. *The Miracle of Lourdes*. New York: Popular Library, 1957.
David-Neel, Alexandra. *Magic & Mystery in Tibet*. New York: Dover, 1971.
Edmunds, Tudor H., and Associates, eds. *Some Unrecognized Factors in Medicine*. Wheaton, Illinois: A Quest Book. Theosophical Publishing House, 1976.
Edwards, Harry. *The Healing Intelligence*. New York: Hawthorne Books, 1971.
Eisenbud, J. *Psi & Psychoanalysis*. New York: Grune & Stratton, 1970.
Furst, Peter T. *Flesh Of The Gods: The Ritual Use Of Hallucinogens*. New York: Praeger, 1972.
Gonzáles-Wippler, Migene. *Santeria: African Magic in Latin America*. New York: Julian Press, 1973.
Hall, Manly P. *Healing: The Divine Art*. Los Angeles. Philosophical Research Society, 1944.
Hammond, Sally. *We Are All Healers*. New York: Harper & Row, 1973.
Hartmann, Franz. *Occult Science In Medicine*. New York: Weiser, reprinted, 1975.
Heindel, Max. *Occult Principles of Health and Healing*. Oceanside, California: Rosicrucian Fellowship Publishing Co., 1938.
Kelsey, Morton T. *Healing and Christianity*. New York: Harper & Row, 1973.
Kiev, A., ed. *Magic Faith and Healing*. New York: Macmillan, 1964.
Kilner, Walter J. *The Human Aura*. New York: Weiser, rev'ed., 1973.
Krippner, Stanley, and Villoldo, Alberto. *The Realms of Healing*. Millbrae, California: Celestial Arts, 1976.
Kruger, Helen. *Other Healers, Other Cures*. New York: Bobbs-Merrill Co., 1974.
Kuhlman, Kathryn. *God Can Do It Again*. New York: Pyramid Family Library, 1969.
LeShan, Lawrence. *The Medium, The Mystic and The Physicist*. New York: Viking Press, 1973.
———. *Toward a General Theory of the Paranormal*. New York: Parapsychological Foundation Monograph #9, 1969.
Long, Max Freedom. *The Secret Science Behind Miracles*. Santa Monica, California: De Vorss, 1948.
———. *The Secret Science at Work*. Santa Monica, California: De Vorss, 1953.
Macdonald, R.G., Hickman, J.L., and Dakin, H.S. *Preliminary Physical Measurements of Psychological Effects Associated with Three Alleged Psychic Healers*. Privately published in 1976 by the authors, available through H.S. Dakin, 3101 Washington Street, San Francisco, California 94115.
Nolen, William A. *Healing: A Doctor in Search of a Miracle*. New York: Random House, 1974.
Oursler, W. *The Healing Power of Faith*. New York: Hawthorne Books, 1957.
Ram Dass, B. *The Only Dance There Is*. Garden City, New York: Doubleday/Anchor, 1974.
Reichenbach, Karl, Baron Von. *Researches on the Vital Force*. Seacaucus, New Jersey: University Books, rev'ed., 1974.
Sherman, Harold. *Wonder Healers of the Philippines*. Santa Monica, California: De Vorss, 1967.
———. *Your Power to Heal*. Greenwich, Connecticut: Fawcett, 1972.
White, John, ed. *Psychic Exploration*. New York: G.P. Putman's Sons, 1974.
Worrall, Ambrose & Olga. *The Gift of Healing*. New York: Harper & Row, 1965.

### Therapeutic Touch

Blofeld, John. *The Tantric Mysticism of Tibet*. New York: E.P. Dutton, 1970.
Eliade, Nurcea. *Yoga: Immortality and Freedom*. Trans. by Will R. Trask. Princeton, N.J.: Princeton University Press, 1969.
Evans-Wentz, W.Y. *Tibetan Yoga*. London: Oxford University Press, 1967.
Feldenkrais, M. *Awareness Through Movement*. New York: Harper & Row, 1972.
———. *Body and Mature Behavior*. New York: International Universities Press, 1973.
Grad, B. "A Telexinatic Effect on Plant Growth II. Experiments Involving Treatment of Saline in Stoppered Bottles," *International Journal of Parapsychology* 6:473-498.
Krieger, D. "Healing by the Laying-on of Hands as a Facilitator of Bioenergetic Change: The Response of *In-Vivo* Human Hemoglobin," *International Journal for Psychoenergetic Systems*, vol. 2, 1976.

———. "Nursing Research for a New Age," *Nursing Times*, 1976.

———. "The Relationship of Touch, with Intent to Help or to Heal Subjects' *In-Vivo* Hemoglobin Values: A Study in Personalized Interaction," *American Nurses Association Ninth Nursing Research Conference*. Kansas City, Missouri: American Nurses Association, 1973.

———. "The Response of *In-Vivo* Human Hemoglobin to an Active Healing Therapy by Direct Laying-on of Hands," *Human Dimensions* **2**:12-15, 1972.

———. "Therapeutic Touch: The Imprimateur of Nursing," *American Journal of Nursing*, pp. 784-787, 1975.

Montagu, Ashley. *Touching*. New York: Columbia University Press, 1971.

Rorvik, D.M. "The Healing Hand of Mr. E.," *Esquire*, February 1974.

Spelteholz-Spanner. *Atlas on Human Anatomy*. Philadelphia: F.A. Davis, rev. ed., 1967.

### Anthroposophical Medicine

Glas, Norbert. *Adolescence and the Diseases of Puberty*. Gloucester, England: Education and Science Publications, 1945.

———. *Kinderkranken als Entwicklungstufen des Menschen*. Vienna, Leipzig, Bern: Verlag fuer Medizin, 1937.

Husemann, Friedrich. *Goethe and the Art of Healing. A Commentary on the Crisis in Medicine*. London: Rudolf Steiner Publishing Co.; New York: The Anthroposophic Press.

Husemann, Friedrich, and Wolff, Otto. *Das Bild Des Menschen als Grundlage der Heilkunst*. 2 volumes. Stuttgart: Verlag Freies Geistesleben. Revised edition, 1974.

Leroi, A. *Cancer as the Disease of Our Time*. London: New Knowledge Books.

———. *The Cell, the Human Organism and Cancer*. London: Anthroposophical Publishing Co. Revised edition, 1951.

———. *Curative Education*. Twelve Lectures, Dornach, June-July, 1924. London: Rudolf Steiner Press, 1972.

———. *Geisteswissenschaftliche Gesichtspunkte zur Therapie*. Nine Lectures, Dornach, April, 1921. Dornach, Switzerland: Verlag der Rudolf Steiner Nachlassverwaltung, 1963.

———. *Geographic Medicine*. Two Lectures, St. Gallen, Switzerland, November, 1917. Spring Valley, New York: Mercury Press, 1976.

———. *The Invisible Man Within Us: Pathology Underlying Therapy*. One Lecture, Dornach, Switzerland, February, 1923. Spring Valley, New York: Mercury Press, 1977.

———. *Meditative Betrachtungen und Antleitungen zur Vertiefung der Heilkunst*. Eight Lectures, Dornach, January, 1924; Five Lectures, Dornach, April, 1924. Dornach, Switzerland: Verlag der Rudolf Steiner Nachlasverwaltung, 1967.

———. *An Occult Physiology*. Eight Lectures, Prague, March, 1911. London: Rudolf Steiner Publishing Co., 1951.

———. *An Outline of Anthroposophical Medical Research*. Abridged report of Two Lectures given in London, 1924. London: Rudolf Steiner Publishing Co., 1939.

———. *Pastoral-Medizinischen Kurs*. Eleven Lectures, Dornach, September, 1924. Dornach, Switzerland: Rudolf Steiner Verlag, 1973.

———. *Pyshiologisch-Therapeutisches auf Grundlage der Geisteswissenschaft*. Eleven Lectures, Stuttgart and Dornach, October, 1920 and October, 1922. Dornach, Switzerland: Rudolph Steiner Verlag, 1975.

———. *Spiritual Science and Medicine*. Twenty Lectures, Dornach, March-April, 1920. London: Rudolf Steiner Publishing Co., 1948. London: Second Impression, Rudolf Steiner Press, 1975.

———. *Ueber Gesundheit and Krankheit. Grundlagen einer geisteswissenschaftlichen Sinneslehre*. Eighteen Lectures before the Workers on the Goetheanum. October, 1923. Dornach, Switzerland: Rudolf Steiner Verlag, 1976.

———. *What Can the Art of Healing Gain Through Spiritual Science?* Three Lectures, Arnheim, Holland, July 1924. London: Anthroposophical Publishing Co., 1950.

Steiner, Rudolf, and Wegman, Ita. *Fundamentals of Therapy—An Extension of the Art of Healing Through Spiritual Knowledge*. London: Rudolf Steiner Press. Third Edition, revised, 1967.

### Edgar Cayce

McGarey, W. *Acupuncture and Body Energies*. Phoenix, Arizona: Gabriel Press, 1973.

———. *Edgar Cayce and the Palma Christi*. Virginia Beach, Virginia: Edgar Cayce Foundation, 1970.

McGarey, W., and Carter, M. *Edgar Cayce on Healing*. New York: Paperback Library, 1972.

McGarey, W., and McGarey, G. *There Will Your Heart Be Also*. Englewood Cliffs, New Jersey: Prentice-Hall, 1975.

Reilly, H.J.W., and Brod, R.H. *The Edgar Cayce Handbook for Health*. New York: Macmillan, 1975.

Stearn, J. *Edgar Cayce–The Sleeping Prophet*. New York: Doubleday, 1967.

Sugrue, T. *There Is a River: The Story of Edgar Cayce*. New York: Dell, 1964.

Windsor, J. "A Holistic Theory of Mental Illness," *A.R.E. Journal, Autumn, 1969*.

## PSYCHOPHYSICAL APPROACHES

### Massage

Bankart, A.S. Blundell. *Manipulative Surgery*. London: Constable & Co., 1932. Reprinted by Health Research, Mokelumne Hill, California.

Burrows, H. Jackson and Coltart W.D. *Treatment by Manipulation*. Reprinted by Health Research, Mokelumne Hill, California, 1970.

Downing, George. *The Massage Book*. New York: Random House Bookworks, 1972.

Kellogg, John Harvey. *The Art of Massage*. Battle Creek, Michigan: Modern Medicine Publishing Co., 1929. Reprinted by Health Research, Mokelumne Hill, California.,

Lake, Thomas T. *Treatment by Neuropathy and The Encyclopedia of Physical and Manipulative Therapeutics*. Reprinted by Health Research, Mokelumne Hill, California, 1972.

Leboyer, Frederick. *Loving Hands*. New York: Alfred A. Knopf, 1976.

Miller, Roberta Delong. *Psyhic Massage*. New York: Harper Colophon, 1975.

Serizawa, Katsusuke. *Massage: The Oriental Method*. Elmsford, New York: Japan Publications, 1972.

White, George Starr. *Zone Therapy*. Columbus, Ohio: I.W. Long Publishing Co., 1917. Reprinted by Health Research, Mokelumne Hill, California.

### Shiatsu

Blate, Michael. *The G-Jo Handbook*. Davie, Florida: Falkynor Books, 1976.

de Langre, Jacques. *The First Book of Do-In*. Magalia, California: 1974, updated and revised, 1976.

Irwin, Yukiko with Wagenvoord, James. *Shiatzu*. Philadelphia: Lippincott.

Namikoshi, Toru. *Shiatsu*. Elmsford, New York: Japan Publications, 1969.

———. *Shiatsu Therapy, Theory and Practice*. Elmsford, New York: Japan Publications, 1974.

Ohashi, Wataru. *Do It Yourself Shiatsu*. New York: E.P. Dutton, 1976.

Serizawa, Katsusuke. *Tsubo: Vital Points for Oriental Therapy*. Elmsford, New York: Japan Publications, 1976.

Warren, Frank Z. *Freedom From Pain Through Acupressure*. New York: Wentworth, 1976.

### Polarity Therapy

Publications of Randolph Stone (may be obtained through Pierre Pannetier, Polarity Therapy, 401 North Glassell Street, Orange, California 92666).

*Energy: The Vital Polarity in the Healing Art*
*The Wireless Anatomy of Man and Its Function*
*Polarity Therapy and Its Triune Function*
*Vitality Balance*
*The Mysterious Sacrum: The Key to Body Structure and Function*
*Appendix to the New Energy Concept of the Healing Art*
*Supplement to the Wireless Anatomy of Man*
*A Series of 25 Charts: Body Balance through Evolutionary Energy Currents*
*A Purifying Diet*
*Health-Building: The Conscious Art of Living Well*
*Summary: A Supplement to Health-Building*
*Easy Stretching Postures for Vitality and Beauty*
*Polarity Therapy Principles and Practice with Particular Attention to the Oft-Neglected Hypotension-Vasodilation Cases*
*Energy Tracing: 1970 Notes and Findings*
*Brief Explanation of the Secrets of the Emerald Tablet of Hermes*
*1971 Private Notes for Students of Polarity Therapy Conventions*

### Sensory Awareness

Selver, Charlotte. *Sensory Awareness and Total Functioning*. Reprinted from *General Semantics Bulletin*. Nos. 20 and 21, 1957. Available through Charlotte Selver Foundation, 32 Cedars Road, Caldwell, New Jersey 07006.

Selver, Charlotte, and Brooks, Charles. *Report on Sensory Awareness*. Reprinted from *Explorations In Human Potentialities*, 1966. Available through Charlotte Selver Foundation, 32 Ceders Road, Caldwell, New Jersey 07006.

Brooks, Charles. *Sensory Awareness: The Rediscovery of Experiencing*. New York: Viking, 1974.

### Alexander

Alexander, F.M. *The Use of the Self*. New York: E.P. Dutton, 1941.

Barlow, Wilfred. *The Alexander Technique*. New York: Alfred A. Knopf, 1973.

Jones, F.P. *Body Awareness in Action*. New York: Schocken Books, 1976.

Maisel, E. *The Alexander Technique*. New York: University Books, 1969.

Tinbergan, N. "Ethology and Stress Diseases," *Science* **185**:20-27, 1974.

Westfeldt, L. *F. Matthias Alexander*. Westport, Connecticut: Associated Booksellers, 1964.

### Rolfing

Feitis, Rosemary. *Ida Rolf Talks about Rolfing and Physical Reality*. New York: Harper and Row, 1978.

Hammann, Kalen. "What Structural Integration (Rolfing) Is an Why it Works," *Osteopathic Physician*, March 1972.

Johnson, Don. *The Protean Body, a Rolfers View of Human Flexibility*. New York: Harper-Colophon, 1977.

Keen, Sam. "Sing the Body Electric/My New Carnality," *Psychology Today*, October 1970.

Rolf, Ida P. *Rolfing: The Integration of the Human Structure* Santa Monica, California: Dennis-Landman, 1977.

———. "Structural Integration: A Contribution to the Under standing of Stress," *Confinia Psychiatrica*, 1973.

Siverman, J. "Stress, Stimulus Intensity Control, and the Struc tural Integration Technique," *Confinia Psychiatrica*, pp. 201 219, 1973.

Turner, Sue. "Structural Integration and Stress," *Aquatic World pp. 20-22, March 1976*.

*Additional articles available through The Rolf Institute, P.O. Box 1868, Boulder, Colorado 80306.*

### Dance Therapy

Bernstein, Penny. *Theory and Methods in Dance-Movemen Therapy*. Dubuque, Iowa: Kendell Hunt, 1972.

Canner, Norma. *And a Time to Dance*. Boston: Beacon Press 1968.

Chaikin, Harris, ed. *Marian Chace: Her Papers*. Columbia Maryland: A.D.T.A., 1975.

Hatcher, Caro, and Mullin, H. *More Than Words*. Pasadena California: Parents for Movement Publications, 1967.

Lefco, Helene. *Dance Therapy*. Chicago: Nelson Hall, 1974.

Mason, Kathlee C., ed. *Dance Therapy–Focus on Dance VII* Washington, D.C.: A.A.H.P.E.R., 1974.

North, Marion. *Personality Assessment through Movement*. London: Macdonald and Evans, 1972.

Pesso, Albert. *Movement in Psycho-Therapy*. New York: N.Y.U. Press, 1969.

Salkin, Jeri. *Body Ego Technique*. Springfield, Illinois: Charles C Thomas, 1973.

Schoop, Trudi, and Mitchell, P. *Won't You Join the Dance?* Palo Alto, California: National Press Books, 1974.

## HUMANISTIC AND TRANSPERSONAL PSYCHOTHERAPIES

### Gestalt

Goldstein, K. *The Organism, a Holistic Approach to Biology Derived from Pathological Data in Man*. Boston: Beacon Pres 1963.

Goodman, P. *Growing Up Absurd*. New York: Random Hous 1960.

———. *Five Years*. New York: Random House, 1966.

Lederman, J. *Anger and the Rocking Chair: Gestalt Awarene with Children*. New York: McGraw-Hill, 1969.

Perls, Fritz. *Ego, Hunger and Aggression*. London: Allen a Unwin, 1947; New York: Random House, 1969.

Perls, Fritz, Hefferline, Ralph F. and Goodman, Paul. *Gesta Therapy*. New York: Julian Press, 1951; New York: Del 1965.

Perls, Laura. The Psychoanalyst and the Critic. *Complex*, No. (summer 1950), 41-47.

———. Notes on the Psychology of Give and Take. *Comple* 1953, 9, 24-30. Also in Pursglove, 118-128.

———. Two Instances of Gestalt Therapy. *Case reports in cli ical psychology*, Kings County Hospital, New York, 195 Also in Pursglove, 42-63.

———. The Gestalt Approach. *Annals of Psychotherapy*, Vo 2, 1961.

———. One Gestalt Therapist's Approach. In Fagen an Shepard, 1970, 125-9.

Polster, Erving and Miriam. *Gestalt Therapy Integrated*. Ne York: Brunner/Mazel, 1973.

Pursglove, P., ed. *Recognitions in Gestalt Therapy*. New Yor Funk and Wagnalls, 1968.

Reich, Wilhelm. *Selected Writings, an Introduction to Orgonomy* New York: Farrar, Straus & Giroux, 1960.

———. *Character Analysis*. New York: Farrar, Straus Giroux, 1961.

———. *Function of the Orgasm*. New York: Farrar, Straus Giroux, 1973.

### Art Therapy

Buck, John N. *The House–Tree–Person Technique: Revised Manual*. Beverly Hills, California: Western Psychological Service 1966.

Burns, Robert C., and Kaufman, S. Harvard. *Actions, Styles, an Symbols in Kinetic Family Drawings (K-F-D): An Interpreti Manual*. New York: Brunner/Mazel, 1972.

Frankl, Victor. *The Will to Meaning: Foundations and Applic tions of Logotherapy*. New York: New American Librar 1969.

Gantt, Linda, and Schmal, Marilyn S. *Art Therapy: A Bibliog raphy, January 1940-June 1973*. Rockville, Maryland: DHE

Publication No. (ADM) 74-51, 1974.
Garai, Josef E. "Art Therapy: Catalyst for Creative Expression and Personality Integration," in *New Approaches to Psychotherapy*. Englewood Cliffs, New Jersey: Prentice-Hall, 1977.
———. "The Humanistic Approach to Art Therapy and Creativity Development." *New-Ways*, vol. 1, no. 2, 1975.
Garai, Selma H., and Garai, Josef E. "Techniques of Family Art Therapy," *Group*, November 1974.
Hammer, Emanuel F. *The Clinical Application of Projective Drawings*. Springfield, Illinois: Charles C. Thomas, 1958.
Harris, Jay, and Joseph, Cliff. *Murals of the Mind: Image of a Psychiatric Community*. New York: International Universities Press, 1973.
Jourard, Sidney M. *The Transparent Self*, rev. ed. New York: Van Nostrand Reinhold, 1971.
Keyes, Margaret F. *The Inward Journey: Art as Psychotherapy for You*. Millbrae, California: Celestial Arts, 1974.
Kramer, Edith. *Art as Therapy with Children*. New York: Schocken Books, 1971.
———. *Art Therapy in a Children's Community*. Springfield, Illinois: Charles C. Thomas, 1958.
Kwiatkowska, Hanna Y. "Family Art Therapy and Family Art Evaluation," *Psychiatry and Art* 3:138-151, 1971.
Machover, Karen. *Personality Projection in the Drawing of the Human Figure: A Method of Personality Investigation*. Springfield, Illinois: Charles C. Thomas, 1949.
May, Rollo. *The Courage to Create*. New York: Norton, 1975.
Naumberg, Margaret. "Art Therapy: Its Scope and Function," in *The Clinical Application of Projective Drawings*, ed. by E.F. Hammer. Springfield, Illinois: Charles C. Thomas, 1958.
———. *Dynamically Oriented Art Therapy: Its Principles and Practice*. New York: Grune and Stratton, 1966.
———. *Psychoneurotic Art: Its Function in Psychotherapy*. New York: Grune and Stratton, 1953.
———. *Schizophrenic Art: Its Meaning in Psychotherapy*. London: Heinemann, 1950.
Rank, Otto. *Art and Artist: Creative Urge and Personality Development*. New York: Alfred A. Knopf, 1932. Reprinted by Agathon Press, New York, 1968 and 1975.
Rhyne, Janie. *The Gestalt Art Experience*. Monterey, California: Brooks/Cole, 1973.
Robbins, Arthur and Sibley, Linda Beth. *Creative Art Therapy*. New York: Brunner/Mazel, 1976.
Shostrom, Everett L. "From Abnormality to Actualization." *Psychotherapy: Theory, Research and Practice*, vol. 10, no. 1, 1973.
Ulman, Elinor, and Dachinger, Penny. *Art Therapy in Theory and Practice*. New York: Schocken Books, 1975.

## Drama Therapy

Anderson, Harold. *Projective Techniques*. Englewood Cliffs, New Jersey: Prentice-Hall, 1964.
Axline, Virginia M. *Play Therapy*. New York: Ballantine Books, 1969.
Brown, George I. *Reach, Touch & Teach*. New York: Viking Press, 1971.
Chiefetz, Dan. *Theatre in My Head*. Boston, Massachusetts: Little, Brown & Co., 1971.
Courtney, Richard. *Play, Drama and Thought*. London: Cassel & Co., 1968.
Heathcothe, Dorothy. *Drama as a Learning Medium*. Washington, D.C.: University Press, 1964; N.E.A., 1976.
King, Nancy. *Giving Form to Feeling*. New York: Drama Book Specialist, 1975.
Koch, Kenneth. *Wishes, Lies and Dreams*. New York: Chelsea House Publisher, 1970.
Lowenfeld, Viktor. *Creative and Mental Growth*. New York: Macmillan, 1947.
Lowndes, Betty. *Creative Movement and Drama*. Boston, Massachusetts: Plays, 1971.
Maslow, Abraham H. *Toward a Psychology of Being*. Princeton, New Jersey: Van Nostrand, 1962.
Mearns, Hugh. *Creative Power*. New York: Dover, 1958.
Moreno, Jacob L. *Psychodrama*. 2 vols. New York: Beacon, 1959.
Piaget, J. *Play, Dreams, and Imitation in Childhood*. New York: Norton, 1951.
Rogers, Carl. *On Becoming a Person*. Boston, Massachusetts: Houghton, Mifflin Co., 1961.
Schattner, Gertrud, and Courtney, Richard, eds. *Drama in Therapy*. New York: Drama Book Specialists (in press).
Shaftel, F., and G. *Role-Playing for Social Values*. Englewood Cliffs, New Jersey: Prentice-Hall, 1967.
Slade, Peter. *Child Drama*. London: University Press, 1954.
Spolin, Viola. *Improvisation for the Theatre*. Evanston, Illinois: Northwestern University Press, 1964.
Ward, Winefred. *Playmaking with Children*. New York: Appleton, 1957.
Way, Brian. *Development Through Drama*. London: Longman, 1967.
Wethered, Audrey G. *Drama and Movement in Therapy*. London: McDonald & Evans, 1973.

## Music Therapy

Adon, Bar, and Leopold, W.F. *Child Language*. Englewood Cliffs, New Jersey: Prentice-Hall, 1971.
Aichorn, August. *Wayward Youth*. New York: Viking, 1935.
Alvin, Juliette. *Music for the Handicapped Child*. London: Oxford University Press, 1965.
Bailey, Philip. *They Can Make Music*. London: Oxford University Press, 1973.
Baruch, Dorothy W. *One Little Boy*. New York: Julian Press, 1952.
Bettelheim, Bruno. *Empty Fortress*. New York: Free Press, 1967.
Bloom, Lois. *Language Development*. Cambridge, Massachusetts: M.I.T. Press, 1970.
Bonny, Helen and Savary, Louis. *Music and Your Mind: Listening with a New Consciousness*. New York: Harper & Row, 1973 (out of print; order from ICM Training Seminars, 417 E. Belvedere, Baltimore, MD 21207).
Bright, Ruth. *Music in Geriatric Care*. New York: St. Martins Press, 1973.
Clark, Linda. *Health, Youth and Beauty Through Color Breathing*. Milbrae, California: Celestial Arts, 1976.
Gaston, E.T., ed. *Music in Thearpy*. New York: Macmillan, 1968.
Green, Hannah. *I Never Promised You a Rose Garden*. New York: Rhinehart & Winston, 1964.
Gribbin, John. *The Jupiter Effect*. New York: Vintage, 1974.
Heline, Corinne. *Color and Music in the New Age*. Oceanside, California: New Age Press, 1964.
———. *Music: The Keynote of Human Evolution*. Oceanside, California: New Age Press, 1965.
———. *Beethoven's Nine Symphonies*. Oceanside, California: New Age Press, 1963.
———. *Esoteric Music of Richard Wagner*. Oceanside, California: New Age Press, 1948.
Kastein and Trace. *The Birth of Language*. Springfield, Illinois: Charles C. Thomas, 1962.
Keyes, Laura Elizabeth. *Toning: The Creative Power of the Voice*. Marina del Rey, California: De Vorss, 1973.
Nordoff, Paul, and Robbins, Clive. *Music Therapy for Handicapped Children*. Spring Valley, New York: Rudolf Steiner Publishing, 1965.
Priestly, M. *Music Therapy in Action*. New York: St. Martins Press, 1975.
Redl, Fritz, and Weiman, David. *Children Who Hate*. Glencoe, Illinois: Free Press, 1951.
Reik, Theodore. *The Haunting Melody*. New York: Grove Press, 1960.
Schwebel, Milton. *Who Can Be Educated?* New York: Grove Press, 1968.
Scott, Cyril. *Misc: Its Secret Influence Throughout The Ages*. London: Theosophical Publishing House, 1937.
Stebbing, Lionel. *Music: Its Occult Basis and Healing Value*. Sussex, England: New Knowledge Books, 1974.
Winckel, Fritz. *Music, Sound and Sensation*. New York: Dover, 1967.
Zuckerkandl, Victor. *Sound and Symbol*. Princeton, New Jersey: Princeton University Press, 1969.

## Hypnosis

Ambrose, Gordon. *Hypnotherapy with Children*. London: Staples, 1956.
Cheek, David, and Lecron, Leslie. *Clinical Hypnotherapy*. New York: Grune & Stratton, 1968.
Craisilneck, Harold, and Hall, James A. *Clinical Hypnosis*. New York: Grune & Stratton, 1975.
Erickson, Milton H. *Advanced Techniques of Hypnosis and Therapy*, ed. by Jay Haley. New York: Grune & Stratton, 1967.
———. *Hypnotic Realities*. New York: Halsted Press, 1977.
Hilgard, Ernest R., and Hilgard, Josephine R. *Hypnosis in the Relief of Pain*. Los Altos, California: William Kaufman, 1975.
Hull, Clark. *Hypnosis and Suggestability*. New York: Appleton Century Crofts, 1933.
Jampolsky, Gerald G. "Hypnotherapy and Kirlian Photography." In *Psychotherapy and Behavior Change*, ed. by Lee McCabe. New York: Grune & Stratton, 1977.
Kroger, William. *Clinical and Experimental Hypnosis*. Philadelphia: Lippincott, 1963.
Lecron, Leslie M., ed. *Experimental Hypnosis*. New York: Macmillan, 1956.
Masters, Robert, and Houston, Jean. *Mind Games: The Guide to Inner Space*. New York: Viking Press, 1972.
Meares, A. *A System of Medical Hypnosis*. New York: Julian Press, 1960.
Shor, Ronald E., and Orne, Martin, eds. *The Nature of Hypnosis: Selected Basic Reading*. New York: Holt, Rhinehart & Winston, 1965.
Wolberg, Louis R. *Hypnosis–Is It for you?* New York: Harcourt, Brace, Javonovich, 1972.

## Humanistic Psychology

Allport, Gordon. *Becoming: Basic Consideration for a Psychology of Personality*. New Haven, Connecticut: Yale University Press, 1955.
Bugental, J.F.T. *Challenges of Humanistic Psychology*. New York: McGraw-Hill, 1967.
Buhler, Charlotte, and Allen, Melanie. *Introduction to Humanistic Psychology*. Monterey, California: Brooks-Cole, 1972.
Giorgi, Amedeo. *Psychology as a Human Science*. New York: Harper, 1970.
Goble, Frank G. *The Third Force: The Psychology of Abraham Maslow*. New York: Grossman Publishers, 1970; Pocketbooks, 1971.
Jourard, Sidney. *Transparent Self*, 2nd ed. New York: Van Nostrand Reinhold, 1971.
———. *Healthy Personality: An Approach from the Viewpoint of Humanistic Psychology*. New York: Macmillan, 1974.
Maslow, Abraham. *Toward a Psychology of Being*, 2nd ed. New York: Van Nostrand Reinhold, 1968.
May, Rollo, et al. *Existence: A New Dimension in Psychiatry and Psychology*. New York: Basic, 1958; Simon & Schuster, 1958.
Rogers, Carl. *On Becoming a Person*. Boston: Houghton Mifflin, 1970.
Severin, Frank T. *Discovering Man in Psychology*. New York: McGraw-Hill, 1973.
Sutich, A.J., and Vich, M.A., eds. *Readings in Humanistic Psychology*. New York: Free Press, 1969.

## Psychosynthesis

Assagioli, Roberto A. *The Act of Will*. New York: Viking, 1974; Baltimore: Penguin, 1974.
———. *Jung and Psychosynthesis*. May be ordered from the Montreal or San Francisco Institutes.
———. *Psychosynthesis: A Manual of Principles and Techniques*. New York: Hobbs-Dorman, 1965; Baltimore: Penguin, 1976.
Crampton, Martha. *An Historical Survey of Mental Imagery Techniques in Psychosynthesis and Description of the Dialogic Imagery Method*. Montreal: Quebec Center for Psychosynthesis, 1974.
———. *Psychosynthesis: Some Key Aspects of Theory and Practice*. Montreal: Quebec Center for Psychosynthesis, 1977.

## Transpersonal Psychology

Anderson, Marianne, and Savary, Louis. *Passages: A Guide for Pilgrims of the Mind*. New York: Harper and Row, 1972.
Assagioli, Roberto. *Psychosynthesis*. New York: Viking Press, 1971.
Burden, Virginia. *The Process of Intuition, A Psychology of Creativity*. Wheaton, Illinois: Theosophical Publishing House, 1975.
DeRopp, Robert S. *The Master Game: Pathways to Higher Consciousness Beyond the Drug Experience*. New York: Dell Publishing Co., 1968.
Grof, Stanislav. *Realms of the Human Unconscious: Observations from LSD Research*. New York: E.P. Dutton & Co., 1976.
Keyes, Ken Jr. *Handbook to Higher Consciousness*. Berkeley, California: Living Love Center, 1975.
LeShan, Lawrence. *How To Meditate: A Guide to Self-Discovery*. Boston: Little, Brown & Co., 1974; New York: Bantam Books, 1975.
Lilly, John C. *The Center of the Cyclone: An Autobiography of Inner Space*. New York: Julian Press, 1972.
Maslow, Abraham H. *The Farther Reaches of Human Nature*. New York: Viking Press, 1972.
Masters, Robert, and Houston, Jean. *Mind Games: The Guide to Inner Space*. New York: Viking Press, 1972.
Naranjo, Claudio. *The One Quest*. New York: Viking Press, 1972; paperback, New York: Ballantine Books, 1973.
Naranjo, Claudio, and Ornstein, Robert. *On the Psychology of Meditation*. New York: Viking Press, 1971.
Ornstein, Robert. *The Psychology of Consciousness*. San Francisco: W.H. Freeman & Co., 1972.
Ostrander, Sheila, and Schroeder, Lynn. *Psychic Discoveries Behind the Iron Curtain*. New York: Bantam Books, 1971.
Ram, Dass with Levin, Stephen. *Grist for the Mill*. Santa Cruz, California: Unity Press, 1977.
Roberts, Jane. *The Nature of Personal Reality: A Seth Book*. Englewood Cliffs, New Jersey: Prentice-Hall, 1974.
Swami Rama, Rudolph Ballentine and Swami Ajaya. *Yoga and Psychotherapy: The Evolution of Consciousness*. Glenview, Illinois: Himilayan Institute, 1976.
Tart, Charles T., ed. *Altered States of Consciousness*. New York: John Wiley & Sons, 1969; paperback, Garden City, New York: Doubleday Anchor Books, 1972.
Trungpa, Chogyam. *Cutting Through Spiritual Materialism*. Berkeley, California: Shambhala, 1973.
Weil, Andrew. *The Natural Mind*. Boston: Houghton, Mifflin, 1972.

## Life, Death, and After Life

Bede. *A History of the English Church and People*. Translated by Leo Sherley-Price. Harmondsworth, England: Penguin Books, 1968.
Choron, Jacques. *Death and Modern Man*. New York: Collier Books, 1964.
———. *Death and Western Thought*. New York: Collier Books, 1964.

Crowther, Duane S. *Life Everlasting*. Salt Lake City, Utah: Book-craft, 1967.

Hallowell, I. "Spirits of the Dead in Salteaux Life and Thought," *Journal of the Royal Anthropologic Institute* **70**:29-51, 1940.

De Quincey, Thomas. *Confessions of an English Opium Eater With Its Sequels Suspiria De Profundis and the English Mail Coach*, Malcolm Elwin, ed. London: McDonald and Co., 1956.

Evans-Wentz, W. Y., ed. *The Tibeten Book of the Dead*. Translated into English by Lama Kazi Dawa-Samdup-s. New York: Oxford University Press, 1960.

Hamilton, Edith, and Cairns, Huntington. "The Republic, Book X," *The Collected Dialogues of Plato*. New York: Bollingen Foundation, 1961.

Heim, A. "Remarks on Fatal Falls." In *Yearbook of the Swiss Alpine Club 1892*, **27**:327-337. Translated by R. Noyes and R. Kichi. *Omega* **3**:45-52, 1972.

James, William. *The Varieties of Religious Experience*. New York: Mentor Books, 1958.

Jung, Carl G. *Memories, Dreams, Reflections*, Aniela Jaff´e, ed., and translated by Richard and Clara Winston. New York: Vintage Books, 1965.

————. *Synchronicity*. Princeton, New Jersey: Princeton University Press, 1973.

Kubler-Ross, Elisabeth. *On Death and Dying*. New York: Macmillan, 1969.

Moody, Raymond A. *Life After Life*. New York: Bantam, 1976.

Noyes, Russell. "The Experience of Dying." *Psychiatry*, Vol. 35, pp. 174-184, 1972.

Noyes, Russell, and Kletti, Roy. "Depersonalization in the Face of Life Threatening Danger: A Description," *Psychiatry*, Vol. 39, pp. 19-27, 1976.

————. "Depersonalization in the Face of Life Threatening Danger: An Interpretation," *Omega* **7**:103-114, 1976.

Osis, Karlis. "Deathbed Observations by Physicians and Nurses," *Parapsychology Monographs*, No. 3, Psychology Foundation, New York, 1961.

————. "What Do the Dying See?" *Newsletter of the American Society for Psychical Research*, **24**, Winter, 1975.

Plato. *The Last Days of Socrates*. Translated by Hugh Tredenick. Baltimore: Penguin Books, 1959.

Ritchie, George. *Return from Tomorrow*. Lincoln, Virginia: Chosen Books (to be published early 1978).

Sabom, Michael B. and Kreutizger, Sarah. "The Experience of Near Death," *Death Education*, **1**:195-203, 1977.

————. "Near Death Experiences," *Journal of the Florida Medical Association*, September, 1977.

Swedenborg, Emanuel. *Heaven and Heaven*. Translated by George Dole. New York: Pillar Books, 1976.

Tylor, Edward B. *Primitive Culture*, Vol. II New York: Henry Holt and Co., 1874.